Updates in Clinical Dermatology

Series Editors

John Berth-Jones
Chee Leok Goh
Howard I. Maibach

More information about this series at http://www.springer.com/series/13203

Stephen K. Tyring
Stephen Andrew Moore
Angela Yen Moore · Omar Lupi

Editors

Overcoming Antimicrobial Resistance of the Skin

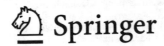

Editors
Stephen K. Tyring
Department of Dermatology
University of Texas Health Science
Center
Houston, TX
USA

Angela Yen Moore
Division of Dermatology
Baylor University Medical Center
Dallas, TX
USA

Arlington Center for Dermatology
Arlington, TX
USA

Arlington Research Center
Arlington, TX
USA

Stephen Andrew Moore
Arlington Center for Dermatology
Arlington, TX
USA

Arlington Research Center
Arlington, TX
USA

Omar Lupi
Immunology
Federal University of Rio de Janeiro
Rio de Janeiro
Brazil

ISSN 2523-8884   ISSN 2523-8892   (electronic)
Updates in Clinical Dermatology
ISBN 978-3-030-68323-8   ISBN 978-3-030-68321-4   (eBook)
https://doi.org/10.1007/978-3-030-68321-4

I would like to dedicate this book to my wonderful wife, Patricia, for her love and patience.

– Stephen K Tyring

I would like to express my boundless appreciation to Dr. Angela Moore whose passion for dermatology has launched me on the trajectory to be a life-long learner of the skin sciences.

I would like to thank Dr. Tyring for his unwavering support and confidence that I could contribute to such a critical work.

– Stephen Andrew Moore

I dedicate this volume to front-line clinicians worldwide who battle microscopic foes and to the next generation who will continue this fight.

– Angela Yen Moore

Preface

Although dermatologists prescribe more antibiotics per provider than any other specialty, *Overcoming Antimicrobial Resistance of the Skin* was written for all healthcare professionals, not just those who prescribe antibiotics. Antimicrobial resistance (AMR) is a public health crisis that existed before the COVID-19 pandemic and unfortunately will continue to be a major problem long after this pandemic has passed. It is an emergent health threat responsible for the death of approximately 35,000 in the United States and approximately 700,000 people globally each year. It is projected that the continued rise in AMR could result in the death of 10,000,000 annually by 2050. In fact, the World Health Organization (WHO) calls AMR one of the most urgent health threats of our time. The AMR crisis does not just involve antibiotic resistance, because similar problems exist for antivirals, e.g., for HIV; antiparasitics, e.g., for malaria; and antifungals, e.g., for *Candida auris*. This book, however, was not written simply to point out the problem, but to focus on possible solutions. In the twenty-first century, it is difficult to imagine the world before antibiotics. In the beginning of the twentieth century, however, dying of sepsis following childbirth or a simple skin infection was common, as were deaths due to pneumonia and meningitis. Although antibiotics only became widely available to the general public in the second half of the twentieth century, as did most currently available vaccines, Dr. Alexander Fleming warned of the potential problem of AMR in his 1954 Nobel Prize address. The solution, however, is not simply new antibiotics nor new methods of killing infectious organisms. The "cure" of an infectious disease is not the global solution, because "it is better to prevent than lament," which means public health measures and vaccines.

The importance of vaccines first gained general knowledge in the late eighteenth century, that is, the smallpox vaccine, and public health measures such as hand washing, clean drinking water, sewage disposal, and pasteurization became more common in the nineteenth century. These measures continue to be of upmost importance in the twenty-first century. Likewise, respiratory precautions, including face masks, quarantines, contact tracing, taking temperatures, asking about symptoms, and social distancing, were advocated and followed during the influenza pandemic of 1918 to 1919. It is sadly ironic that such precautions are not followed more closely during the current COVID-19 pandemic.

The political and economic effects of infectious diseases, like the effects on morbidity and mortality, are striking. Countries undergoing political and economic crisis, for example, Venezuela, often experience collapse of their healthcare systems. The "Black Death" in the form of *Yersinia pestis* not only killed millions of people between 1335 and 1368, it also had disastrous effects on Europe's economy and trade. It also contributed to the collapse of the Chinese, Russian, Persian, and Mongol empires. Like the 1918 to 1919 influenza pandemic, the COVID-19 pandemic has left millions of people globally unemployed. Ironically, the influenza pandemic enabled a presidency, while the COVID-19 pandemic helped destroy a presidency.

The evolution of AMR is now outpacing the development of new countermeasures. This situation threatens patient care, economic growth and security, public health, agriculture, and national security. Agreements and legislation have formed to address the AMR issues, and billions of dollars have been spent. Overcoming AMR is no longer a matter of finding new mechanisms of action. Many other factors to consider include biofilms and the microbiome as well as costs. Phytocompounds are being investigated further. New drug delivery systems are being tested, including use of nanoparticles. Newly discovered cellular pathways, for example, the MHC class II transactivator (CIITA) gene plus CD74, can be explored to block viral infections. Bacteriophages, once the subject of fictional cures, are now being used to overcome AMR.

All of these innovations, however, will be insufficient without public health measures, including vaccines. As the world awaits COVID-19 vaccines, fewer children are being vaccinated against other infections. According to the WHO, >80,000,000 children less than 1 year old could miss routine vaccinations due to the pandemic. Measles deaths worldwide have swelled to their highest level in 23 years. Due to lack of vaccination, 30,000 to 60,000 people, mostly adults, die each year of non-pandemic influenza just in the United States. Lack of vaccination against preventable diseases ultimately leads to further antimicrobial use and accelerates AMR. Antimicrobial overuse during the COVID-19 pandemic could also further AMR. UNICEF and GAVI have found that routine vaccinations are stalled in at least 68 countries. In developed countries, unfounded fear of vaccines by adults will prevent children from receiving available vaccines. The messenger RNA vaccines against COVID-19 are reported to be 95% effective and will be given as two doses. Because not everyone will or can receive these vaccines, 70% to 90% of susceptible individuals will need to be vaccinated to achieve herd immunity. Even then, public health measures, for example, hand washing, face masks, and social distancing, will still need to be maintained to achieve control of the pandemic.

As seen from the COVID-19 pandemic, understanding newly emerging diseases is crucial for all healthcare workers. We have learned many critical lessons: build resilient health systems with trust in science and public health agencies; invest in biomedical research and development; focus on equity and evidence-based facts; and trust and fund global healthcare institutions, because infectious diseases do not respect national borders. The emergence of novel infectious diseases is a public health threat, further exacerbated by AMR. Antimicrobials have allowed for huge strides in public health over the last century, but danger of resistance is a real and major concern that must be addressed immediately. Therefore, it is imperative that healthcare workers have an understanding of emerging infectious diseases and AMR.

Houston, TX, USA   Stephen K. Tyring

Acknowledgments

I would like to thank Yasmin Khalfe, who not only contributed several chapters to this book, but also helped me proofread the entire book, removing mistakes and overlaps as well as filling in gaps.

– Steven K. Tyring

I would like to acknowledge Asja Rehse and the Springer team for equipping me with the resources and research necessary to bring this project to fruition.

– Stephen Andrew Moore

I must express my profound gratitude to my research mentor and friend Dr. Stephen Tyring who has set the standard of excellence in investigating and understanding the miraculous cutaneous organ and the ways microbes would derail its purpose.

– Angela Yen Moore

Contents

Contributors

Divya R. Bhamidipati, MD, DTM&H Division of Infectious Diseases, Department of Medicine, Emory University School of Medicine, Atlanta, GA, USA

Yelena Dokic, BS School of Medicine, Baylor College of Medicine, Houston, TX, USA

Sahira Farooq, BS McGovern Medical School and UT Health, Houston, TX, USA

Fabio Francesconi, MD, PhD Dermatology Section - Federal University of the State of Amazonas (UFAM), Manaus, Brazil

Dermatologist - Hospital de Medicina Tropical, Manaus, Brazil

Valeska Francesconi, MD, PhD Dermatology Section - State University of Amazonas, Manaus, Brazil

Dermatologist - Hospital de Medicina Tropical, Manaus, Brazil

Saira George, MD MD Anderson Cancer Center, Department of Dermatology, Houston, TX, USA

Alex Panizza Jalkh, MD, MSc Dermatologist - FMTHVD/State University of Amazonas, Manaus, Brazil

Joseph Jebain, MD Center for Clinical Studies, Houston, TX, USA

Chetan Jinadatha, MD, MPH Infectious Diseases Section, Central Texas Veterans Health Care System, Department of Internal Medicine, Temple, TX, USA

Eleanor Johnson, BA School of Medicine, Baylor College of Medicine, Houston, TX, USA

Yasmin Khalfe, BA, MD School of Medicine, Baylor College of Medicine, Houston, TX, USA

Emily Limmer, BS University of Texas Southwestern Medical Center, Dallas, TX, USA

Omar Lupi, MD, MSc, PhD Associate Professor of Dermatology - Federal University of the State of Rio de Janeiro (UNIRIO), Rio de Janeiro, Brazil

Immunology Section - Federal University of Rio de Janeiro (UFRJ), Rio de Janeiro, Brazil

Titular Professor & Chairman - Policlinica Geral do Rio de Janeiro (PGRJ), Rio de Janeiro, Brazil

Ibero Latin American College of Dermatology (CILAD), Buenos Aires, Argentina

International League of Dermatological Societies (ILDS), London, UK

Angela Yen Moore, MD Division of Dermatology, Baylor University Medical Center, Dallas, TX, USA

Arlington Center for Dermatology, Arlington, TX, USA

Arlington Research Center, Arlington, TX, USA

Stephen Andrew Moore Arlington Center for Dermatology, Arlington, TX, USA

Arlington Research Center, Arlington, TX, USA

Audrey H. Nguyen Department of Dermatology, Emory University School of Medicine, Atlanta, GA, USA

Harrison P. Nguyen, MD, MBA, MPH, DTM&H Department of Dermatology, Emory University School of Medicine, Atlanta, GA, USA

Crystal E. Nwannunu, BS, MD Candidate 2020 McGovern Medical School, University of Texas Health Science Center, Houston, TX, USA

Shravya Reddy Pothula, BS Biology School of Medicine, Baylor College of Medicine, Houston, TX, USA

Radhika A. Shah, BS, MS Texas A&M University College of Medicine – Baylor University Medical Center, Dallas, TX, USA

Texas A&M University, Dallas, TX, USA

Alfredo Siller Jr., MD Baylor Scott and White Medical Center, Department of Internal Medicine, Temple, TX, USA

Natalie Skopicki Department of Dermatology, Emory University School of Medicine, Atlanta, GA, USA

Ritu Swali, MD Department of Dermatology, University of Nebraska Medical Center, Omaha, NE, USA

Stephen K. Tyring, MD, PhD Department of Dermatology, University of Texas Health Science Center, Houston, TX, USA

Center for Clinical Studies, Houston, TX, USA

Jiasen Wang, MD McGovern Medical School, Department of Internal Medicine, Houston, TX, USA

Claire Wiggins, BS Baylor College of Medicine, Houston, TX, USA

Julie H. Wu, MD New York University School of Medicine, Department of Dermatology, New York, NY, USA

Part I

Emerging Bacterial Resistance to Antibiotics

Mechanisms of Bacterial Resistance

Radhika A. Shah

Abbreviations

2-DOS	2-Deoxystreptamine
ABC	ATP-binding cassette
ABC-F	ATP-binding cassette family
AG	Aminoglycoside
AME	Aminoglycoside-modifying enzymes
ARE	Antibiotic resistance
CAMP	Cationic antimicrobial peptide
CAT	Chloramphenicol acetyltransferase
CDC	Centers for Disease Control and Prevention
DAP	Daptomycin
DHFR	Dihydrofolate reductase
DHPS	Dihydropteroate synthase
Erm	Erythromycin ribosomal methylation
LPS	Lipopolysaccharide
MDR	Multidrug-resistant
MEGA	Macrolide efflux genetic assembly
MGE	Mobile genetic elements
MLS_B	Macrolide-lincosamide-streptogramin B
MRSA	Methicillin-resistant *Staphylococcus aureus*
MSSA	Methicillin-sensitive *Staphylococcus aureus*
MurA	UDP-*N*-acetylglucosamine enolpyruvyl transferase
OM	Outer membrane
OptrA	Oxazolidinone and phenicol transferable resistance A
PABA	Para-aminobenzoic acid
PBP	Penicillin-binding protein
PMBN	Polymyxin B nonapeptide
QRDR	Quinolone resistance-determining region
RMTase	RNA methyltransferase
RNAP	RNA polymerase
RPP	Ribosomal protection protein
rRNA	Ribosomal ribonucleic acid
SAM	S-adenosyl-L-methionine
SCC*mec*	Staphylococcal chromosomal cassette *mec*
SSTI	Skin and soft tissue infections
TMP-SMX	Trimethoprim-sulfamethoxazole
UDP-MurNAc	UDP-*N*-acetylmuramic acid
UNAG	UDP-*N*-acetylglucosamine
Vat	Virginiamycin acetyltransferase
Vgb	Virginiamycin gene B
VISA	Vancomycin intermediate *Staphylococcus aureus*
VRE	Vancomycin-resistant *Enterococci*

The original version of this chapter was revised. The correction to this chapter can be found at https://doi.org/10.1007/978-3-030-68321-4_17.

R. A. Shah (✉)
Texas A&M University College of Medicine - Baylor University Medical Center, Dallas, TX, USA
e-mail: radhikashah23@exchange.tamu.edu

Introduction

Antibiotics first achieved widespread use during World War II in the 1940s; however, antibiotic resistance has quickly emerged as a global health crisis over the past several years [1, 2]. The rate at which bacteria are gaining resistance far exceeds that of new drug discovery, placing not only those with infectious diseases at greater risk but also those undergoing immunosuppression by organ transplantation, chemotherapy, or dialysis [3]. Medical and agricultural applications are increasing resistance in both arenas [3]. Eighteen antibiotic-resistant pathogens have recently been identified by the Centers for Disease Control and Prevention (CDC) in their 2019 report as "urgent," "serious," or "concerning" threats to human health (CDC).

Antibiotic resistance is defined as the ability of certain pathogens, including bacteria and fungi, to evade antibiotics designed to kill them (CDC). The number of infections and deaths due to antibiotic-resistant pathogens has fallen since the CDC's Antibiotic Resistance (AR) Threats report was first released in 2013; however, current estimates of almost 2.9 million antibiotic-resistant infections every year prompt investigation into the concept of the antibiotic "resistome" [3]. To begin this investigation, we will discuss resistance in the context of antibiotic targets and biochemical mechanisms of resistance [4].

Origins of Resistance

In 1940, the first antibiotic-resistant bacteria produced penicillinases, which destroyed penicillin [5–7]. Penicillin was first discovered in 1928 by Alexander Fleming, a bacteriologist in London who observed the antibacterial properties of what we now know as penicillin, originally just a fungal contaminant in a petri dish. Years later, scientists could purify the drug and determine its b-lactam structure comprising a four-membered b-lactam ring. The mechanism of action of penicillin antibiotics involves the inhibition of transpeptidase and cross-linking of peptidoglycan via imitation of the last two D-alanine residues [6].

In the decades following the discovery of penicillin, widespread use led to the development of resistant strains of bacteria that produced penicillinases and prompting development of semisynthetic b-lactamase-resistant penicillins [6]. Besides the development of such semisynthetic antimicrobial drugs as methicillin, the discovery of cephalosporin antibiotics in 1945 allowed temporary circumvention around penicillin resistance due to its altered beta-lactam structure [8]. The cephalosporin family of antibiotics includes several generations of drugs, including cephalexin, ceftriaxone, and cefepime, whose spectrum of activity against Gram-negative bacteria increases with each generation.

Resistance to b-lactam antibiotics is mediated by b-lactamase enzymes, which result in the inactivation of cell wall synthesis of bacteria [6]. The enzymes are encoded by genes, known as resistance factors, residing on the bacterial chromosome or plasmids. Specifically, b-lactamases catalyze hydrolysis of the b-lactam bond in the ring structure, producing acidic derivatives that lack antimicrobial properties [9]. Resistance to b-lactam antibiotics will be discussed in further detail later in this chapter.

Mechanisms

The means by which bacteria avoid being targeted by antibiotics comprise an array of simple to complex mechanisms. The simplest and most basic method of resistance involves inherent mutations in the bacterial target gene, preventing binding of the mutant protein by the antibiotic [10]. This type of resistance is inevitable due to intrinsic integrity restrictions of DNA synthesis and can result from just a single gene modification. The acquisition of genes encoding proteins that weaken antibiotic binding to molecular targets can also contribute to de novo bacterial resistance [11]. In addition, molecular targets can be modified by enzymes to block drug binding [12].

Other mechanisms involve lowering an antibiotic's concentration via enzymatic or chemical modification [13]. Efflux pumps along with other transport alterations to decrease permeability can reduce the intracellular concentration of these drugs, to increase resistance to antibiotics [14, 15]. Finally, if an antibiotic target comprises an entity other than a single gene product, resistance to these drugs is attained via retrieval of pre-existing diversity in cell structures and altering their biosynthesis through global cell adaptations (Table 1.1) [16, 17].

Table 1.1 Mechanisms of bacterial resistance by class

Antibiotic class	Mechanisms	Resistant bacteria
Tetracyclines	Target protection	*Campylobacter, Staphylococcus, Streptococcus, Enterococcus*
	Efflux pumps	*Staphylococcus, Streptococcus, Enterococcus, Enterobacter*
Macrolides	Target protection	*Staphylococcus*
	Target site mutation	*Mycobacterium avium, Helicobacter pylori, Streptococcus pneumoniae*
	Enzymatic alteration of target	*Staphylococcus, Enterococcus, Bacteroides*
	Destruction of antibiotic	*Staphylococcus, Enterococcus*
	Efflux pumps	*Staphylococcus*, some Gram-negative species
Lincosamides	Target protection	*Staphylococcus*
	Target site mutation	*Mycobacterium avium, Helicobacter pylori, Streptococcus pneumoniae*
	Enzymatic alteration of target	*Staphylococcus, Enterococcus, Bacteroides*
Oxazolidinones	Target protection	*Streptococcus*
	Target site mutation	*Staphylococcus, Streptococcus, Enterococcus*
	Enzymatic alteration of target	*Staphylococcus, Streptococcus*
Phenicols	Target protection	*Enterococcus*
	Target site mutation	*Escherichia coli, Bacillus subtilis*
	Enzymatic alteration of target	*Staphylococcus, Streptococcus, Enterococcus*
	Chemical alteration of antibiotic	*Staphylococcus, Streptococcus, Enterococcus*
Pleuromutilins	Target protection	*Staphylococcus, Streptococcus, Enterococcus*
	Enzymatic alteration of target	*Staphylococcus, Enterococcus*
Streptogramins	Target protection	Group A – *Staphylococcus, Streptococcus, Enterococcus* Group B – *Staphylococcus, Streptococcus, Enterococcus*
	Enzymatic alteration of target	*Staphylococcus, Streptococcus, Enterococcus*
Aminoglycosides	Target site mutation	*Mycobacterium tuberculosis*
	Enzymatic alteration of target	Actinomycetes
	Chemical alteration of antibiotic	*Salmonella enterica, Klebsiella pneumoniae, Legionella pneumophila*
Rifampin	Target site mutation	*Mycobacterium tuberculosis*
Quinolones	Target site mutation	*Staphylococcus, Enterococcus*
	Target protection	
Glycopeptides	Target site mutation	*Staphylococcus, Streptococcus, Enterococcus*
	Global cell adaptations	*Staphylococcus*
Beta-lactams	Complete replacement/bypass of target site	*Staphylococcus*
	Destruction of antibiotic	*Escherichia coli*
	Decreased permeability	*Escherichia coli*
Sulfonamides	Complete replacement/bypass of target site	*Staphylococcus, Escherichia coli*
Epoxides	Destruction of antibiotic	*Escherichia coli, Pseudomonas aeruginosa, Streptococcus*
Lipopeptides	Global cell adaptations	*Staphylococcus, Enterococcus*

Alteration of Bacterial Proteins Serving as Antimicrobial Targets (Changes in Target Sites)

One of the prime targets of antibiotics is the bacterial ribosome [18], a macromolecular machine for manufacturing proteins, that includes several ribosomal proteins along with three ribosomal RNAs (rRNAs) – 16S, 23S, and 5S [19]. Protein synthesis is a three-step process, including initiation, elongation, and termination, of which elongation is most commonly targeted by antibiotics [18]. Elongation involves the translocation of amino acids to the growing peptide across the A-, P-, and E-sites, resulting in the formation of a single polypeptide. When protein synthesis comes to a halt due to targeting by antibiotics, bacterial cells cannot proliferate. For this reason, they possess certain mechanisms, either innate or acquired, against certain classes of antibiotics to evade targeting, including target protection (Table 1.2) or modification of the target site [18].

Target Protection

Tetracyclines

Tetracyclines, a group of antibiotics first introduced in the 1940s, possess a broad spectrum of activity against both Gram-positive and Gram-

negative bacteria and can be divided into two groups – typical tetracyclines, such as tetracycline, doxycycline, and minocycline, and atypical tetracyclines. Ribosomal protection via Tet(O) and Tet(M) proteins in these bacteria promotes resistance to the typical tetracyclines, as this group of antibiotics act via binding of the 30S ribosomal subunit and subsequent inhibition of the elongation phase of protein synthesis [20, 21]. These ribosomal protection proteins (RPPs) were initially derived from *Campylobacter jejuni* and *Streptococcus* species. They exhibit their protective function due to their similarity in sequence to ribosomal elongation factors, EF-G and EF-Tu [22]. Since both elongation factors belong to the superfamily of GTPases, the RPPs accordingly possess GTPase activity and can hydrolyze GTP in a ribosome-dependent manner [23, 24]. Two mechanisms may explain Tet(O)-mediated tetracycline resistance – (1) a conformational change induced by tetracycline may lead to the binding of Tet(O) to the ribosome and (2) tetracycline may bind ribosomes with open A-sites, which may be the preferred substrate for Tet(O) as opposed to ribosomes with occupied A-sites [25, 26]. The presence of GTP and its subsequent hydrolysis via Tet(O) and Tet(M) allows these RPPs to dislodge tetracyclines from the 30S subunit, preventing its inhibitory action on protein synthesis and conferring resistance.

Table 1.2 Resistance through target protection

Antibiotic class	Mechanism	Type	Bacteria
Tetracyclines	Tet(O)- and Tet(M)-mediated protection	Ribosomal protection proteins (RPPs)	Gram-positive and Gram-negative species
Macrolides	vga(A)-, msr(A)-, msr(C)-, msr(D)-, and msr(E)-mediated protection	ARE ABC-F proteins	Gram-positive species
Lincosamides	vga(A)-, vga(C)-, vga(E)-, vga(D)-, vga(B)-, sal(A)-, eat(A)-, lsa(A)-, lsa(C)-, lsa(B)-, and lsa(E)-mediated protection	ARE ABC-F proteins	Gram-positive species
Oxazolidinones	optr(A)-mediated protection	ARE ABC-F proteins	Gram-positive species
Phenicols	optr(A)-mediated protection	ARE ABC-F proteins	Gram-positive species
Pleuromutilins	vga(A)-, vga(C)-, vga(E)-, vga(D)-, vga(B)-, sal(A)-, eat(A)-, lsa(A)-, lsa(C)-, lsa(B)-, and lsa(E)-mediated protection	ARE ABC-F proteins	Gram-positive species
Streptogramins (group A)	vga(A)-, vga(C)-, vga(E)-, vga(D)-, vga(B)-, sal(A)-, eat(A)-, lsa(A)-, lsa(C)-, lsa(B)-, and lsa(E)-mediated protection	ARE ABC-F proteins	Gram-positive species
Streptogramins (group B)	msr(A)-, msr(C)-, msr(D)-, and msr(E)-mediated protection	ARE ABC-F proteins	Gram-positive species

A novel tetracycline antibiotic, sarecycline (Seysara), has achieved widespread use and recognition in recent years to treat moderate-to-severe acne via a narrow spectrum of antimicrobial activity targeting *C. acnes* and clinically relevant Gram-positive bacteria, including organisms with high-level resistance to the macrolide erythromycin, while having a limited activity against enteric Gram-negative bacteria, a major constituent of the gut microflora [27]. In addition to its anti-inflammatory and anti-bacterial efficacy, sarecycline boasts an improved safety profile, causing less nausea, diarrhea, dizziness, vertigo, and photosensitivity compared to tetracycline, doxycycline, and minocycline [28]. Its mechanism of action involves extension of the C7 group of the sarecycline into the mRNA channel on the small ribosomal subunit, giving way for the drug to interact with the A-site codon in mRNA [29]. This interaction leads to additional stabilization, greater affinity, and increased inhibitory effect of the antibiotic. Due to its narrow spectrum of activity and rational structural design, resistance is less likely to be encountered [27, 30]. It is currently the only antibiotic used in the treatment of acne with a low resistance claim on its label; *Cutibacterium acnes* displays a low propensity for the development of resistance to sarecycline, with spontaneous mutation frequencies being 10^{-10} at 4-8 x MIC. The main mechanism by which bacteria develop resistance against tetracycline-class drugs is ribosomal protection and efflux pump [31]. The hydrolytic activity of the Tet(M) protein in bacteria causes tetracyclines to display an elevated MIC, resulting in decreased susceptibility and ultimately, resistance. An association between broad-spectrum tetracycline antibiotics, especially doxycycline, and gastrointestinal disorders, such as inflammatory bowel disease (IBD) and irritable bowel syndrome (IBS), has been reported in the literature [32–34]. The etiology of this association is still unclear, but it is reported that the broad-spectrum antibiotics' effects may alter the human microbiome to the extent of causing disease. It is important to consider this possibility when prescribing broad-spectrum tetracycline-class antibiotics, especially in long-term treatment of acne, for which doxycycline and minocycline are commonly used.

Macrolides

Macrolides have been used clinically since the 1950s, as the first-generation erythromycin was discovered around that time [35]. Second-generation macrolides, which include clarithromycin and azithromycin, showcased superior pharmacological properties and were introduced later in the 1980s [35, 36]. The emergence of resistance further provoked the development of ketolides, a newer generation of macrolides [37]. Their mechanism of action is similar to that of the tetracyclines; however, rather than binding the 30S subunit of the ribosome, the macrolides bind the 23S rRNA of the 50S subunit of the ribosome to block protein synthesis [38]. The ATP-binding cassette (ABC) family of proteins plays a role in resistance to macrolides by Gram-positive bacteria via ribosomal protection [39]. The ABC-F proteins consist of a single polypeptide grouped together with two ABC domains and are involved in a variety of functions within the cell, including DNA repair, enzyme regulation, and translational control [40]. The particular subgroup of the ABC-F proteins possessed by Gram-positive bacteria responsible for mediating resistance to macrolides and other antibiotics that act on the 50S ribosomal subunit are known as the antibiotic resistance (ARE) ABC-F proteins. The mechanism by which resistance against macrolides is conferred was recently discovered when studying the *vga*(A) determinant of the ARE ABC-F protein class found in *Staphylococcus* species. It was found that this determinant, in addition to msr(A), msr(C), msr(D), and msr(E) found in other species, reduced susceptibility to various classes of antibiotics, including macrolides, though vga(A) has only been previously associated with lincosamide, pleuromutilins, and group A streptogramin resistance [39, 41]. Based on the protein's ability to trigger dissociation of several structurally different classes of antibiotics, its mechanism was determined to be ribosomal protection [39].

Lincosamides

The lincosamide class of antibiotics is structurally composed of L-proline substituted by a 4'-alkyl chain connected to a lincosamine by an amide bond [42, 43]. Lincomycin and clindamycin are two antibiotics in this class, which target anaerobic bacteria, streptococci, and staphylococci [44]. Lincomycin was first isolated from *Streptomyces lincolnensis*, and its chlorinated derivative, clindamycin, has shown superior antibacterial activity, making it a viable option for clinical application [45]. The mechanism of action of these antibiotics, just like macrolides, involves the inhibition of protein synthesis by binding the 23S rRNA of the 50S ribosomal subunit and inhibiting translocation [45]. To evade this, bacteria employ a ribosomal protection mechanism similar to that of macrolides, which involves the ARE ABC-F protein class. The specific determinants conferring resistance to the lincosamides include the Vga, Lsa, Sal, and Vsl homologues [46]. These homologues protect the ribosome via the displacement of the antibiotic [39, 46, 47].

Oxazolidinones

Oxazolidinones, particularly linezolid, were first introduced in 1996 and approved by the Food and Drug Administration in 2000 after their antibacterial effects had been studied [48]. Linezolid, particularly, has since been identified as a lead compound, exhibiting pharmacological parameters proposing its value as a starting point for therapeutics development [48, 49]. It is commonly used in the treatment of diseases caused by various Gram-positive bacteria, including vancomycin-resistant *Enterococci* (VRE) species, such as *Enterococcus faecium*, hospital-acquired pneumonia caused by *Staphylococcus aureus*, and community-acquired pneumonia caused by *Streptococcus pneumoniae* [49]. Unlike the antibiotic classes already discussed, this class attacks bacteria by binding both the 30S and 50S ribosomal subunits, preventing the formation of the initiation complex and ultimately decreasing the rate of translation [49, 50]. Although linezolid has been utilized successfully in the treatment of several multidrug-resistant (MDR) organisms, resistance to oxazolidinones is concerning. Resistance through ribosomal protection occurs by dissociation of the antibiotic due to the oxazolidinone and phenicol transferable resistance A (OptrA) determinant of the ARE ABC-F class of proteins via binding of the peptidyl transferase A site [47, 51, 52].

Phenicols

Chloramphenicol was first isolated in 1947, claiming its title as the first phenicol antibiotic and first natural product containing a nitro group [53]. Other phenicols, including thiamphenicol and florfenicol, are rarely used in humans but are sometimes employed in veterinary medicine [53]. Chloramphenicol's spectrum of activity ranges across various classes of Gram-positive and Gram-negative bacteria, but the serious adverse effects associated with its use, such as dose-independent aplastic anemia, dose-dependent bone marrow suppression, and gray baby syndrome in neonates and infants, have downgraded its status as a promising antimicrobial agent [54, 55]. Due to this, actual clinical use to treat infections is very limited [53]. Its mechanism of action is like that of many other antibiotics, through binding of the 50S ribosomal unit to inhibit the elongation step of translation. Just like the antibiotic classes already discussed, one mechanism by which bacteria evade the actions of phenicols is via ribosomal protection. The same determinant of the ARE ABC-F class of proteins which confers resistance to oxazolidinones, OptrA, also confers resistance to the phenicol class of antibiotics by dissociating the antibiotic from its ribosomal target [46].

Pleuromutilins

Like phenicols, pleuromutilins were discovered as natural antimicrobial agents in the early 1950s [56]. From these, tiamulin and valnemulin, two semisynthetic pleuromutilins, were created. The pleuromutilins possess activity against anaerobic Gram-negative and Gram-positive bacteria in particular. Although tiamulin and valnemulin are exclusively utilized in veterinary medicine, retapamulin was the first pleuromutilin approved for human use as a topical treatment in 2007 [53, 56–59]. Furthermore, lefamulin was the first pleuromutilin developed for use in the intravenous and oral forms to treat systemic infections [58]. The mechanism by which pleuromutilins exhibit their bacteriostatic activity is via inhibition of peptide bond formation through binding of the V domain of the 50S ribosomal subunit, thereby interfering with proper positioning of the CCA ends of tRNAs for peptide transfer in the A- and P-sites [58, 60]. It has also been postulated that the pleuromutilins may also act via inhibition of the initiation step of translation [58, 61]. Although resistance is rarely a concern in this class of antibiotics, it does exist. The manner by which the target classes of bacteria evade the pleuromutilins is via ribosomal protection. Vga/Lsa/Sal/Vml, the same ARE ABC-F protein homologues that confer resistance to lincosamides, confer resistance to pleuromutilin antibiotics through interaction with the ribosome and displacement of the bound drug [46, 47].

Quinolones

The quinolones are a synthetic class of antibiotics rather than being isolated from living organisms. The first quinolone, nalidixic acid, was derived from chloroquine, an anti-malarial drug, and through further manipulation and addition of a fluorine atom, fluoroquinolones were developed [62, 63]. Newer-generation fluoroquinolones exhibit improved coverage against Gram-positive and Gram-negative organisms, and they include ciprofloxacin, levofloxacin, and moxifloxacin [62]. These antibiotics exert their bactericidal effects via inhibition of the bacterial DNA gyrase and topoisomerase IV, which, in turn, inhibits DNA replication [62]. Their extensive Gram-positive and Gram-negative coverage makes them a desirable treatment option for many infectious processes. Although their effects as antibiotics are outstanding, they may still succumb to bacterial resistance via two mechanisms, one of which is target protection.

Target protection is plasmid-mediated and was first reported in 1998. The responsible gene, *qnrA*, was identified by PCR in 2002 and found at low frequency on plasmids in Gram-negative isolates [64]. This gene encodes a pentapeptide repeat protein (PRP), QnrA1, which binds to topoisomerase II and competes with DNA by protecting DNA gyrase and topoisomerase IV

from inhibitory quinolone activity [65]. Other PRPs responsible for quinolone resistance include QnrB1 and QnrS1. PRPs contain domains composed of tandem repeats of amino acid sequences. In a study involving Qnr-type determinants from *Vibrio parahaemolyticus*, it was shown that a single amino acid substitution significantly enhanced resistance to quinolone antibiotics when the gene was cloned and expressed in *Escherichia coli* [65, 66].

Streptogramins

The streptogramin family of antibiotics consists of two substances which are chemically unrelated: streptogramin A and streptogramin B. The A group are polyunsaturated mactolactones, and they belong to the polyketide family of antibiotics. The B group, on the other hand, are cyclic hexadepsipeptides of the nonribosomal peptide antibiotic family [67, 68]. This family of antibiotics, which was patented by Merck in 1957, gets its name from the strain from which it was isolated, *Streptomyces graminofaciens* [67, 69]. Although initially targeted for use in animal production, the streptogramin family of antibiotics, particularly pristinamycin, was finally introduced into human therapy. Pristinamycin covers a wide range of Gram-positive pathogens and a few Gram-negative pathogens, including drug-resistant organisms [67, 70]. Streptogramin A and streptogramin B have moderate bacteriostatic activity through inhibition of protein synthesis, and they both act on the 50S subunit of the ribosome, and while the A type prevents binding of the amino acyl-tRNA, the B type inhibits peptide elongation by releasing the peptidyl-tRNA [67, 71]. Several mechanisms of resistance to streptogramins have been described in the literature (Fig. 1.1); however, not much is known about ribosomal protection. Different transporter genes that code for ABC transporters, such as varL, varM, and varS, have been implicated in this particular mechanism and confer resistance to streptogramin antibiotics [67, 72, 73].

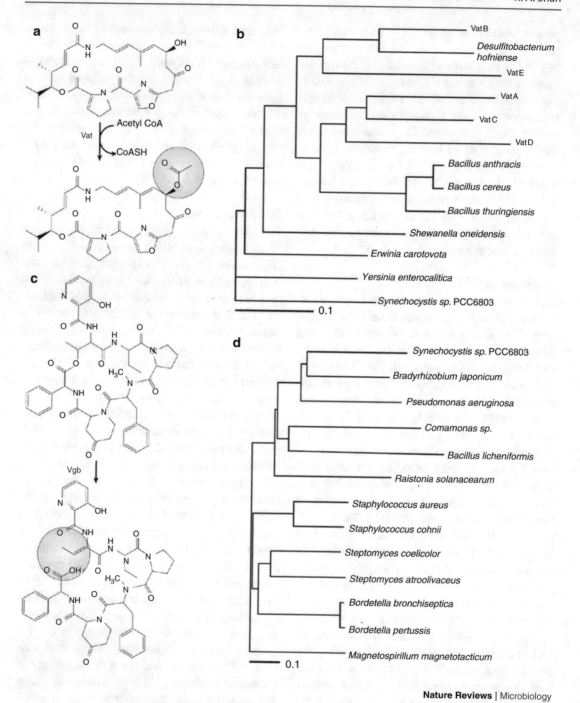

Nature Reviews | Microbiology

Fig. 1.1 Resistance to streptogramin A antibiotics occurs via acetylation of a hydroxyl group. (a) Chemical modification of pristinamycin is catalyzed by virginiamycin acetyltransferase (Vat) enzymes. (b) Various homologues and orthologues of Vat enzymes, which are found in clinically resistant strains of bacteria, are also widely distributed in several environmental bacterial species. (c) Resistance to streptogramin B antibiotics is catalyzed by virginiamycin resistance gene B (Vgb) enzymes through cleavage of the cyclic depsipeptide of pristinamycin IA. (d) Various homologues and orthologues of Vgb genes are found in the genomes of environmental bacteria. The sequence alignments of amino acids were constructed using Clustal W. The trees do not represent a phylogenetic analysis, but they convey the sequence relationship among the enzymes [74].

Modification of Target Site

More commonly than ribosomal protection, modification of target sites is employed by many pathogens to evade the bacteriostatic or bactericidal effects of antibiotics. Since antibiotics typically bind their targets with high affinity, any changes to the target structure that prevent binding by the antibiotic but preserve function can confer resistance [75]. These changes in the target structure can be achieved in several ways, including point mutations in genes encoding target sites, enzymatic alterations of binding sites, and replacement or bypass of target sites [76].

Mutations

Aminoglycosides

The aminoglycoside (AG) class of antibiotics was introduced in the clinical setting in the 1940s. The first AG, streptomycin, was isolated from *Streptomyces* griseus, and it was the first antibiotic successfully used to treat tuberculosis [77]. Due to its success, several other AGs were subsequently discovered and used in clinical practice to target Gram-positive and Gram-negative pathogens, including neomycin, gentamicin, and tobramycin. In addition to severe adverse effects related to these drugs, including ototoxicity and nephrotoxicity, widespread use inevitably led to the development of resistance against these antibiotics, leading to attempts to counter this through the development of semi-synthetic second-generation AGs, such as amikacin. Like many other classes of antibiotics, AGs act via inhibition of protein synthesis. These drugs bind to the 16S rRNA of the 30S ribosomal subunit with high affinity, altering the structure and ultimately promoting mistranslation and error-prone protein synthesis [78, 79].

Other ways by which AGs inhibit protein synthesis is through inhibition of initiation and elongation [76, 77]. Resistance to these drugs is achieved most commonly via modification of the bacterial target site through mutations [79, 80]. These mutations can occur in the *rrs* gene, which codes for the 16S rRNA, hindering AG binding [80]. Many of the mutations, however, are lethal and not very common. A viable mutant, A1408G, disrupts the hydrogen bonding interaction between 2-deoxystreptamine (2-DOS) AGs, such as neomycin B and gentamicin, and the helix 44 (h44) nucleotide A1408. This mutation has been found in some resistant strains of *Mycobacterium tuberculosis* [80, 81]. Another mutation leading to resistance in *M. tuberculosis* is the rspL mutation, which affects the S12 protein and leads to high-level resistance to streptomycin. This mutation interferes with tRNA selection through conformational distortions of the decoding site, impairing GTPase activation of Ef-Tu [82].

Macrolides

In addition to ribosomal protection, bacteria can confer resistance to macrolides via mutations in their target sites. As mentioned earlier, macrolides act on the 23S rRNA of the 50S ribosomal subunit, so mutations altering this part of the ribosome can lead to resistance to these antibiotics. Mutants of the ribosome observed in macrolide-lincosamide-streptogramin B (MLS_B) antibiotics include base substitutions in domain II or V of 23S rRNA and ribosomal proteins, such as L4 and L22 [83–85]. Since macrolides primarily interact with A2058 and A2059 of the 23S rRNA, mutations in these nucleotides confer resistance to these antibiotics. In addition, insertion, deletion, and missense mutations in genes encoding L4 and L22 proteins of the ribosome can lead to resistance to macrolide antibiotics.

The L4 and L22 proteins consist of globular surface domains and elongated "tentacles," which are able to extend into the large ribosomal subunit's core and line part of the peptide exit tunnel. As a result of these mutations, rRNA processing and ribosome assembly are affected, making the bacterial ribosome a nonviable target for macrolide antibiotics [86–88].

Phenicols

Unlike resistance to macrolides via target mutation, resistance to phenicols is rarely achieved through this mechanism; however, it has been reported in the literature. Mutations in major ribosomal protein gene clusters have been observed in *Escherichia coli* and *Bacillus subtilis*, resulting in resistance to phenicol antibiotics [54, 89]. In addition, in a similar mechanism of resistance to that affecting macrolide antibiotics, mutations in the gene coding for 23S rRNA can also confer resistance to phenicols [54, 90, 91]. An explanation why this type of resistance is rarely seen against phenicol antibiotics is the lethality of the mutations themselves, rendering the ribosomes nonfunctional [54].

Rifampin

Rifampin, discovered in Italy in 1965 and applied in clinical practice in the United States in 1971, is an established first-line drug utilized in the treatment of tuberculosis. The drug is derived from rifamycin SV, which itself is semisynthetically derived from rifamycin B, a complex macrocyclic antibiotic [92]. Through binding and inactivation of bacterial DNA-dependent RNA polymerase (RNAP) paired with intracellular penetration, rifampin is able to execute its bactericidal effects against a wide spectrum of pathogens, including Gram-positive and Gram-negative species as well as *Chlamydia* and *Legionella* species [92, 93]. Resistance to rifampin occurs primarily through target mutation involving the *rpoB* gene coding for the b-subunit of the RNAP. The region affected is known as the *Rif*

site and resides between amino acid positions 500 and 575. As a result of this mutation, rifampin's binding affinity for RNAP decreases, ultimately leading to resistance [93, 94]. Although binding affinity of rifampin for RNAP is decreased, catalytic activity of the RNAP is preserved, allowing transcription to occur normally [95].

Lincosamides

Lincosamides, particularly clindamycin, interact with the 23S rRNA of the 50S ribosomal subunit primarily at the A2058 and A2059 sites. Mutant strains of *Mycobacterium smegmatis* were created via transformation with plasmid pMV361 to observe and detail the exact mechanism of resistance conferred to clindamycin. Susceptibility of these mutant strains were subsequently tested, and it was found that an A-to-G mutation at site 2058 conferred a high level of resistance to clindamycin, whereas an A-to-G mutation at site 2059 conferred a lower level of resistance [96].

Quinolones

The quinolones are a synthetic class of antibiotics rather than being isolated from living organisms. The first quinolone, nalidixic acid, was derived from chloroquine, an anti-malarial drug, and through further manipulation and addition of a fluorine atom, fluoroquinolones were developed [97]. Newer-generation fluoroquinolones exhibit improved coverage against Gram-positive and Gram-negative organisms, and they include ciprofloxacin, levofloxacin, and moxifloxacin [97]. These antibiotics exert their bactericidal effects via inhibition of the bacterial DNA gyrase and topoisomerase IV, which, in turn, inhibits DNA replication [97, 98]. Their extensive Gram-positive and Gram-negative coverage makes them a desirable treatment option for many infectious processes. Although their effects as antibiotics are outstanding, they may still succumb to bacterial resistance via two mechanisms, one of which is target mutation. Amino acid substitutions at the quinolone resistance-determining regions (QRDR) of corresponding genes account for mutations in the bacterial DNA replication enzymes. In mutations affecting DNA gyrase, substitutions occur at the *gyrA* and *gyrB* genes, while substitutions occur at *parC* and *parE* in mutations affecting DNA topoisomerase IV [99]. In Gram-positive organisms, *parC* is usually the first gene to undergo mutation to target topoisomerase IV; however, in Gram-negative organisms, mutations in *gyrA* confer protection for the bacteria through DNA gyrase [99, 100]. The QRDR corresponds to particular regions on the DNA-binding surfaces of affected enzymes, and mutations here reduce the antibiotic's binding affinity for the enzymes, thereby conferring resistance [98]. It has been found that resistance to fluoroquinolones occurs in a stepwise fashion with progressively more mutations, increasing resistance [100].

Oxazolidinones

Since oxazolidinones, such as linezolid and tedizolid, interact with the 23S rRNA, mutations here lead to resistance of several Gram-positive organisms, such as enterococci, to these drugs by decreasing binding affinity [101] (Fig. 1.2). As mentioned earlier, oxazolidinones exert their bacteriostatic effects by inhibiting the initiation of translation and translocation of the peptidyl-tRNA from the A-site to the P-site [102]. Most mutations in the 23S rRNA involve G to U substitutions in the peptidyl-transferase region at position 2576, affecting the P-site. This particular mutation has been observed in vancomycin-resistant enterococci, resulting in a decrease in linezolid sensitivity [103]. Other 23S rRNA modifications have been observed in *E. coli*, including mutations closer to the A-site at positions 2032 and 2447 [104].

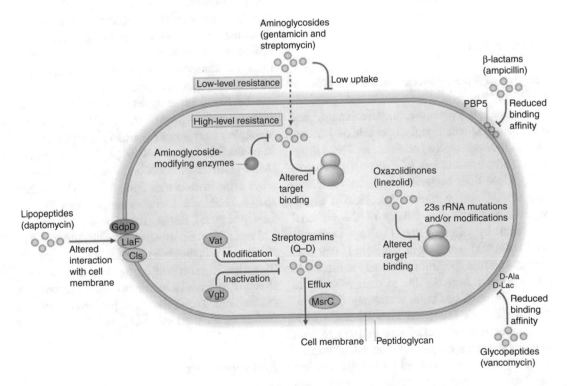

Fig. 1.2 Main mechanisms of enterococcal antibiotic resistance

Enterococci possess both intrinsic and extrinsic antibiotic resistance mechanisms, which are shown here. Resistance to ampicillin in *Enterococcus faecium* occurs through the production of penicillin-binding protein 5 (PBP5), which has a low affinity for b-lactam antibiotics. In addition, these bacteria exhibit low-level resistance to aminoglycoside antibiotics due to decreased uptake of the polar molecules. On the other hand, high-level resistance to aminoglycosides can also occur through the acquisition of modifying enzymes, leading to altered target binding. The peptidoglycan synthesis pathway is affected in resistance to glycopeptide antibiotics, such as vancomycin. In resistance to streptogramin quinupristin-dalfopristin (Q-D) antibiotics, several pathways are implicated, including drug modification via Vat, drug inactivation via Vgb, and drug efflux via ABC proteins [102]. Although rare, resistance to the oxazolidinone antibiotic, linezolid, involves 23S rRNA-binding site mutations. Daptomycin resistance involves altered cell membrane interactions [103].

Glycopeptides

The glycopeptide antibiotics consist of a group of cyclic or polycyclic non-ribosomal peptides, which include vancomycin, teicoplanin, and other semisynthetic lipoglycopeptide derivatives, such as dalbavancin and oritavancin. These drugs act as substrate binders of cell-wall precursors and achieve their bactericidal effects via inhibition of cell-wall synthesis. Specifically, glycopeptides prevent cross-linking of the bacterial cell wall by binding the D-alanyl-D-alanine (D-Ala-D-Ala) terminus of the lipid II cell wall precursor. Their spectrum of activity is limited to Gram-positive bacteria due to their inability to traverse through the outer membrane in Gram-negative species [104]. Of significance, vancomycin was first used clinically in 1955 to treat infections caused by penicillin-resistant staphylococci [104]. It was not until 1987 that the first case of a vancomycin-resistant strain was reported [105, 106]. While Gram-negative species of bacteria are intrinsically resistant to the action of glycopeptides due to the outer membrane's capacity to block the passages of large, complex molecules, Gram-positive species possess different mechanisms to evade death, including target mutation. Several mutations in genetic loci contribute to a thickened cell wall, which serves as the target of glycopeptide antibiotics.

Enzymatic Alteration

Macrolides, Lincosamides, and Streptogramin B

A well-known mechanism of resistance employed by some bacterial species is an erythromycin ribosomal methylation (*erm*) gene-encoded enzymatic methylation of the ribosome. Methylation occurs on an adenine residue in position A2058 of domain V of the 23S rRNA of the 50S ribosomal subunit, thus impairing binding of the antibiotic molecule to its target and ultimately leading to resistance. Since macrolides, lincosamides, and streptogramin B interact with the same binding site on the ribosome, *erm* gene expression confers cross-resistance across antibiotic classes through plasmids and transposons in pathogenic bacteria [76, 107]. These genes, specifically *erm(A)* and *erm(C)*, can be found in staphylococci. While *erm(A)* is predominantly found in methicillin-resistant *Staphylococcus aureus* (MRSA), *erm(C)* is found in methicillin-susceptible *Staphylococcus aureus* (MSSA). In streptococci and enterococci, *erm(B)* plays a role in resistance through methylation. The specific antibiotics in these classes induce the *erm* family of genes, leading to the production of Erm and methylase and subsequent methylation of 23S rRNA [107]. In the absence of an inducer, a mRNA transcript is generated along with a secondary structure that works to conceal the upstream *erm* binding site. Translation then proceeds normally, preventing the production of Erm [76].

Aminoglycosides

Aminoglycosides (AGs) can also succumb to bacterial resistance via enzymatic alteration. The 16S ribosomal subunit contains RNA methyltransferases (RMTases), which modify the AG-binding site and prevent AG from binding [108]. These RMTases, which include RmtB and ArmA, were isolated from *actinomycetes*, the same organisms from which AGs were originally isolated, and in order to protect ribosomes from AG inhibition, these organisms produce the RMTases to methylate their own 16S rRNA [82]. They can be found in food products, which suggest food as a vehicle for the spread of AG resistance [109]. Other bacterial species can acquire the RMTases by uptake of a plasmid which contains the RMTase gene as well as other potential resistance genes. The mechanism by which RMTases confer resistance is through methylation of a nucleotide, either the N7 position of nucleotide G1405 or the N1 position of A1408, in the AG-binding site of the 16S rRNA. Unfortunately, because of the RMTases' ability to confer resistance to clinically useful antibiotics, such as amikacin, the increasing prevalence of bacterial possession of RMTases poses a sizeable threat [81].

Oxazolidinones, Phenicols, Pleuromutilins, and Streptogramin A

Another plasmid-borne determinant, the *cfr* gene, confers resistance to oxazolidinones, such as linezolid. This gene has been found in several human pathogens, including *S. aureus*, *E. faecalis*, *E. faecium*, and Gram-negative bacteria [110]. The gene codes for the Cfr enzyme, which belongs to the S-adenosyl-L-methionine (SAM) methylase family and also confers resistance to the phenicol, pleuromutilin, and streptogramin A classes of antibiotics. The Cfr enzyme functions similarly to Erm, as it is responsible for the methylation which occurs at position A2503 of the 23S rRNA of the 50S ribosomal subunit. This methylation results in a decreased binding affinity of the antibiotic for the bacteria and ultimately leads to bacterial resistance [76, 110]. It is important to note, however, that tedizolid, another oxazolidinone antibiotic, is not affected by this mechanism of resistance [76].

Complete Replacement or Bypass of Target Site

Beta-Lactams

β-lactams are the most widely used class of antibiotics. Benzyl penicillin was first discovered in the 1920s. Since then, countless derivatives and other β-lactam classes, including cephalosporins, monobactams, and carbapenems, have been discovered [111]. As each new class was developed, the spectrum of activity also increased to enhance coverage and address resistance. The β-lactams are bactericidal and act via interruption of bacterial cell-wall synthesis through covalent binding to penicillin-binding proteins (PBPs) [76, 111]. These proteins are enzymes which play a role in the final steps of peptidoglycan cross-linking, or transpeptidation, in Gram-positive and Gram-negative bacteria [111]. Resistance to β-lactams, particularly in *S. aureus*, is achieved through the acquisition of a foreign gene, *mecA*, which is found in a DNA fragment known as the staphylococcal chromosomal cassette *mec* (SCC*mec*). The *mecA* gene encodes PBP2a, which has a low affinity for all β-lactams and renders most of these drugs useless against resistant bacteria, such as MRSA [112]. The action of *mecA* is mediated by a two-component regulatory system, including the repressor protein, MecI, and a signal transducer, MecR1. Upon detection of β-lactams in the environment, MecR1 triggers a signal transduction cascade, removing MecI from its DNA-binding site and allowing transcription of *mecA* [76, 112].

Sulfonamides

Sulfonamides, the first commercially available class of antibiotics, were first used clinically in the 1930s. In this class, sulfamethoxazole and sulfadiazine have proven to be the most useful agents. Trimethoprim, on the other hand, was first used clinically in the 1960s [113]. Used in combination, trimethoprim and sulfamethoxazole have a synergistic effect. Both drugs act antagonistically against enzymes in the folic acid synthesis pathway. Sulfamethoxazole inhibits dihydropteroate synthase (DHPS), preventing the formation of dihydrofolate from para-aminobenzoic acid (PABA). Trimethoprim inhibits dihydrofolate reductase (DHFR), preventing the formation of tetrahydrofolate from dihydro-folate [113]. Unlike resistance to β-lactams and glycopeptides, resistance to trimethoprim-sulfamethoxazole (TMP-SMX) involves increased production of the antimicrobial target, which would overwhelm the antibiotic due to an increased number of targets [76]. The overpro-duction of DHPS and DHFR occurs via muta-tions in the promoter regions of DNA encoding these enzymes, resulting in their increased pro-duction and subsequent negative impact on the ability of TMP-SMX to inhibit folate production [113].

Enzymatic Degradation of Antimicrobial Drugs (Modifications of the Antibiotic Molecule)

Resistance to certain antibiotic drugs can be achieved through bacterial modification or degra-dation of the antibiotic, as bacteria encode sev-eral enzymes that can perform these actions [114]. Mechanisms of modification include acet-ylation, phosphorylation, glycosylation, and hydroxylation, and these impede the binding of corresponding drugs to their ribosomal targets [115]. On the other hand, bacteria can encode enzymes that lead to degradation or destruction of the antibiotic molecule, such as β-lactamases and macrolide esterases [116–118].

Chemical Alterations of the Antibiotic

Aminoglycosides
The presence of aminoglycoside (AG)-modifying enzymes (AMEs) in bacteria confers resistance to the AG class of antibiotics via covalent modifi-cation of the hydroxyl or amino groups of the drug. These enzymes can be found in mobile genetic elements (MGEs) as well as on chromo-somes in certain species of bacteria, and they are acquired by pathogenic bacteria via horizontal gene transfer [81]. The AMEs consist of acetyl-transferases, adenyl transferases, and phos-photransferases [76]. AG acetyltransferases belong to the GCN5 family of proteins and are classified based on their regiospecificity of enzyme action on the AG structure. These enzymes carry out their function by binding to the A-site on the 16S rRNA of the ribosome, resulting in an impairment of the codon-anticodon decoding mechanism. This leads to aberrant pro-tein synthesis, consequent impaired translation fidelity, and, ultimately, resistance to these drugs [119, 120].

Phenicols
One mechanism of resistance to chloramphenicol involves enzymatic alteration through the expres-sion of chloramphenicol acetyltransferases (CATs) in bacteria. Several *cat* genes are expressed in both Gram-positive and Gram-negative bacteria and can be classified according to the level of resistance conferred. Type A CATs confer high-level resistance to chloramphenicol, whereas Type B CATs confer low-level resis-tance [53]. The trimeric acetyltransferases act by acetylating hydroxyl groups of chloramphenicol, rendering the drug unable to bind the 50S ribo-somal subunit of bacteria appropriately [89–91].

Destruction of the Antibiotic Molecule

Beta-Lactams
Resistance to β-lactams has been studied intensely since the first-reported production of penicillinase by *E. coli* [111]. The enzymes con-ferring resistance to the β-lactam antibiotics are collectively known as the β-lactamases, and the molecular mechanisms contributing to the development of resistance via hydrolytic cleav-age include the action of an active site Ser nucleophile or activation of water via a zinc ion center (Fig. 1.3). Genes encoding β-lactamases can be found on either the bacterial chromo-

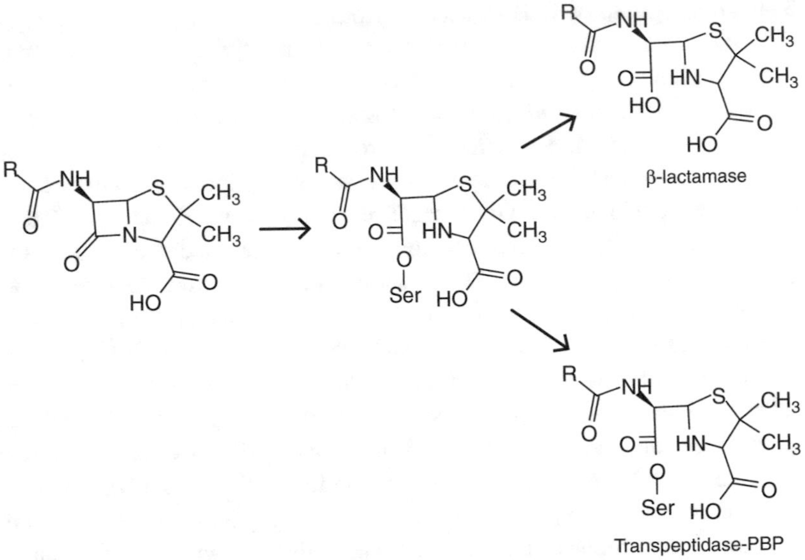

Fig. 1.3 The acylation of b-lactam antibiotics occurs via the action of transpeptidases and b-lactamases. While transpeptidases are subsequently trapped, b-lactamases lead to deacylation and hydrolysis [121].

some or on plasmids. Chromosomal β-lactamases are universal throughout a particular bacterial species, but β-lactamases encoded by plasmids are variable and transferable across species [116, 118]. This transferable resistance creates an issue when an infectious process warrants the use of a β-lactam antibiotic as first-line therapy, such as penicillin or cephalosporin, as options become limited. For example, cephalosporins are commonly used in the treatment of skin and soft tissue infections (SSTIs) due to their extended coverage and wide spectrum of activity, but the increasing prevalence of resistance now poses a threat to this easily accessible, cost-effective therapy. The β-lactamases are particularly prevalent in Gram-negative pathogens. The Ser-β-lactamases utilize a covalent catalytic mechanism similar to that of Ser proteinases and esterases, which involves a ring-opening nucleophilic attack on the lactam ring followed by hydrolytic cleavage of the enzyme intermediate. As a result, β-lactam antibiotics are rendered unable to inhibit bacterial cell-wall synthesis.

Macrolides

Macrolide antibiotics are formed cyclically via an ester bond resulting from the final ring-forming step, which is catalyzed by a thioesterase [119]. This ester bond serves as the target for macrolide resistance enzymes, the first of which was reported in an isolate of *E. coli* in the 1980s [120]. The macrolide resistance enzymes, such as erythromycin esterases, lead to high levels of resistance, although the utilization of these enzymes by bacteria is not a common drug resistance mechanism [117]. The genes encoding these esterases can be found on MGEs, concerning for widespread resistance in the microbial community [114].

Epoxides

Fosfomycin, a phosphoenolpyruvate (PEP) analogue produced by various *Streptomyces* species, was discovered in the late 1960s. Its bactericidal mechanism of action involves inhibition of an enzyme-catalyzed reaction in bacterial cell-wall synthesis [122]. Specifically, fosfomycin disrupts the formation of the peptidoglycan precursor UDP-*N*-acetylmuramic acid (UDP-MurNAc), which is the first step of biosynthesis in the cytoplasm. The enzyme UDP-*N*-acetylglucosamine enolpyruvyl transferase (MurA) is involved in peptidoglycan synthesis through the transfer of the enolpyruvyl portion of the PEP to the

3′-hydroxyl group of UDP-*N*-acetylglucosamine (UNAG). MurA has been found to contain an active site harboring a thiol group of a cysteine at position 115 in *E. coli* to which fosfomycin binds, inactivating the enzyme and preventing cell wall synthesis. The drug is active against both Gram-positive and Gram-negative pathogens, especially *Enterococcus* species, *Staphylococcus epidermidis*, *E. coli,* and *Shigella* species [123].Resistance to fosfomycin occurs due to the destruction of the drug through the ring opening by either water or a thiol-containing co-substrate. FosA, a fosfomycin resistance enzyme, is encoded on resistance plasmids in Gram-negative bacteria and acts by catalyzing the fosfomycin epoxide ring opening utilizing the thiolate of glutathione as the reactive nucleophile [124]. Plasmids found in Gram-positive bacteria possess a gene, *fosB*, which codes for an enzyme with a similar function [103, 125].

Changes in Membrane Permeability to Antibiotics

Oftentimes, resistance to antibiotics is mediated by the inability of the drug to reach its target due to changes in membrane permeability, through either decreased permeability or presence of efflux pumps. The outer membrane (OM) of Gram-negative bacteria adds an extra layer of protection to the organism and comprises a lipid bilayer containing pore-forming porins [126]. Resistance due to decreased permeability can be achieved by different means, including porin-mediated and lipid-mediated mechanisms. On the other hand, resistance due to efflux pumps occurs in Gram-positive and Gram-negative pathogens and involves the extrusion of the antibiotic out of the cell [65].

Decreased Permeability

Some antibiotic drugs, such as β-lactams, cross the bilayer using the pore-forming porins, while other drugs, such as macrolides and other hydrophobic drugs, cross the bilayer via diffusion.

Therefore, any changes to the porin structure or the lipids which make up the bilayer can decrease permeability and resistance [126]. The OM of Gram-negative bacteria comprises the phospholipid and lipopolysaccharides (LPS). Lipopolysaccharide molecules consist of three separate parts, including lipid A, a short core oligosaccharide, and O-antigen. Certain Gram-negative bacteria expressing a full-length LPS have an intrinsic resistance to hydrophobic antibiotics [126]. On the other hand, membrane-permeabilizing antibiotics, such as Tris/EDTA, polymyxin B, and polymyxin B nonapeptide (PMBN), can increase sensitivity of bacteria like *E. coli* and *Salmonella typhimurium* to the hydrophobic drugs through the release of LPS into the growing medium and resultant replacement by glycerophospholipids. This replacement results in a patchy bilayer with greater permeability to lipophilic compounds [126, 127]. However, resistant mutants have been isolated from the aforementioned Gram-negative pathogens [126, 128]. These mutants contain substitutions in their LPS molecules which lower the negative charge, resulting in a decreased repulsion between molecules and reduced sensitivity to polymyxin B and PMBN [127, 128]. When considering porin-mediated resistance, the ability or rate of entry of antibiotics must be taken into account, as any decrease in these can lead to resistance. Functional changes or loss of porins results in acquired resistance. *OmpF*, a major porin, has been implicated in several reports of changes in porin expression contributing to resistance [129, 130]. Major porin-based mechanisms of bacterial resistance include the following: (1) outer membrane alterations due to loss of porins or replacement of major porins by other porins and (2) altered function due to mutations which result in reduced permeability [126, 129].

Beta-Lactams

Loss of the *OmpF* porin is implicated in isolates of *E. coli* resistant to β-lactam antibiotics [130]. In a study of these β-lactam-resistant mutants of *E. coli*, *OmpF* porins could not be located, although the growth medium favored expression of the encoding gene. The mutants instead over-produced the *OmpC* porin, which was found to produce a less efficient channel compared to that of *OmpF*. This replacement resulted in decreased permeability of β-lactams and, ultimately, resistance to these drugs [131, 132]. In addition to a loss of porins, mutations affecting porin function can also confer resistance to antibiotics. Loop 3 of different porins inserts into the interior portion of porin channels to form the constriction zone [130–132]. When a G-to-D mutation occurs in loop 3 of the *OmpF/OmpC*-like protein of *Enterobacter aerogenes*, a loss of conductance in the porin results, leading to decreased susceptibility to β-lactams [130–132].

Efflux Pumps

Another mechanism by which bacteria may become resistant to antibiotics is through their ability to expel toxic compounds out of the cell. One of the first examples of this was described in the 1980s, demonstrating *E. coli's* efflux system and its ability to clear the cytoplasm of tetracycline [133]. Efflux pumps can be found in both Gram-positive and Gram-negative pathogens and are classified into five major families: (1) the major facilitator superfamily; (2) the small multidrug resistance superfamily; (3) the resistance-nodulation-cell-division family; (4) the ATP-binding cassette family; and (5) the multidrug and toxic compound extrusion family [134].

Tetracyclines

A classic example of efflux pump-mediated resistance involves tetracycline antibiotics. Tet efflux pumps, which belong to the major facilitator superfamily, utilize proton exchange to generate energy for extruding tetracyclines. They are encoded by *tet* genes in MGEs of many Gram-negative organisms [65]. Working against a concentration gradient, efflux proteins exchange protons for a tetracycline-cation complex, and, as a result, the intercellular concentration of tetracycline is reduced [135]. It is important to note that the efflux pumps decrease susceptibility tetracycline and doxycycline, whereas minocycline and

tigecycline remain unaffected [65]. Other transport systems besides those that are tetracycline-specific can extrude tetracyclines via MDR efflux pumps, such as AcrAB-TolC and MexAB-OprM in *Enterobacteriaceae* and *P. aeruginosa*, respectively [136, 137].

Macrolides

Efflux pumps conferring resistance to the macrolide class of antibiotics are encoded by *mef* genes, including *mefE* and *mefA*. The Mef pumps can be found in *Streptococcus* species as well as other Gram-positive organisms. While MefA is typically carried in transposons found in the bacterial chromosome, MefE resides in the macrolide efflux genetic assembly (MEGA) element, a fragment of DNA on the chromosome [65]. Other efflux pumps, which belong to the ABC transporter family, also contribute to macrolide resistance in Gram-positive pathogens. MsrA, a plasmid-borne determinant, is responsible for macrolide resistance in *Staphylococcus epidermidis*, and MsrC, a chromosomally encoded protein, is responsible for low-level macrolide resistance in *Enterococcus faecalis* [65, 138].

Global Cell Adaptations

Aside from the complex, sophisticated mechanisms that bacteria have developed over time in response to an attack by molecules and competition of nutrients, some species have developed resistant phenotypes to antibiotics, such as daptomycin and vancomycin, through a global cell adaptive response [65].

Lipopeptides

Daptomycin (DAP), a lipopeptide antibiotic, executes its bactericidal effect by disrupting the homeostasis of the cell envelope. This class of antibiotics is related to cationic antimicrobial peptides (CAMPs), which are produced by the innate immune system. Certain bacterial species, such as *E. faecalis*, have developed mechanisms to withstand action by these CAMPs and protect the cell envelope (Fig. 1.2). A DAP-resistant strain of *E. faecalis* was studied using whole-genome sequencing, and changes in a three-component regulatory system, LiaFSR, were discovered. LiaFSR regulates the stress response for the cell envelope in Gram-positive bacteria. The system was first described in *Bacillus subtilis* and consists of three proteins: (1) LiaF, a transmembrane protein which acts as a negative regulator of the system; (2) LiaS, a histidine kinase protein which phosphorylates the response regulator; and (3) LiaR, the response regulator. An isoleucine deletion at position 177 of LiaF was shown to increase the MIC of DAP and abolish DAP's bactericidal activity. Another regulatory system, YycFG, has been implicated in DAP resistance in *S. aureus* and enterococci. The mechanism underlying resistance through this regulatory system is not well-understood, but it seems to involve alteration in cell-wall metabolism through changes in surface charge, producing electrostatic repulsion of the positively charged DAP-calcium complex from the cell envelope and, eventually, resistance [65].

Glycopeptides

S. aureus isolates possessing an intermediate susceptibility to vancomycin (VISA) exhibit distinct metabolic characteristics phenotypically, including an increase in fructose utilization, increased fatty acid metabolism, decrease in glutamate availability, and increased expression of cell wall synthesis genes. These global adaptations seem to result in a reduced autolytic activity along with a thickened cell wall. In addition, an increased amount of free D-Ala-D-Ala dipeptides contributes to the reduced autolytic activity. The adaptations result in a "trapping" of the antibiotic in the outermost layers of the cell wall and prevent the drug from entering the cell to reach its target. As a result of this phenomenon, the fidelity of bacterial cell wall synthesis and cross-linking of the peptidoglycan structure remains unchanged [65].

Emerging Antibiotic Resistance

In early 2020, an increasing number of cases of antibiotic-resistant *Neisseria meningitidis* serogroup Y (NmY) was reported to the CDC, including isolates resistant to penicillin and ciprofloxacin. Further investigation and whole-genome testing of 2097 samples from patients with invasive meningococcal disease between 2011 and 2020 found 33 isolates containing the $bla_{rob-1}\beta$-Lactamase Enzyme Gene[a] conferring resistance to penicillin, while 11 of these isolates contained a gene conferring ciprofloxacin resistance. Although these 11 isolates showed susceptibility to third-generation cephalosporins, the typical first-line agents utilized in treatment of bacterial meningitis, susceptibility of meningococcal isolates to penicillin should be appropriately evaluated prior to transition of treatment to penicillin or ampicillin. Susceptibility testing is also beneficial in guiding healthcare providers' choices in medication prophylaxis for close contacts [139–142].

In the context of acne vulgaris, an emerging resistance to broad-spectrum antibiotics has been reported. Broad-spectrum antibiotics are active against both Gram-positive and Gram-negative bacteria, and are much more likely to select for resistant strains. The use of broad-spectrum antibiotics in acne has been associated with dysbiosis of the skin and gut microflora [139]. In many countries, over 50% of *C. acnes* strains isolated from acne patients were resistant strains. In a study of antibiotic susceptibility to *C. acnes* strains isolated from Israeli acne patients, resistance rates were highest for erythromycin (25.0%), followed by doxycycline (19.4%), clindamycin (16.7%), minocycline (11.1%), and tetracycline (8.3%) [143]. In another study conducted in Jordan (2020), 37% of *C. acnes* isolates obtained from acne patients were found to be resistant to doxycycline [144]. Resistance to *C. acnes* has shown to be correlated with therapeutic failure in acne vulgaris [145].

Low-dose or "sub-antimicrobial" dose of doxycycline has been used in rosacea and acne vulgaris, with the intention to only utilize the anti-inflammatory effect of the antibiotic. However, contrary to the common belief, recent studies demonstrated that low-dose antibiotic exposure leads to the development of high-level resistance [146–148].

Conclusion

Although antibiotic resistance has become a global health crisis due to the inability to treat infections caused by particular pathogens, its development can be viewed as a natural phenomenon following the principles of Darwinian evolution. Considering the duration over which bacterial organisms have inhabited our planet, the clinical application of antibiotics is a relatively recent development. However, the lack of appropriately implemented antibiotic stewardship practices in the clinical setting are greatly contributing to the phenomenon of resistance by the following means: (1) unclear instructions on proper self-administration of antibiotics; (2) the use of sub-antimicrobial dose of antibiotics; (3) the use of over-prescription of antibiotics for minor bacterial infections; and (4) the use of broad-spectrum antibiotics for narrow-spectrum indications such as acne and Gram-positive cutaneous infections. Unfortunately, these resistant pathogens have not just one mechanism of evading the bactericidal and bacteriostatic effects by antibacterial drugs, but several to avoid the actions of the various classes of antibiotics. These mechanisms include changes in target sites, enzymatic degradation, changes in membrane permeability, and global cell adaptations. With a clearer and a greater understanding of the particular mechanisms of resistance, spectrum of antibiotic activity, an increase in research, and antibiotic stewardship, the public health threat of bacterial resistance might be counteracted.

References

1. Rasch RFR. Ancient history and new frontiers: infectious diseases. Nurs Clin North Am. 2019;54(2):xv–xvi.

2. Sultan I, Rahman S, Jan AT, Siddiqui MT, Mondal AH, Haq QMR. Antibiotics, resistome and resistance mechanisms: a bacterial perspective. Front Microbiol. 2018;9:2066.

3. Perry J, Waglechner N, Wright G. The prehistory of antibiotic resistance. Cold Spring Harb Perspect Med. 2016;6(6):a025197.

4. Waglechner N, Wright GD. Antibiotic resistance: it's bad, but why isn't it worse? BMC Biol. 2017;15(1):84.

5. Bondi A, Dietz C. Bacterial penicillinase; production, nature, and significance. J Bacteriol. 1946;51:125.

6. Lobanovska M, Pilla G. Penicillin's discovery and antibiotic resistance: lessons for the future? Yale J Biol Med. 2017;90(1):135–45.

7. Abraham EP, Chain E. An enzyme from bacteria able to destroy penicillin. 1940. Rev Infect Dis. 1988;10(4):677–8.

8. Bo G. Giuseppe Brotzu and the discovery of cephalosporins. Clin Microbiol Infect. 2000;6(Suppl 3):6–9.

9. Sutherland R. The nature of the insensitivity of Gram-negative bacteria towards penicillins. J Gen Microbiol. 1964;34:85–98.

10. Campbell EA, Korzheva N, Mustaev A, et al. Structural mechanism for rifampicin inhibition of bacterial rna polymerase. Cell. 2001;104(6):901–12.

11. Brakhage AA, Al-abdallah Q, Tüncher A, Spröte P. Evolution of beta-lactam biosynthesis genes and recruitment of trans-acting factors. Phytochemistry. 2005;66(11):1200–10.

12. Shivakumar AG, Dubnau D. Characterization of a plasmid-specified ribosome methylase associated with macrolide resistance. Nucleic Acids Res. 1981;9(11):2549–62.

13. Abdelwahab H, Martin del Campo JS, Dai Y, Adly C, El-sohaimy S, Sobrado P. Mechanism of Rifampicin inactivation in Nocardia farcinica. PLoS One. 2016;11(10):e0162578.

14. Piddock LJ. Clinically relevant chromosomally encoded multidrug resistance efflux pumps in bacteria. Clin Microbiol Rev. 2006;19(2):382–402.

15. Pagès JM, James CE, Winterhalter M. The porin and the permeating antibiotic: a selective diffusion barrier in Gram-negative bacteria. Nat Rev Microbiol. 2008;6(12):893–903.

16. Hasper HE, Kramer NE, Smith JL, et al. An alternative bactericidal mechanism of action for lantibiotic peptides that target lipid II. Science. 2006;313(5793):1636–7.

17. Handwerger S, Pucci MJ, Volk KJ, Liu J, Lee MS. Vancomycin-resistant Leuconostoc mesenteroides and Lactobacillus casei synthesize cytoplasmic peptidoglycan precursors that terminate in lactate. J Bacteriol. 1994;176(1):260–4.

18. Wilson DN. Ribosome-targeting antibiotics and mechanisms of bacterial resistance. Nat Rev Microbiol. 2014;12(1):35–48.

19. Poehlsgaard J, Douthwaite S. The bacterial ribosome as a target for antibiotics. Nat Rev Microbiol. 2005;3(11):870–81.

20. Connell SR, Tracz DM, Nierhaus KH, Taylor DE. Ribosomal protection proteins and their mechanism of tetracycline resistance. Antimicrob Agents Chemother. 2003;47(12):3675–81.

21. Oliva B, Chopra I. Tet determinants provide poor protection against some tetracyclines: further evidence for division of tetracyclines into two classes. Antimicrob Agents Chemother. 1992;36(4):876–8.

22. Sanchez-pescador R, Brown JT, Roberts M, Urdea MS. Homology of the TetM with translational elongation factors: implications for potential modes of tetM-conferred tetracycline resistance. Nucleic Acids Res. 1988;16(3):1218.

23. Burdett V. Tet(M)-promoted release of tetracycline from ribosomes is GTP dependent. J Bacteriol. 1996;178(11):3246–51.

24. Trieber CA, Burkhardt N, Nierhaus KH, Taylor DE. Ribosomal protection from tetracycline mediated by Tet(O): Tet(O) interaction with ribosomes is GTP-dependent. Biol Chem. 1998;379(7):847–55.

25. Connell SR, Trieber CA, Dinos GP, Einfeldt E, Taylor DE, Nierhaus KH. Mechanism of Tet(O)-mediated tetracycline resistance. EMBO J. 2003;22(4):945–53.

26. Grossman TH. Tetracycline antibiotics and resistance. Cold Spring Harb Perspect Med. 2016;6(4):a025387.

27. Zhanel G, Critchley I, Lin LY, Alvandi N. Microbiological profile of Sarecycline, a novel targeted spectrum tetracycline for the treatment of acne vulgaris. Antimicrob Agents Chemother. 2019;63(1):e01297–18.

28. Moore A, Green LJ, Bruce S, et al. Once-daily oral sarecycline 1.5 mg/kg/day is effective for moderate to severe acne vulgaris: results from two identically designed, phase 3, randomized, double-blind clinical trials. J Drugs Dermatol. 2018;17(9):987–96.

29. Batool Z, Lomakin IB, Polikanov YS, Bunick CG. Sarecycline interferes with tRNA accommodation and tethers mRNA to the 70S ribosome. Proc Natl Acad Sci U S A. 2020;117(34):20530–7.

30. Haidari W, Bruinsma R, Cardenas-de la garza JA, Feldman SR. Sarecycline review. Ann Pharmacother. 2020;54(2):164–70.

31. Speer BS, Shoemaker NB, Salyers AA. Bacterial resistance to tetracycline: mechanisms, transfer, and clinical significance. Clin Microbiol Rev. 1992;5(4):387–99.

32. Margolis DJ, Fanelli M, Hoffstad O, Lewis JD. Potential association between the oral tetracycline class of antimicrobials used to treat acne and inflammatory bowel disease. Am J Gastroenterol. 2010;105(12):2610–6.

33. Nguyen LH, Örtqvist AK, Cao Y, et al. Antibiotic use and the development of inflammatory bowel disease: a national case-control study in Sweden. Lancet Gastroenterol Hepatol. 2020;5(11):986–95.

34. Lee TW, Russell L, Deng M, Gibson PR. Association of doxycycline use with the development of gastroenteritis, irritable bowel syndrome and inflammatory bowel disease in Australians deployed abroad. Intern Med J. 2013;43(8):919–26.

35. Vázquez-laslop N, Mankin AS. How macrolide antibiotics work. Trends Biochem Sci. 2018;43(9):668–84.

36. Bryskier A, et al. Macrolides – chemistry, pharmacology and clinical uses. Blackwell Science LTd; 1993.

37. Bryskier A. Telithromycin--an innovative ketolide antimicrobials. Jpn J Antibiot. 2001;54 Suppl A:64–9.

38. Fyfe C, Grossman TH, Kerstein K, Sutcliffe J. Resistance to macrolide antibiotics in public health pathogens. Cold Spring Harb Perspect Med. 2016;6(10):a025395.

39. Sharkey LK, Edwards TA, O'neill AJ. ABC-F proteins mediate antibiotic resistance through ribosomal protection. MBio. 2016;7(2):e01975.

40. Davidson AL. Structure function and evolution of bacterial ATP-binding cassette systems. Microbiol Mol Biol Rev. 2008;72(2):317–64.

41. Di Giambattista M, Engelborghs Y, Nyssen E, Cocito C. Kinetics of binding of macrolides, lincosamides, and synergimycins to ribosomes. J Biol Chem. 1987;262(18):8591–7.

42. Feßler AT, Wang Y, Wu C, Schwarz S. Mobile lincosamide resistance genes in staphylococci. Plasmid. 2018;99:22–31.

43. Bryskier A, Lincosamines A, Bryskier, editors. Antimicrobial agents: antibacterials and antifungals. Washington D.C.: ASM Press; 2005. p. 592–603.

44. Smieja M. Current indications for the use of clindamycin: a critical review. Can J Infect Dis. 1998;9(1):22–8.

45. Spížek J, Řezanka T. Lincosamides: chemical structure, biosynthesis, mechanism of action, resistance, and applications. Biochem Pharmacol. 2017;133:20–8.

46. Ero R, Kumar V, Su W, Gao YG. Ribosome protection by ABC-F proteins-molecular mechanism and potential drug design. Protein Sci. 2019;28(4):684–93.

47. Kerr ID, Reynolds ED, Cove JH. ABC proteins and antibiotic drug resistance: is it all about transport? Biochem Soc Trans. 2005;33(Pt 5):1000–2.

48. Ford CW, Zurenko GE, Barbachyn MR. The discovery of linezolid, the first oxazolidinone antibacterial agent. Curr Drug Targets Infect Disord. 2001;1(2):181–99.

49. Hashemian SMR, Farhadi T, Ganjparvar M. Linezolid: a review of its properties, function, and use in critical care. Drug Des Devel Ther. 2018;12:1759–67.

50. Batts DH. Linezolid--a new option for treating gram-positive infections. Oncology (Williston Park). 2000;14(8 Suppl 6):23–9.

51. Wang Y, Lv Y, Cai J, et al. A novel gene, optrA, that confers transferable resistance to oxazolidinones and

phenicols and its presence in Enterococcus faecalis and Enterococcus faecium of human and animal origin. J Antimicrob Chemother. 2015;70(8):2182–90.

52. Bender JK, Cattoir V, Hegstad K, et al. Update on prevalence and mechanisms of resistance to linezolid, tigecycline and daptomycin in enterococci in Europe: Towards a common nomenclature. Drug Resist Updat. 2018;40:25–39.

53. Schwarz S, Shen J, Kadlec K, et al. Lincosamides, Streptogramins, Phenicols, and Pleuromutilins: mode of action and mechanisms of resistance. Cold Spring Harb Perspect Med. 2016;6(11):1027037.

54. Schwarz S, Kehrenberg C, Doublet B, Cloeckaert A. Molecular basis of bacterial resistance to chloramphenicol and florfenicol. FEMS Microbiol Rev. 2004;28(5):519–42.

55. Shaw WV. Chloramphenicol acetyltransferase: enzymology and molecular biology. CRC Crit Rev Biochem. 1983;14(1):1–46.

56. Novak R, Shlaes DM. The pleuromutlin antibiotics: a new class for human use. Curr Opin Investig Drugs. 2010;11(2):182–91.

57. Giguère S. Lincosamides, pleuromutilins, and streptogramins. In: Giguère S, Prescott JF, Dowling PM, editors. Antimicrobial therapy in veterinary medicine. 5th ed. Hoboken: Wiley; 2013. p. 199–210.

58. Paukner S, Riedl R. Pleuromutilins: potent drugs for resistant bugs-mode of action and resistance. Cold Spring Harb Perspect Med. 2017;7(1):a027110.

59. Paukner S, Sader HS, Ivezic-schoenfeld Z, Jones RN. Antimicrobial activity of the pleuromutilin antibiotic BC-3781 against bacterial pathogens isolated in the SENTRY antimicrobial surveillance program in 2010. Antimicrob Agents Chemother. 2013;57(9):4489–95.

60. Schlünzen F, Pyetan E, Fucini P, Yonath A, Harms JM. Inhibition of peptide bond formation by pleuromutilins: the structure of the 50S ribosomal subunit from Deinococcus radiodurans in complex with tiamulin. Mol Microbiol. 2004;54(5):1287–94.

61. Hunt E. Pleuromutlin antibiotics. Drugs Future. 2000;25:1163–8.

62. Bolon MK. The newer fluoroquinolones. Infect Dis Clin N Am. 2009;23(4):1027–51.

63. Andriole VT. The quinolones: past, present, and future. Clin Infect Dis. 2005;41(Suppl 2):S113–9.

64. Hooper DC, Jacoby GA. Topoisomerase inhibitors: fluoroquinolone mechanisms of action and resistance. Cold Spring Harb Perspect Med. 2016;6(9):a025320.

65. Rodríguez-martínez JM, Briales A, Velasco C, Conejo MC, Martínez-martínez L, Pascual A. Mutational analysis of quinolone resistance in the plasmid-encoded pentapeptide repeat proteins QnrA, QnrB and QnrS. J Antimicrob Chemother. 2009;63(6):1128–34.

66. Saga T, Kaku M, Onodera Y, Yamachika S, Sato K, Takase H. Vibrio parahaemolyticus chromosomal qnr homologue VPA0095: demonstration by transformation with a mutated gene of its potential to reduce quinolone susceptibility in Escherichia coli. Antimicrob Agents Chemother. 2005;49(5):2144–5.

67. Mast Y, Wohlleben W. Streptogramins - two are better than one! Int J Med Microbiol. 2014;304(1):44–50.

68. Barrière JC, Berthaud N, Beyer D, Dutka-malen S, Paris JM, Desnottes JF. Recent developments in streptogramin research. Curr Pharm Des. 1998;4(2):155–80.

69. Charney J, Fisher WP, Curran C, Machlowitz RA, Tytell AA. Streptogramin, a new antibiotic. Antibiot Chemother (Northfield). 1953;3(12):1283–6.

70. Stille W, Brodt H-R, Groll AH, Just-Nübling G. Antibiotika-Therapie: Klinik und Praxis der antiinfektiösen Behandlung 3-7945-2160-9. Schattauer Verlag; 2005.

71. Cocito C, Di Giambattista M, Nyssen E, Vannuffel P. Inhibition of protein synthesis by streptogramins and related antibiotics. J Antimicrob Chemother. 1997;39:7–13.

72. Lee CK, Kamitani Y, Nihira T, Yamada Y. Identification and in vivo functional analysis of a virginiamycin S resistance gene (varS) from Streptomyces virginiae. J Bacteriol. 1999;181:3293–7.

73. Pulsawat N, Kitani S, Nihira T. Characterization of biosynthetic gene cluster for the production of virginiamycin M, a streptogramin type A antibiotic, in Streptomyces virginiae. Gene. 2007;393:31–42.

74. Wright GD. The antibiotic resistome: the nexus of chemical and genetic diversity. Nat Rev Microbiol. 2007;5(3):175–86.

75. Blair JM, Webber MA, Baylay AJ, Ogbolu DO, Piddock LJ. Molecular mechanisms of antibiotic resistance. Nat Rev Microbiol. 2015;13(1):42–51.

76. Munita JM, Arias CA. Mechanisms of antibiotic resistance. Microbiol Spectr. 2016;4(2):10.

77. Becker B, Cooper MA. Aminoglycoside antibiotics in the 21st century. ACS Chem Biol. 2013;8(1):105–15.

78. Kotra LP, Haddad J, Mobashery S. Aminoglycosides: perspectives on mechanisms of action and resistance and strategies to counter resistance. Antimicrob Agents Chemother. 2000;44(12):3249–56.

79. Krause KM, Serio AW, Kane TR, Connolly LE. Aminoglycosides: an overview. Cold Spring Harb Perspect Med. 2016;6(6):a027029.

80. Davis BD. Mechanism of bactericidal action of aminoglycosides. Microbiol Rev. 1987;51(3):341–50.

81. Garneau-tsodikova S, Labby KJ. Mechanisms of resistance to aminoglycoside antibiotics: overview and perspectives. Medchemcomm. 2016;7(1):11–27.

82. Maus CE, Plikaytis BB, Shinnick TM. Molecular analysis of cross-resistance to capreomycin, kanamycin, amikacin, and viomycin in Mycobacterium tuberculosis. Antimicrob Agents Chemother. 2005;49(8):3192–7.

83. Demirci H, Wang L, Murphy FV, et al. The central role of protein S12 in organizing the structure of the decoding site of the ribosome. RNA. 2013;19(12):1791–801.

84. Pechère JC. Macrolide resistance mechanisms in Gram-positive cocci. Int J Antimicrob Agents. 2001;18(Suppl 1):S25–8.

85. Vester B, Douthwaite S. Macrolide resistance conferred by base substitutions in 23S rRNA. Antimicrob Agents Chemother. 2001;45(1):1–12.

86. Franceschi F, Kanyo Z, Sherer EC, Sutcliffe J. Macrolide resistance from the ribosome perspective. Curr Drug Targets Infect Disord. 2004;4(3):177–91.

87. Zaman S, Fitzpatrick M, Lindahl L, Zengel J. Novel mutations in ribosomal proteins L4 and L22 that confer erythromycin resistance in Escherichia coli. Mol Microbiol. 2007;66(4):1039–50.

88. Diner EJ, Hayes CS. Recombineering reveals a diverse collection of ribosomal proteins L4 and L22 that confer resistance to macrolide antibiotics. J Mol Biol. 2009;386(2):300–15.

89. Baughman GA, Fahnestock SR. Chloramphenicol resistance mutation in Escherichia coli which maps in the major ribosomal protein gene cluster. J Bacteriol. 1979;137(3):1315–23.

90. Anderson LM, Henkin TM, Chambliss GH, Bott KF. New chloramphenicol resistance locus in Bacillus subtilis. J Bacteriol. 1984;158(1):386–8.

91. Ettayebi M, Prasad SM, Morgan EA. Chloramphenicol-erythromycin resistance mutations in a 23S rRNA gene of Escherichia coli. J Bacteriol. 1985;162(2):551–7.

92. Vesely JJ, Pien FD, Pien BC. Rifampin, a useful drug for nonmycobacterial infections. Pharmacotherapy. 1998;18(2):345–57.

93. Morris AB, Brown RB, Sands M. Use of rifampin in nonstaphylococcal, nonmycobacterial disease. Antimicrob Agents Chemother. 1993;37(1):1–7.

94. Landick R, Stewart J, Lee DN. Amino acid changes in conserved regions of the beta-subunit of Escherichia coli RNA polymerase alter transcription pausing and termination. Genes Dev. 1990;4(9):1623–36.

95. Singh A, Grover S, Sinha S, Das M, Somvanshi P, Grover A. Mechanistic principles behind molecular mechanism of rifampicin resistance in mutant RNA polymerase beta subunit of mycobacterium tuberculosis. J Cell Biochem. 2017;118(12):4594–606.

96. Poehlsgaard J, Pfister P, Böttger EC, Douthwaite S. Molecular mechanisms by which rRNA mutations confer resistance to clindamycin. Antimicrob Agents Chemother. 2005;49(4):1553–5.

97. Jacoby GA. Mechanisms of resistance to quinolones. Clin Infect Dis. 2005;41(Suppl 2):S120–6.

98. Hawkey PM. Mechanisms of quinolone action and microbial response. J Antimicrob Chemother. 2003;51(Suppl 1):29–35.

99. Pan XS, Ambler J, Mehtar S, et al. Involvement of topoisomerase IV and DNA gyrase as ciprofloxacin targets in Streptococcus pneumoniae. Antimicrob Agents Chemother. 1996;40(10):2321–6.

100. Ferrero L, Cameron B, Crouzet J. Analysis of gyrA and grlA mutations in stepwise-selected ciprofloxacin-resistant mutants of Staphylococcus aureus. Antimicrob Agents Chemother. 1995;39(7):1554–8.

101. Swaney SM, Aoki H, Ganoza MC, Shinabarger DL. The oxazolidinone linezolid inhibits initiation of protein synthesis in bacteria. Antimicrob Agents Chemother. 1998;42:3251–5.

102. Raad II, Hanna HA, Hachem RY, Dvorak T, Arbuckle RB, Chaiban G, Rice LB. Clinical-use-associated decrease in susceptibility of vancomycin-resistant Enterococcus faecium to linezolid: a comparison with quinupristin–dalfopristin. Antimicrob Agents Chemother. 2004;48:3583–5.

103. Xiong L, Kloss P, Douthwaite S, Andersen NM, Swaney S, Shinabarger DL, Mankin AS. Oxazolidinone resistance mutations in 23S rRNA of Escherichia coli reveal the central region of domain V as the primary site of drug action. J Bacteriol. 2000;182:5325–31.

104. Zeng D, Debabov D, Hartsell TL, et al. Approved Glycopeptide antibacterial drugs: mechanism of action and resistance. Cold Spring Harb Perspect Med. 2016;6(12):a026989.

105. Arias CA, Murray BE. The rise of the Enterococcus: beyond vancomycin resistance. Nat Rev Microbiol. 2012;10(4):266–78.

106. Mccormick MH, Mcguire JM, Pittenger GE, Pittenger RC, Stark WM. Vancomycin, a new antibiotic. I. Chemical and biologic properties. Antibiot Annu. 1955;3:606–11.

107. Leclercq R. Mechanisms of resistance to macrolides and lincosamides: nature of the resistance elements and their clinical implications. Clin Infect Dis. 2002;34(4):482–92.

108. Wachino J, Arakawa Y. Exogenously acquired 16S rRNA methyltransferases found in aminoglycoside-resistant pathogenic Gram-negative bacteria: an update. Drug Resist Updat. 2012;15(3):133–48.

109. Granier SA, Hidalgo L, San Millan A, et al. ArmA methyltransferase in a monophasic Salmonella enterica isolate from food. Antimicrob Agents Chemother. 2011;55(11):5262–6.

110. Diaz L, Kiratisin P, Mendes RE, Panesso D, Singh KV, Arias CA. Transferable plasmid-mediated resistance to linezolid due to cfr in a human clinical isolate of Enterococcus faecalis. Antimicrob Agents Chemother. 2012;56(7):3917–22.

111. Bush K, Bradford PA. β-Lactams and β-lactamase inhibitors: an overview. Cold Spring Harb Perspect Med. 2016;6(8):a025247.

112. Chambers HF, Deleo FR. Waves of resistance: Staphylococcus aureus in the antibiotic era. Nat Rev Microbiol. 2009;7(9):629–41.

113. Huovinen P. Resistance to trimethoprim-sulfamethoxazole. Clin Infect Dis. 2001;32(11):1608–14.

114. Wright GD. Bacterial resistance to antibiotics: enzymatic degradation and modification. Adv Drug Deliv Rev. 2005;57(10):1451–70.

115. Kapoor G, Saigal S, Elongavan A. Action and resistance mechanisms of antibiotics: a guide for clinicians. J Anaesthesiol Clin Pharmacol. 2017;33(3):300–5.

116. Poole K. Resistance to beta-lactam antibiotics. Cell Mol Life Sci. 2004;61(17):2200–23.

117. Nakamura A, Nakazawa K, Miyakozawa I, et al. Macrolide esterase-producing Escherichia coli clinically isolated in Japan. J Antibiot. 2000;53(5):516–24.

118. Williams JD. Beta-lactamases and beta-lactamase inhibitors. Int J Antimicrob Agents. 1999;12(Suppl 1):S3–7.

119. Donadio S, Staver MJ, Mcalpine JB, Swanson SJ, Katz L. Modular organization of genes required for complex polyketide biosynthesis. Science. 1991;252(5006):675–9.

120. Barthélémy P, Autissier D, Gerbaud G, Courvalin P. Enzymic hydrolysis of erythromycin by a strain of Escherichia coli. A new mechanism of resistance. J Antibiot. 1984;37(12):1692–6.

121. Palzkill T. Metallo-β-lactamase structure and function. Ann N Y Acad Sci. 2013;1277:91–104.

122. Skarzynski T, Mistry A, Wonacott A, Hutchinson SE, Kelly VA, Duncan K. Structure of UDP-N-acetylglucosamine enolpyruvyl transferase, an enzyme essential for the synthesis of bacterial peptidoglycan, complexed with substrate UDP-N-acetylglucosamine and the drug fosfomycin. Structure. 1996;4(12):1465–74.

123. Falagas ME, Vouloumanou EK, Samonis G, Vardakas KZ. Fosfomycin. Clin Microbiol Rev. 2016;29(2):321–47.

124. Llaneza J, Villar CJ, Salas JA, Suarez JE, Mendoza MC, Hardisson C. Plasmid-mediated fosfomycin resistance is due to enzymatic modification of the antibiotic. Antimicrob Agents Chemother. 1985;28(1):163–4.

125. Etienne J, Gerbaud G, Fleurette J, Courvalin P. Characterization of staphylococcal plasmids hybridizing with the fosfomycin resistance gene fosB. FEMS Microbiol Lett. 1991;68(1):119–22.

126. Delcour AH. Outer membrane permeability and antibiotic resistance. Biochim Biophys Acta. 2009;1794(5):808–16.

127. Nikaido H. Molecular basis of bacterial outer membrane permeability revisited. Microbiol Mol Biol Rev. 2003;67(4):593–656.

128. Dame JB, Shapiro BM. Use of polymyxin B, levallorphan, and tetracaine to isolate novel envelope mutants of Escherichia coli. J Bacteriol. 1976;127(2):961–7.

129. Fernández L, Hancock RE. Adaptive and mutational resistance: role of porins and efflux pumps in drug resistance. Clin Microbiol Rev. 2012;25(4):661–81.

130. Harder KJ, Nikaido H, Matsuhashi M. Mutants of Escherichia coli that are resistant to certain beta-lactam compounds lack the ompF porin. Antimicrob Agents Chemother. 1981;20(4):549–52.

131. Koebnik R, Locher KP, Van gelder P. Structure and function of bacterial outer membrane proteins: barrels in a nutshell. Mol Microbiol. 2000;37(2):239–53.

132. Dé E, Baslé A, Jaquinod M, et al. A new mechanism of antibiotic resistance in Enterobacteriaceae induced by a structural modification of the major porin. Mol Microbiol. 2001;41(1):189–98.

133. Mcmurry L, Petrucci RE, Levy SB. Active efflux of tetracycline encoded by four genetically different tetracycline resistance determinants in Escherichia coli. Proc Natl Acad Sci U S A. 1980;77(7):3974–7.

134. Piddock LJ. Clinically relevant chromosomally encoded multidrug resistance efflux pumps in bacteria. Clin Microbiol Rev. 2006;19(2):382–402.

135. Roberts MC. Update on acquired tetracycline resistance genes. FEMS Microbiol Lett. 2005;245(2):195–203.

136. Visalli MA, Murphy E, Projan SJ, Bradford PA. AcrAB multidrug efflux pump is associated with reduced levels of susceptibility to tigecycline (GAR-936) in Proteus mirabilis. Antimicrob Agents Chemother. 2003;47(2):665–9.

137. Dean CR, Visalli MA, Projan SJ, Sum PE, Bradford PA. Efflux-mediated resistance to tigecycline (GAR-936) in Pseudomonas aeruginosa PAO1. Antimicrob Agents Chemother. 2003;47(3):972–8.

138. Poole K. Efflux-mediated antimicrobial resistance. J Antimicrob Chemother. 2005;56(1):20–51.

139. Thompson KG, Rainer BM, Antonescu C, Florea L, Mongodin EF, Kang S, Chien AL. Minocycline and its impact on microbial dysbiosis in the skin and gastrointestinal tract of acne patients. Ann Dermatol. 2020;32(1):21–30.

140. Dreno B, Thiboutot D, Gollnick H, Bettoli V, Kang S, Leyden JJ, Shalita A, Torres V. Antibiotic stewardship in dermatology: limiting antibiotic use in acne. Eur J Dermatol. 2014;24(3):330–4.

141. Tan HH, Tan AW, Barkham T, Yan XY, Zhu M. Community-based study of acne vulgaris in adolescents in Singapore. Br J Dermatol. 2007;157(3):547–51.

142. Dessinioti C, Katsambas A. Propionibacterium acnes and antimicrobial resistance in acne. Clin Dermatol. 2017;35(2):163–7.

143. Sheffer-Levi S, Rimon A, Lerer V, Shlomov T, Coppenhagen-Glazer S, Rakov C, Zeiter T, Nir-Paz R, Hazan R, Molcho-Pessach V. Antibiotic susceptibility of Cutibacterium acnes strains isolated from Israeli Acne patients. Acta Derm Venereol. 2020;100(17):adv00295. https://doi.org/10.2340/00015555-3654.

144. Alkhawaja E, Hammadi S, Abdelmalek M, Mahasneh N, Alkhawaja B, Abdelmalek SM. Antibiotic resistant Cutibacterium acnes among acne patients in Jordan: a cross sectional study. BMC Dermatol. 2020;20(1):1–9.

145. EADY EA, Cove JH, Holland KT, Cunliffe WJ. Erythromycin resistant propionibacteria in antibiotic treated acne patients: association with therapeutic failure. Br J Dermatol. 1989; 121(1):51–7.

146. Andersson DI, Hughes D. Microbiological effects of sublethal levels of antibiotics. Nat Rev Microbiol. 2014;12(7):465–78.

147. Wistrand-Yuen E, Knopp M, Hjort K, Koskiniemi S, Berg OG, Andersson DI. Evolution of high-level resistance during low-level antibiotic exposure. Nat Commun. 2018;9(1):1–2.

148. Armstrong AW, Hekmatjah J, Kircik LH. Oral Tetracyclines and Acne: a systematic review for dermatologists. J Drugs Dermatol. 2020;19(11):s6–13.

Emerging Bacterial Infections

2

Crystal E. Nwannunu

Abbreviations

ACA	Acrodermatitis chronica atrophicans
CDC	Centers for Disease Control and Prevention
EID	Emerging infectious disease
ELISA	Enzyme-linked immunosorbent assay
EM	Erythema migrans
PCR	Polymerase chain reaction
RMSF	Rocky Mountain spotted fever
TIBOLA	Tick-borne lymphadenopathy
TMP-SMZ	Trimethoprim-sulfamethoxazole
VAP	Ventilator-associated pneumonia
WHO	World Health Organization

Introduction

Emerging infectious diseases (EIDs) include infections that have clinically presented among humans recently or have rapidly increased in incidence or geographic distribution [1]. In this chapter, we aim to provide a cohesive review of the cutaneous and non-cutaneous clinical mani-festations, diagnostic workup recommendations, and management tools for these emerging dermatological bacterial infections.

Emerging Bacterial Infections

Acinetobacter baumannii

Nosocomial-Associated Infections

Acinetobacter baumannii is an opportunistic gram-negative aerobic pathogen and encompasses a group of three bacteria (*A. baumannii*, *A. nosocomialis*, and *A. pitti*). This bacterium is found in soil and water and is primarily a nosocomially acquired infection [2–4]. It has been shown to colonize areas of the skin, wound, and mucous membranes, including the respiratory and gastrointestinal tract [3]. *Acinetobacter baumannii* has a high incidence among immunocompromised individuals, predominantly individuals who have experienced a prolonged (>90 days) hospital stay [3, 4]. Due to its ability to survive on artificial surfaces for an extended period of time, this bacterium has increased in incidence with multidrug resistance [2–4].

The rise of *A. baumannii* infections, predominately reported in the United Kingdom and United States, possibly relates to the return home of colonized and infected injured members of the military forces after deployment to war zones in the desert [3]. The dry and desert conditions experienced in geographic locations such as Iraq

The original version of this chapter was revised. The correction to this chapter can be found at https://doi.org/10.1007/978-3-030-68321-4_17.

C. E. Nwannunu (✉)
McGovern Medical School, University of Texas Health Science Center, Houston, TX, USA

© Springer Nature Switzerland AG 2021, corrected publication 2022
S. K. Tyring et al. (eds.), *Overcoming Antimicrobial Resistance of the Skin*, Updates in Clinical Dermatology, https://doi.org/10.1007/978-3-030-68321-4_2

provide an ideal physiologic environment for the robust growth of *A. baumannii*.

Cutaneous manifestations of this disease include skin and soft tissue infections such as cellulitis, skin abscesses, and necrotizing fasciitis. Most infections initially begin as a break in the skin, evolving to a well-demarcated erythematous and edematous form of cellulitis. At this stage, the lesion is known to have a "peau d' orange" appearance [2, 3]. The cellulitis advances to a sandpaper-like presentation, with numerous coalescing clear vesicles overlying the lesion. Hemorrhagic bullae can occur in areas of skin disruptions, where a visible necrotizing process is observed. If these symptoms are left untreated, individuals are at risk of bacteremia, septicemia, and death [2, 3] (Figs. 2.1 and 2.2).

Prolonged periods of hospitalization with the use of mechanical ventilation increase the risk of ventilator-associated pneumonia (VAP) by *A. baumannii*. Hospital-acquired pneumonia outbreaks have been attributed to colonized hands and poor hygiene among healthcare professionals. *Acinetobacter* is also a pathogen known to cause sepsis and post neurosurgical meningitis. External ventricular drains used in neurosurgery are thought to serve as a potential site for this opportunistic infection [3].

Diagnosis of *A. baumannii* is made by culturing the bacteria from the individual's sputum, blood, wound, skin and soft tissue, or cerebrospinal fluid. Histopathology from skin and soft tissue biopsies can be performed for further analysis in the diagnostic workup [2, 4, 6] (Fig. 2.3).

Broad-spectrum carbapenems, such as imipenem, are often the drug of choice for suspected *Acinetobacter* infections. Although *A. baumannii* has a high rate of antibiotic resistance, antibiotic therapy is recommended after antimicrobial susceptibility testing is performed. Polymyxins also should be considered when resistance to carbapenems is present [2–4].

Rickettsial Diseases

Cat Flea Rickettsiosis
Rickettsia felis, an emerging gram-negative vector-borne bacterium, is the causative agent for cat flea rickettsiosis. As the name entails, this pathogen is primarily transmitted by the cat flea, *Ctenocephalides felis*. First identified as a spo-

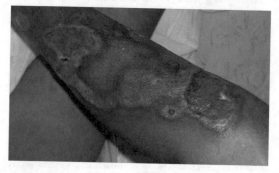

Fig. 2.1 The "peau d' orange" appearance seen in *Acinetobacter baumannii* skin and soft tissue infections. (Reproduced with permission of Ref. [2])

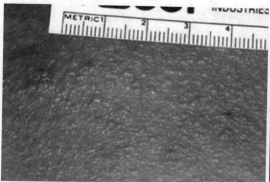
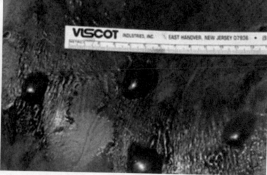

Fig. 2.2 (Left) Cellulitis of the skin reveals mild erythema, sandpaper-like appearance covered by coalescing vesicles. (Right) Hemorrhagic bullae, complication of this infection if left untreated. (From Ref. [5])

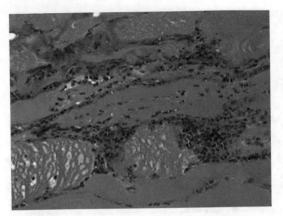

Fig. 2.3 Histopathology analysis of soft tissue biopsy revealed presence of bacteria and necrosis of subcutaneous fascia caused by *Acinetobacter baumannii*. Consistent with necrotizing fasciitis

radic disease in the United States in the early 1990s, *Rickettsia felis* has now been identified throughout the world and now a common cause of fever in Africa [2, 7].

Non-cutaneous clinical manifestations of cat flea rickettsiosis include fever, fatigue, myalgia, and headache. Cutaneous symptoms typically include a maculopapular rash and an eschar at the site of inoculation [2, 8]. The rash is described as pruritic and can present on the chest, abdomen, or lower extremities and can be indistinguishable from murine typhus, another flea-borne infection [2]. The maculopapular rash, like other rickettsioses, appears 3–5 days after the acute fever. Less than half of infected individuals develop a rash [2, 8]. The eschar site is characterized by the presence of localized inflammation and necrotic skin.

The gold standard for rickettsial diagnosis is serology utilizing immunofluorescence assay. Although this diagnostic modality is more readily accessible, it is nonspecific for species identification and differentiation [2]. Preferred diagnostic protocols include polymerase chain reaction (PCR) of the eschar biopsy specimen or Western blot [2, 8]. These preferred approaches can help differentiate *R. felis* from other mimicking febrile illnesses.

Due to its clinical similarities with other febrile illnesses and limited access to appropriate laboratory tests, *R. felis* is often difficult to diagnose and most likely underreported [8]. Prompt empiric administration of doxycycline 100 mg orally or intravenously twice a day for adults, and 2.2 mg per kg orally or intravenously twice a day for children who weigh less than 100 lb. (45.4 kg) is the treatment of choice for this cat flea rickettsiosis and most rickettsial diseases [2]. Although the optimal duration of therapy has not been established, a 5-day to 7-day course is generally recommended after the fever subsides.

Tick-Borne Lymphadenopathy

Tick-borne lymphadenopathy (TIBOLA) is predominately caused by *Rickettsia slovaca* and less commonly *R. rioja* and *R. raoultii*. Its vector is the Dermacentor tick. TIBOLA is an emerging infection, as the second most common rickettsial disease in Europe following Mediterranean spotted fever. This disease frequently occurs in colder seasons, in contrast to Mediterranean spotted fever that occurs primarily during the summer [9].

Clinical findings include a vector tick bite in the scalp area that results in an eschar with erythema and edema. These lesions can last up to 1 to 2 months, followed by regional lymphadenopathy characterized as painful and localized in the cervical or occipital regions [2]. Common additional symptoms include fever, headache, and asthenia, followed by scarring alopecia [9]. Rarely, myalgia, vertigo, and rash have been reported (Fig. 2.4).

TIBOLA can be diagnosed clinically by the unique scalp eschar (Fig. 2.5). To obtain a more definitive diagnosis, PCR from skin biopsies or swab specimens of the eschar can be performed [2, 10]. Common nonspecific laboratory abnormalities observed in infected individuals include elevated transaminases, C-reactive protein, sedimentation rate, leukocytosis, or leukopenia [9].

Empiric antibiotic treatment in TIBOLA with doxycycline (100 mg twice daily) is recommended, with use of ciprofloxacin and azithromycin or clarithromycin when doxycycline is contraindicated [8] (Table 2.1).

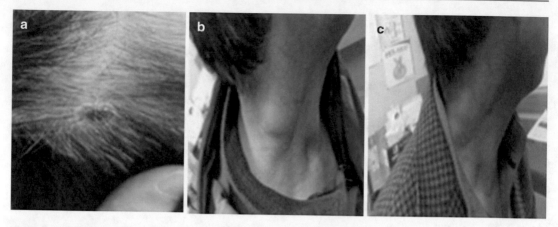

Fig. 2.4 Inoculation site of scalp eschar followed by the progression of cervical lymphadenopathy in patient with TIBOLA. (**a**) Inoculation site of tick bite. (**b**) Regional lymphadenopathy presenting in the cervical region. (**c**) Resolution of lympadenopathy as compared to initial presentation seen in (**b**)

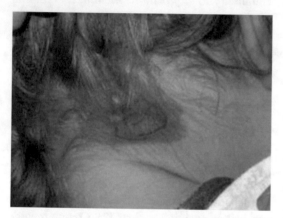

Fig. 2.5 Scalp eschar is used to diagnose TIBOLA clinically as it is a characteristic cutaneous finding. (Reproduced with permission of Ref. [2])

Burkholderia pseudomallei

Melioidosis
Burkholderia pseudomallei is a soil-dwelling Gram-negative bacterium that is the causative agent of melioidosis. Its mode of transmission is through direct contact with contaminated water and soil. This can occur by inhalation, inoculation, or ingestion of the bacteria. Melioidosis, also called Whitmore's disease, predominates in tropical climates including Southeast Asia, South Asia, Southern China, and Northern Australia [2, 11–14]. *Burkholderia pseudomallei* has recently emerged in such new areas as South America and Africa. Most cases reported outside of endemic

regions such as the United States are acquired due to recent travel to an endemic region [2].

Non-cutaneous symptoms of this disease include fever, cough, chest pain, abdominal discomfort, bone pain, and joint pain. Melioidosis is also associated with pneumonia and septic arthritis. Cutaneous signs can present as an ulcer, pustule, or crusted erythematous lesion (Figs. 2.6 and 2.7). Cutaneous manifestations are reported less often as compared to systemic symptoms.

Diabetes has been documented as the most common risk factor in individuals who acquired melioidosis, with additional risk factors including chronic obstructive pulmonary disease and alcoholism [11–14]. This disease is considered an opportunistic infection but doesn't seem to be associated with HIV/AIDS patients [13].

Due to this disease's variation in clinical presentation, melioidosis can be difficult to diagnose clinically and requires a definitive laboratory diagnostic workup. This can be done by collecting blood, sputum, urine, or skin cultures. Isolation of *B. pseudomallei* from a clinical specimen remains the gold standard. Isolation of the organism in a selective media such as Ashdown's media is desirable but not always necessary [2, 11, 14] (Fig. 2.8).

Management of melioidosis requires two phases of intensive antibiotic treatment, the acute phase and the eradication phase. In the acute phase, parenterally intravenous administration of ceftazidime, meropenem, or imipe-

Table 2.1 Summary of rickettsial diseases

Disease	Species	Characteristic cutaneous finding	Definitive diagnosis	Recommended treatment
Cat flea rickettsiosis	*Rickettsia felis*	Eschar at site inoculation +/− maculopapular rash	PCR of eschar; serology (Western blot)	Doxycycline
TIBOLA	*Rickettsia slovaca, Rickettsia rioja and Rickettsia raoultii*	Scalp eschar and regional lymphadenopathy	PCR of eschar biopsy	Doxycycline Alternatives: ciprofloxacin, azithromycin, clarithromycin

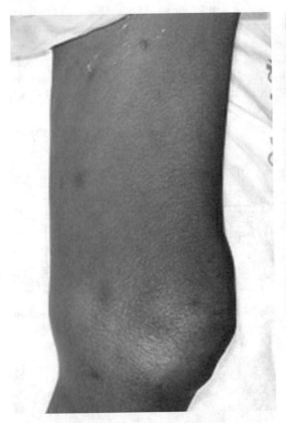

Fig. 2.6 Cutaneous pustules and abscesses of melioidosis on lower extremity. (Reproduced with permission of Ref. [2])

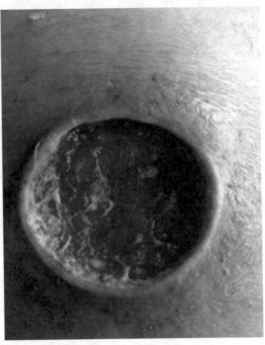

Fig. 2.7 Melioidosis ulcer on left thigh (after incision and drainage). (From Ref. [14])

nem is given for 10–14 days. The eradication phase follows and includes oral antibiotic therapy with trimethoprim-sulfamethoxazole (TMP-SMZ) for 3–6 months. Patients with cutaneous melioidosis have been successfully treated with oral antibiotics alone, with a generally good prognosis, with or without incision and drainage of the lesion [11, 13].

Borrelia mayonii

Lyme Borreliosis

Lyme disease (*Lyme borreliosis*) is a multisystem illness that is endemic in temperate regions of the northern hemisphere. Lyme borreliosis is caused by a gram-negative spirochete *Borrelia burgdorferi* in North America and *B. afzelii* or *B. garinii* in Europe and Asia. Transmitted by the *Ixodes* tick, it is the most common vector-borne infection in the United States and Europe [2, 15]. Recently, *Borrelia mayonii* has been identified as

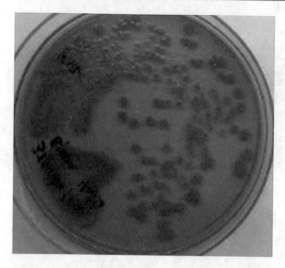

Fig. 2.8 Isolated colonies of *B. pseudomallei* on growth media. (From Ref. [14])

in Stage 2, erythema migrans lesions disseminate throughout the skin (Fig. 2.10). Systemic neurological symptoms, including meningitis and cranial neuropathy and cardiac involvement such as atrioventricular block and myocarditis, have been also documented to occur in Stage 2. In the chronic phase of Stage 3, acrodermatitis chronica atrophicans (ACA), a late cutaneous manifestation, occurs months to years after initial inoculation. Lesions appear on the extensor surfaces of distal extremities with an increased presence in cooler temperature settings (Fig. 2.11). Noncutaneous signs and symptoms during these stages involve mostly neurological pathology such as radiculopathy and cognitive defects. Pathologic joint involvement occurs across all three stages [2, 15, 16]. According to the CDC,

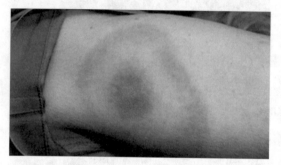

Fig. 2.9 Classic "bulls' eye" target rash present in early stages of Lyme disease

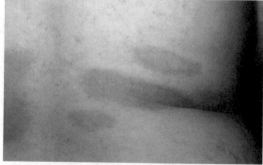

Fig. 2.10 Disseminated erythema migrans. Common cutaneous sign during Stage 2 of Lyme disease course

a new pathogenic spirochete to cause Lyme disease in North America [16]. Current evidence suggests that *B. mayonii* is concentrated in the upper Midwestern region.

B. mayonii produces a similar clinical constellation of symptoms and signs to that caused by *B. burgdorferi*. Multisystemic symptoms of Lyme disease typically progress over the course of three stages. In Stage 1, erythema migrans locally manifests at sites where the tick bite occurs. Often this lesion presents as a target or "bull's eye" appearance and is regarded as the pathognomonic manifestation of Lyme disease (Fig. 2.9). This cutaneous sign typically can last up to 3 weeks after inoculation and is accompanied by constitutional symptoms. Weeks to months later

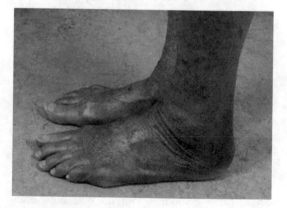

Fig. 2.11 Acrodermatitis chronica atrophicans (ACA) presents as red-bluish discoloration commonly on the extensor distal extremities

Table 2.2 Stages of Lyme borreliosis (Lyme disease)

Stage	Type	Time since initial inoculation	Characteristic cutaneous findings	Additional manifestations
1	Localized	Up to 3 weeks	Primary erythema migrans (erythema chronicum migrans) "Bull's eye appearance"	Constitutional symptoms and joint involvement
2	Disseminated	Weeks to months	Secondary erythema migrans	Neurological and joint cardiac involvement
3	Chronic	Months to years	Acrodermatitis chronica atrophicans	Neurological and joint involvement

unlike *B. burgdorferi*, *B. mayonii* can cause additional symptoms of nausea and vomiting (Table 2.2).

The diagnosis of early Lyme disease is based on clinical findings and history of possible exposure to the vector, since blood antibody levels are measuredly low in the first 4 weeks of infection. However, in the disseminated and chronic stages, a diagnosis using a two-tier serologic testing strategy can be made with an ELISA followed by a Western blot test. To diagnose *B. mayonii*, physicians are recommended to perform PCR testing. This is due to the ability of *B. mayonii* to proliferate readily, and individuals infected have been shown to have a high concentration in their blood [2, 17].

With skin manifestations being an early sign in Lyme disease, diagnosis of these lesions followed by appropriate treatment can prevent the major systemic complications of the disease. Currently, antibiotic therapy is the standard of treatment and is most effective early in the course of the disease. The recommended antibiotic regimen is doxycycline twice daily for 14–21 days for patients with EM. To address patients with disseminated disease or ACA, a longer course of about 3–4 weeks is advised. Alternative antibiotic therapies that can be used include azithromycin, amoxicillin, and cefuroxime [2, 15, 16].

Mycobacterial Infections

Mycobacterium ulcerans (Buruli Ulcer)

Mycobacterium ulcerans, better known as Buruli ulcer, is a slow-growing mycobacterium. This mycobacterium is the third most common mycobacterial infection in the world following tuberculosis and Hansen's disease. Although according to the Centers for Disease Control and Prevention it is unknown how this bacterium is transmitted, it is hypothesized that transmission occurs via direct contact of an open wound and contaminated soil [2, 18].

Mycobacterium ulcerans is endemic to Central Africa, French Guiana, Peru, Bolivia, and Mexico [18]. Most individuals affected by this disease are children and farmers who reside in rural areas near wetlands. This disease has been noted to be spreading with new cases reported in Australia, Asia, and Central and South America. New emerging cases have even been documented in regions of the Bellarine and Mornington Peninsula in Australia [18–21] (Figs. 2.12 and 2.13).

This disease typically presents as one or more firm, nontender, subcutaneous nodules. More commonly presenting on the upper and lower extremities, these lesions enlarge and rupture, leading to ulcers (Fig. 2.14). The toxin produced by this bacterium causes necrosis of the skin and soft tissue [18].

Diagnosis of *Mycobacterium ulcerans* is clinical but can be substantiated by histological examination, acid-fast staining, tissue cultures, and PCR. The histological examination will show necrotizing panniculitis with a sparse inflammatory infiltrate. The acid-fast stain will display a high number of bacilli in the necrotic fat from the lesion. New advancing PCR diagnostic tools allow long-distance transportation of specimens and have been seen to be most efficient in confirmation of diagnoses in remote areas [2, 18, 21].

Until 2004, *Mycobacterium ulcerans* could only be treated by surgical debridement of all

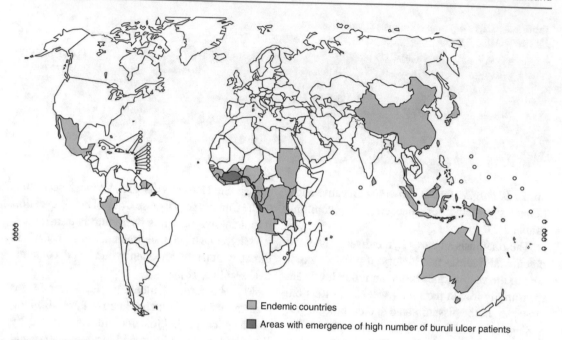

Fig. 2.12 Highlighted countries endemic to and countries with increasing emergence *Mycobacterium ulcerans*. (From Ref. [22])

necrotic tissue and skin grafting [21]. This was effective for early lesions but impractical on large lesions that presented due to delay in proper diagnosis. To address the management of larger lesions, the WHO recommends an 8-week combination antibiotic therapy of rifampicin (10 mg/kg/day) and streptomycin (15 mg/kg/day). Alternative antibiotic combinations of rifampicin (10 mg/kg/day) with clarithromycin (15 mg/kg/day) or moxifloxacin (400 mg/day) have been used, but the effectiveness has not yet been proven in randomized trials [20, 21]. Most ulcers can heal without treatment but run the risk of possible complications including limb deformity, functional disability, and secondary infection [18, 21] (Figs. 2.15 and 2.16).

Bartonella bacilliformis

Verruga Peruana

Bartonella bacilliformis is a gram-negative, aerobic proteobacterium. Infection with *B. bacilliformis* can lead to Carrion's disease. Carrion's disease presents as an acute febrile systemic disease (Oroya fever) and a chronic cutaneous eruptive disease (verruga peruana). This bacterial infection is a vector-borne disease transmitted to humans by the same vector involved in leishmaniasis, the *Lutzomyia verrucarum* sand fly [23]. Although this infection was thought to only occur in the Peruvian Andes, it has been reported more recently in other South American countries within the Amazon basin including Ecuador and Colombia [24].

Non-cutaneous manifestations of Carrion's disease include fever, headache, muscle aches, severe hemolytic anemia, and abdominal pain secondary to hepatomegaly. Cutaneous manifestations present as reddish, purple skin lesions that can progress to nodules. These angiomatous nodules have the potential to bleed, ulcerate, or become filled with pus (pustules). They present commonly on the face, arms, and legs and less commonly on the trunk and abdomen. Proper diagnostic measures are advised, since lesions present clinically identical to those of bacillary angiomatosis [23, 24] (Fig. 2.17).

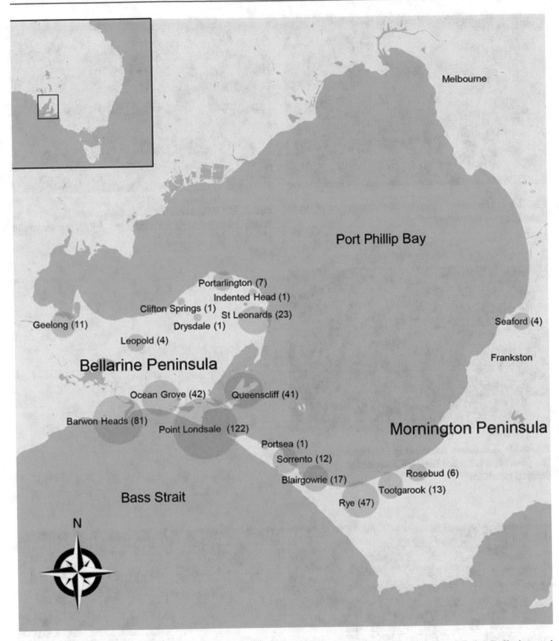

Fig. 2.13 Reported cases of *Mycobacterium ulcerans* in the new emerging endemic region of the Bellarine and Mornington Peninsula in Australia. (From Ref. [19])

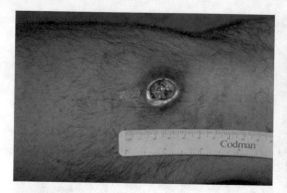

Fig. 2.14 Ulcerative stage of *Mycobacterium ulcerans* presenting on the extremity

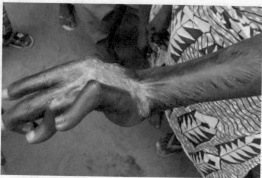

Fig. 2.16 Permanent limb disfigurement displayed in poorly managed patient infected by *Mycobacterium ulcerans*

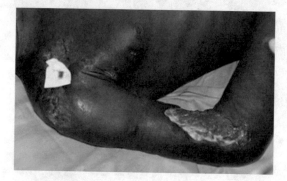

Fig. 2.15 Secondary infection in Mycobacterium ulcerans presents a potential high risk in patients who receive delayed treatment

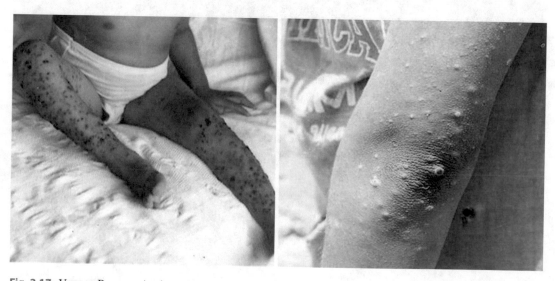

Fig. 2.17 Verruga Peruana: Angiomatous nodules on the lower extremities of an individual infected with *Bartonella bacilliformis.* (From Ref. [25])

According to the CDC, Carrion's disease can be diagnosed via blood culture or direct observation of the bacteria in peripheral blood smears during the acute phase of the infection [26]. Histologic examination of an angiomatous skin lesion reveals histiocytic endothelial proliferation. In contrast to bacillary angiomatosis, bacteria are rarely seen on the hematoxylin-eosin stain. Early diagnosis and treatment are imperative as this infection carries a high mortality rate, causing death to 40–85% of infected humans who do not receive treatment during the acute febrile phase [2, 24].

Chloramphenicol is the recommended treatment of choice for Oroya fever due to frequent co-infection with salmonella [23, 24]. Treatment for verruga peruana traditionally is streptomycin (15–20 mg/kg/day intramuscularly) for 10 days. In the eruptive phase, oral rifampin (10 mg/kg/day) for 10–14 days has become the drug regimen of choice. In untreated individuals with verruga peruana, symptoms can persist from months to years or even self-resolve [2, 23, 24].

Conclusion

Due to evolving migration, increased travel, and climate change, bacterial pathogens once confined to specific endemic areas have been able to expand their opportunities for exposure. Recognizing these once rare diseases can help advance a more thorough differential diagnosis when faced with dermatological manifestations of infectious disease. It is necessary to increase the awareness and provide a more consistent diagnostic plan, as these emerging bacterial infections commonly present with varied and multisystem clinical manifestations. This knowledge will aid in improved and more reliable diagnostic skills among healthcare professionals, allowing the ability to provide early appropriate treatment. This intervention aims to decrease and ultimately prevent the fatal complications associated with many of these emerging bacterial infections.

References

1. Vouga M, Greub G. Emerging bacterial pathogens: the past and beyond. Clin Microbiol Infect. 2016;22(1):12–21.
2. Nawas ZY, Tong Y, Kollipara R, Peranteau AJ, Woc-Colburn L, Yan AC, Lupi O, Tyring SK. Emerging infectious diseases with cutaneous manifestations: viral and bacterial infections. J Am Acad Dermatol. 2016;75(1):1–6.
3. Howard A, O'Donoghue M, Feeney A, Sleator RD. Acinetobacter baumannii: an emerging opportunistic pathogen. Virulence. 2012;3(3):243–50.
4. Montefour K, Frieden J, Hurst S, Helmich C, Headley D, Martin M, et al. *Acinetobacter baumannii*: an emerging multidrug-resistant pathogen in critical care. Crit Care Nurse. 2008;28:15–25. quiz 26
5. Sebeny PJ, Riddle MS, Petersen K. Acinetobacter baumannii skin and soft-tissue infection associated with war trauma. Clin Infect Dis. 2018;47(4):444–9.
6. Guerrero DM, Perez F, Conger NG, Solomkin JS, Adams MD, Rather PN, Bonomo RA. Acinetobacter baumannii-associated skin and soft tissue infections: recognizing a broadening spectrum of disease. Surg Infect. 2010;11(1):49–57.
7. Brown LD, Macaluso KR. Rickettsia felis, an emerging flea-borne rickettsiosis. Curr Trop Med Rep. 2016;3(2):27–39.
8. Yazid Abdad M, Stenos J, Graves S. Rickettsia felis, an emerging flea-transmitted human pathogen. Emerg Health Threats J. 2011;4(1):7168.
9. Silva-Pinto A, de Lurdes Santos M, Sarmento A. Tick-borne lymphadenopathy, an emerging disease. Ticks Tick Borne Dis. 2014;5(6):656–9.
10. Rieg S, Schmoldt S, Theilacker C, Wölfel S, Kern WV, Dobler G. Tick-borne lymphadenopathy (TIBOLA) acquired in Southwestern Germany. BMC Infect Dis. 2011;11(1):167.
11. Princess I, Ebenezer R, Nagarajan Ramakrishnan AK, Nandini S, Thirunarayan MA. Melioidosis: an emerging infection with fatal outcomes. Indian J Crit Care Med. 2017;21(6):397.
12. Volpe-Chaves CE, Rodrigues AC, Lacerda ML, de Oliveira CT, Castilho SB, Franciscato C, de Oliveira Santos IC, Assef AP, Roever L. Melioidosis, an emerging infectious disease in the Midwest Brazil: a case report. Medicine. 2019;98(16):e15235.
13. Wolf J. Melioidosis: the most neglected tropical disease: American Society for Microbiology. Washington, DC:20036.
14. Achappa B, Madi D, Vidyalakshmi K. Cutaneous melioidosis. J Clin Diagn Res. 2016;10(9):WD01.
15. Vasudevan B, Chatterjee M. Lyme borreliosis and skin. Indian J Dermatol. 2013;58(3):167.
16. Steere AC, Strle F, Wormser GP, Hu LT, Branda JA, Hovius JW, Li X, Mead PS. Lyme borreliosis. Nat Rev Dis Primers. 2016;2(1):1–9.

17. Moyer MW. New Cause for Lyme Disease Complicates Already Murky Diagnosis [Internet]. Scientific American. Scientific American; 2016 [cited 2020Feb6]. Available from: https://www.scientificamerican.com/article/new-cause-for-lyme-disease-complicates-already-murky-diagnosis1/.

18. Bravo F, Sanchez MR. New and re-emerging cutaneous infectious diseases in Latin America and other geographic areas. Dermatol Clin. 2003;21(4):655–8.

19. Tai AY, Athan E, Friedman ND, Hughes A, Walton A, O'Brien DP. Increased severity and spread of Mycobacterium ulcerans, Southeastern Australia. Emerg Infect Dis. 2018;24(1):58.

20. Treatment [Internet]. World Health Organization. World Health Organization; 2016 [cited 2020Jan12]. Available from: https://www.who.int/buruli/disease/treatment/en/.

21. Converse PJ, Nuermberger EL, Almeida DV, Grosset JH. Treating Mycobacterium ulcerans disease (Buruli ulcer): from surgery to antibiotics, is the pill mightier than the knife? Future Microbiol. 2011;6(10):1185–98.

22. van der Werf TS, Stienstra Y, Johnson RC, Phillips R, Adjei O, Fleischer B, Wansbrough-Jone MH, Johnson PDR, Portaels F, van der Graaf WTA, Asiedu K. Mycobacterium ulcerans disease. Bull World Health Organ. 2005;83:785–91.

23. Bartonellosis [Internet]. NORD (National Organization for Rare Disorders). Available from: https://rarediseases.org/rare-diseases/bartonellosis/.

24. Rolain JM, Brouqui P, Koehler JE, Maguina C, Dolan MJ, Raoult D. Recommendations for treatment of human infections caused by Bartonella species. Antimicrob Agents Chemother. 2004;48(6):1921–33.

25. Garcia-Quintanilla M, Dichter AA, Guerra H, Kempf VAJ. Carrion's disease: more than a neglected disease. Parasit Vectors. 2019;12:141.

26. Centers for Disease Control and Prevention. Bartonella infection (cat scratch disease, trench fever, and Carrión's disease). For Veterinarians. Disponível em: https://www.cdc.gov/bartonella/veterinarians/index.html. Acedido a. 2015;12.

Re-emerging Bacterial Infections of the Skin

Natalie Skopicki, Audrey H. Nguyen, Yelena Dokic, Eleanor Johnson, Divya R. Bhamidipati, and Harrison P. Nguyen

Abbreviations

ABC	ATP-binding cassette
APIC	Association for Professionals in Infection Control and Epidemiology
ASP	Antibiotic stewardship program
AUR	Antimicrobial Use and Resistance Module
CDC	Centers for Disease Control and Prevention
CMS	Centers for Medicare and Medicaid Services
DAP	Daptomycin
DDT	Dichlorodiphenyltrichloroethane
DHFR	Dihydrofolate reductase
DHPS	Dihydropteroic acid synthase
EPA	Environmental Protection Agency
FDA	Food and Drug Administration
HAI	Identifying Healthcare-Associated Infections
MATE	Multidrug and toxic compound extrusion
MDR	Multidrug resistant
MF	Major facilitator
MRSA	Methicillin-resistant S. aureus
NHSN	National Healthcare Safety Network
PBP	Penicillin-binding protein
RIF	Rifampicin
RMSF	Rocky Mountain spotted fever
RND	Resistance-nodulation-division
SAAR	Standardized antimicrobial administration ratio
SHEA	Society for Healthcare Epidemiology of America
SMR	Small multidrug resistance
STAAR	Strategies to Address Antimicrobial Resistance
STI	Sexually transmitted infection
TMP-SMX	Trimethoprim-sulfamethoxazole
VISA	Vancomycin-resistant *S. aureus*

Natalie Skopicki and Audrey H. Nguyen contributed equally with all other contributors.

N. Skopicki · A. H. Nguyen · H. P. Nguyen (✉)
Department of Dermatology, Emory University School of Medicine, Atlanta, GA, USA

Y. Dokic · E. Johnson
School of Medicine, Baylor College of Medicine, Houston, TX, USA

D. R. Bhamidipati
Division of Infectious Diseases, Department of Medicine, Emory University School of Medicine, Atlanta, GA, USA

Why Do Bacterial Infections Re-emerge?

Re-emerging infections are diseases that were formerly major public health problems, subsequently declined, but have since reappeared in a

© Springer Nature Switzerland AG 2021
S. K. Tyring et al. (eds.), *Overcoming Antimicrobial Resistance of the Skin*, Updates in Clinical Dermatology, https://doi.org/10.1007/978-3-030-68321-4_3

significant proportion of the population [1, 2]. Why do these bacterial diseases re-emerge? A combination of microbiological evolutionary mechanisms and systematic misuse of antibiotics have led to the emergence of multidrug-resistant (MDR) bacteria [3]. MDR pathogens lead to higher rates of mortality in comparison to their susceptible counterparts and cost an estimated $20 billion in the USA alone [4–6]. Antibiotic-resistant infections cause over 35,000 deaths annually in the USA [7] and are predicted to cause 300 million premature deaths by 2050 and a global loss of $100 trillion [8].

Mechanisms of Resistance

Bacteria can develop resistance by mutating existing genes or by acquiring new genes from other strains or species [9]. Horizontal gene transfer is the movement of genetic information between related or unrelated organisms [10]. Specifically, the acquisition of pathogenicity islands, or blocks of genes within the chromosome that code for pathogenic traits [11], is the source of increased virulence of MDR bacteria. There are three main mechanisms of horizontal gene transfer: transformation, transduction, and conjugation (Fig. 3.1). Transformation is the incorporation of exogenous, naked DNA into the bacterial genome through a breakage-and-insertion process [12]. Approximately 1% of bacterial species evolve via transformation [13]. Phage-mediated transduction relies on a virus to transfer genetic material from one bacterium to another [14]. Clinically, however, bacterial transduction is rare; only about one in 10,000 phages carry donor bacterium DNA. Conjugation involves the transfer of genetic material through direct cell-to-cell contact between fertility factor positive (F⁺) and fertility factor negative bacteria (F⁻) [15]. Generally, this genetic material is a mobile genetic element such as a plasmid or transposon [16], DNA sequences that can "jump" from one location within a genome to another. Chromosome-to-chromosome conjugation has also been described [17].

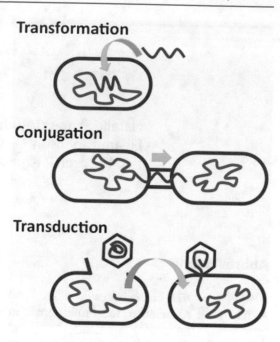

Fig. 3.1 Schematic depicting the three mechanisms of horizontal gene transfer: transformation, conjugation, and transduction [90]

Four general mechanisms can cause resistance to antibiotics: inactivation or modification of the antibiotic, alteration of the target site of the antibiotic that reduces its binding capacity, modification of metabolic pathways to circumvent the antibiotic effect or reduction in intracellular antibiotic accumulation by decreasing the permeability, and increasing the efflux of the antibiotic [18].

Bacteria can produce enzymes capable of altering or destroying antibiotics. Enzymes that modify antibiotics do so by catalyzing the addition of a moiety to the compound. This structural change weakens the avidity between antibodies and antigens, therefore reducing the antibiotic's efficacy or inactivating it. These chemical alterations are achieved through reactions such as acetylation (aminoglycosides, chloramphenicol, streptogramins), phosphorylation (aminoglycosides, chloramphenicol), and adenylation (aminoglycosides, lincosamides) [17]. Most antibiotics affected by this chemical alteration act by inhibiting ribosomal protein synthesis [19]. An example of destroying the antibiotic is β-lactam resistance, attributed to the presence of β-lactamases. By hydrolyzing the amide bond of the β-lactam ring, these enzymes destroy the antibiotic and render it ineffective [20].

Another mechanism of antibiotic resistance is the evolution of measures designed to limit antibiotic activity in bacterial pathogens, specifically by decreasing membrane permeability and producing efflux pumps. Since most antibiotics act on intracellular or periplasmic targets, they first must pass through bacterial cell membranes to reach their destinations [17]. To prevent this, bacteria have evolved three main mechanisms of decreased membrane permeability: shifts in the types of expressed porins, changes in the number of porins, and impaired porin function [21]. Porin alteration reduces antibiotic penetration because antimicrobial compounds are subsequently unable to utilize these water-filled channels to diffuse across the cytoplasmic membrane [22]. Changes in membrane permeability typically confer low-level resistance and are often exhibited in conjunction with other mechanisms of antibiotic resistance [21].

Bacteria can remove antimicrobials from intracellular environments through efflux pumps and transport proteins that actively pump out toxic compounds (in this case, most antibiotics in clinical use) [23]. These systems can be substrate-specific, such as with *tet* determinants for tetracycline, or act on a broader range of substrates (found in MDR bacteria) [24]. Efflux pumps are grouped into one of the five major families according to structure, energy source, substrate range, and distribution in bacteria. These classifications are the major facilitator (MF) family, the small multidrug resistance (SMR) family, the resistance-nodulation-division (RND) family, the ATP-binding cassette (ABC) family, and the multidrug and toxic compound extrusion (MATE) family [23]. Macrolide resistance is a pertinent example of the efflux mechanism. Encoded by *erm*, *mef*, or *msr* genes [25], these pumps can be found in organisms such as staphylococci, streptococci, and enterococci. Efflux pumps that confer macrolide resistance are often RND, ABC, or MF transporters [26].

Bacteria can also develop antibiotic resistance by interfering with the target site through target protection or modification, which decreases target site affinity for the antimicrobial agent. Bacterial mechanisms for target protection function by removing antibiotics from the target site or preventing antibiotics from effectively binding to the target site. Tetracycline resistance determinants *tet*(M) and *tet*(O) are classic examples of this phenomenon. Using GTP as their energy source, these ribosome protection genes remove and release tetracycline from its binding site on ribosomes, allowing for normal protein synthesis. *tet*(M) accomplishes this by acting on domain IV of the 16S rRNA and the tetracycline-binding site. This interaction not only dislodges the tetracycline but also prevents it from rebinding due to changes in ribosomal conformation [27]. *tet*(O) exhibits a similar mechanism involving competition for and alteration of the shape of tetracycline's inhibitory site [28]. Plasmid-mediated fluoroquinolone resistance by the quinolone resistance protein Qnr also uses a target protection mechanism. Qnr competes with quinolone for binding sites on DNA gyrase and topoisomerase IV. By obstructing the binding of quinolone, Qnr prevents the formation and stabilization of lethal gyrase-cleaved DNA-quinolone complexes, which inhibit transcription and replication [29]. Several *qnr* alleles code for this target protection mechanism. Though they confer low levels of resistance, *qnr* genes can promote highly resistant isolates by increasing the fitness of mutants with point mutations in DNA gyrase and/or topoisomerase IV encoding genes [30].

Target site modification is one of the most common mechanisms for the development of antibiotic resistance in bacterial pathogens. These changes are accomplished via mutations in target-site encoding genes, enzymatic alteration, or replacement/bypass of the target site. Bacterial genome modifications as a result of mutations confer structural changes in proteins and/or the cell that decrease antibiotic efficacy.

Rifampicin (RIF) resistance operates through this strategy. Single-step point mutations in the *rpoB* gene (which codes for the β subunit of RNA polymerase) translate to amino acid substitutions that induce structural changes in the RIF-binding site. Due to decreased drug avidity, RIF is unable to properly inhibit RNA transcription. These mutations, however, preserve the catalytic activity of RNA polymerase [31].

Another example of this mutational resistance pathway is resistance to oxazolidinones, of which linezolid resistance is the most well described. Mechanisms for developing linezolid resistance include changes in the genes encoding domain V of the 23S rRNA in the 50S ribosomal subunit and/or ribosomal proteins L3 (*rplC*) and L4 (*rplD*), of which the former occurs most frequently. The most common mutations associated with these pathways are base substitutions, such as a transition from guanine to thymine at nucleotide 2576 for domain V modification. Overall, these processes decrease drug affinity for its target on the A site of bacterial ribosomes [32].

Enzyme-catalyzed modification of target sites also promotes antibiotic resistance by preventing antimicrobials from effectively binding to their target sites. Consequently, these drugs cannot exert their mechanisms of action. A clinically relevant example of enzymatic alteration is macrolide resistance due to the methylation of the ribosome by enzymes encoded by *erm* (erythromycin ribosomal methylation) genes. The addition of one or two methyl groups to the adenine residue of domain V of the 23rRNA impairs the binding of the macrolide to its target. Furthermore, since the binding sites of lincosides and streptogramin B antibiotics overlap with those of macrolides, bacterial pathogens that express *erm* genes can become resistant to all three members of the MLS$_B$ group (constitutive resistance) [26, 33]. This phenotype, however, compromises bacterial fitness because the methylated ribosome cannot synthesize proteins as efficiently. To address this, most bacterial pathogens exhibit inducible MLS$_B$ resistance. In the presence of antibiotics, *erm* genes transcribe an mRNA that can be translated into a methylase to effect rapid resistance. In the absence of antibiotics, this transcript becomes inactivated, allowing the bacterial ribosome to synthesize proteins normally [34].

Instead of modifying the target site, bacteria can evolve new structures that accomplish the original target's biochemical functions without being inhibited by antimicrobials. They can also overproduce the antibiotic target so that enough antibiotic-free structures remain to carry out cellular processes. The mechanism for methicillin resistance in *S. aureus* is an example of target site replacement. Methicillin and other β-lactams inhibit penicillin-binding proteins (PBPs), enzymes that catalyze the transglycosylation and transpeptidation (cross-linking) of peptidoglycan. If peptidoglycan cross-bridges do not form, the cell wall will weaken and lyse, causing the cell to die. MRSA circumvents antibiotic inhibition through the acquisition of foreign gene *mecA*, which encodes PBP2a. When expressed, PBP2a, which has a low affinity for β-lactams, can take over the cross-linking reactions of host PBPs and maintain bacterial cell-wall synthesis (Fig. 3.2) [35].

An example of a target bypassing mechanism is trimethoprim-sulfamethoxazole (TMP-SMX) resistance. This antibiotic works by blocking folate synthesis, impairing the production of purines and certain amino acids. Specifically, TMP inhibits dihydrofolate reductase (DHFR), while SMX inhibits dihydropteroic acid synthase (DHPS), two major enzymes involved in folate synthesis. In response to TMP-SMX, bacteria develop mutations in the promoter region of DNA that code for these enzymes. The genetic changes lead to the overproduction of DHFR and DHPS, effectively overwhelming the antibiotic and allowing for continued folate production [36, 37].

Daptomycin (DAP) is a calcium ion-dependent lipopeptide antibiotic that functions by disrupting cell envelope homeostasis with respect to the phospholipids of the cell membrane. To protect themselves against the bactericidal activity of DAP, some bacteria have developed changes in the regulatory systems that govern cell envelope stress responses [38]. For example, a deletion of an isoleucine at position 177 of LiaF (part of the three-component regulatory system LiaFSR) is the most common mutation associated with DAP

Fig. 3.2 Methicillin-resistant *Staphylococcus aureus* (MRSA) bacteria as seen by a colorized scanning electron micrograph (SEM). The cross-linking reactions are maintained, and the cell walls are visible. (Source: https://www.cdc.gov/mrsa/community/photos/photo-mrsa-1.html [91])

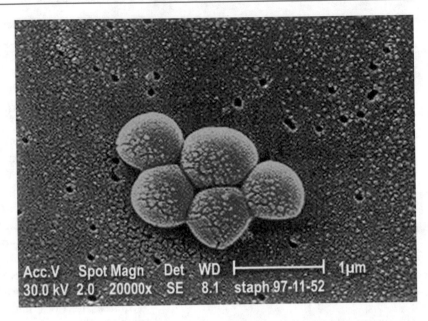

resistance (DAP-R) in *Enterococcus faecalis* [39]. In *S. aureus*, an accumulation of polymorphisms in the two-component system YycFG, which regulates cell membrane composition, has contributed to DAP-R. Another adaptive change involves enzymes that metabolize cell membrane phospholipids. For example, in *S. aureus*, the enzyme MprF (encoded by *mprF*) is responsible for the lysinylation of peptidoglycan, which causes the cell membrane to become positively charged. Mutations in *mprF* enhance the DAP-R phenotype by increasing the function of MprF. This increases the relative charge of the bacterial membrane, allowing it to repel calcium-complexed DAP [40].

S. aureus populations with intermediate vancomycin resistance (VISA) usually evolve this phenotype through an accumulation of genetic modifications in genes forming cell envelope homeostasis regulatory systems, most notably YycFG, VraSR, and GraRS [41]. Other VISA strains exhibit mutations in *rpoB*, which encodes the β-subunit of RNA polymerase [42]. Though the specific mechanisms by which these changes lead to vancomycin resistance are unclear, VISA strains typically exhibit one or more of the following metabolic characteristics: increased fructose utilization, increased fatty acid metabolism, impaired acetate metabolism and tricarboxylic acid cycle, decreased glutamate availability, and increased expression of cell-wall synthesis genes [41, 43]. These phenotypes have been hypothesized to prevent vancomycin from reaching its target [17].

Environmental and Sociodemographic Factors

Environmental conditions, sociodemographic changes, and behavioral factors are also important contributors to re-emergence. Human modification of the environment through industrialization, agriculture, or other practices has led to the re-emergence of bacterial infectious diseases by increasing exposure to vector populations. For example, the construction of dams creates ideal breeding grounds for mosquitoes and allows for the spread of mosquito-borne diseases [44]. Cultivated land attracts animals, which bring along arthropod vectors. The re-emergence of Rocky Mountain spotted fever in the Southwestern USA and Mexico is perpetuated in areas with large numbers of brown dog ticks (*Rhipicephalus sanguineus*), which are often found near human settlements [45].

High-risk sexual activity, migration and travel, and economic and social circumstances that limit access to healthcare have also resulted in the re-emergence of some infections, such as syphilis [46]. In particular, syphilis has re-emerged in high-risk groups, such as men who have sex with men, which is of concern because syphilitic lesions can lead to increased spread of other infections, such as human immunodeficiency virus. Additionally, with increased travel and migration, there has been an increase in cases of syphilis. For instance, rapid economic development has led to mass migrations of young individuals from rural to urban settings. Studies have shown that these migrants are less likely to have health insurance and are more likely to engage in sexually transmitted infection (STI)-associated behaviors such as low condom use and multiple sexual partners [46].

Examples of Re-emerging Bacterial Infections

Recognizing specific infections as public health challenges is important to preventing further spread. In dermatology, *Staphylococcus aureus*, *Treponema pallidum*, *and Rickettsia* spp. are notable re-emerging bacterial diseases.

Staphylococcus aureus

Staphylococcus aureus, one of the most common infectious organisms in humans, is a Gram-positive, coagulase-positive, spherical bacilli that forms clusters [47]. It is highly adaptable, colonizing many areas of the body, including the skin, glands, and mucous membranes such as the nares and gastrointestinal tract [47]. This organism causes a variety of infections, such as skin and soft tissue infections, lower respiratory tract infections, bacteremia, endocarditis, and osteomyelitis [47]. Skin and soft tissue infections can range from mild infections, such as impetigo, to abscesses and cellulitis [48]. Studies have shown that most cases of bacteremia originate from a patient's skin flora and that nasal carriage is a risk factor for developing an infection [49]. Another risk factor for bacteremia is medical instrumenta-

tion, such as central lines [47, 50]. In developed countries, *S. aureus* is the leading cause of bloodstream infections [51]. Aside from infections, *S. aureus* also causes a variety of toxin-mediated diseases. These include toxic shock syndrome, staphylococcal foodborne disease, and scalded skin syndrome [47].

Antibiotic resistance emerged quickly among the *S. aureus* species. Only 2 years after the introduction of penicillin, many isolates began producing beta-lactamase [47, 49]. Methicillin was developed to combat this evolution, but *S. aureus* again developed resistance, this time, by altering its penicillin-binding protein (PBP) [47]. This gave rise to what is now known as methicillin-resistant *S. aureus* (MRSA) (Fig. 3.3). Originally, MRSA was typically associated with hospital-acquired infections, but now it is also emerging as a significant cause of community-associated infections [47].

Impetigo and other minor skin infections can be treated with topical mupirocin 2% ointment. All abscesses should be incised and drained. Systemic antibiotics are indicated if there are signs or symptoms of systemic illness, the patient is toward the extremes of age, or the patient is immunodeficient. Non-purulent cellulitis should be treated with a beta-lactam such as cephalexin. Purulent cellulitis can be treated with clindamycin or doxycycline. Complicated skin and soft tissue infections may require the use of vancomycin [48].

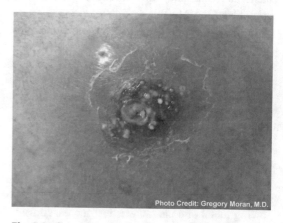

Fig. 3.3 Cutaneous abscess due to MRSA located on the back of a patient. (Source: https://www.cdc.gov/mrsa/community/photos/photo-mrsa-9.html [92])

Treponema pallidum

Syphilis is an infection that is caused by the spirochete *Treponema pallidum* and is spread through two primary mechanisms: sexual contact and vertical transmission from mother to fetus during pregnancy. There are four stages of syphilis, for which skin manifestations vary. These skin manifestations can thus help direct therapy by conveying the stage of the disease. Primary syphilis is characterized by a painless chancre on the genitalia with regional lymphadenopathy (Fig. 3.4). The chancre appears as an indurated ulcer [46]. If unnoticed, the disease may progress to secondary syphilis, which is characterized by a disseminated skin eruption accompanied by generalized lymphadenopathy. This papulosquamous rash presents with pink or red lesions that are 0.2 to 2 cm and usually found on the palms of

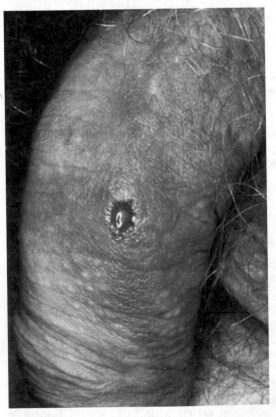

Fig. 3.4 Primary syphilis due to *Treponema pallidum* causing a painless chancre on a patient's penis. (Source: CDC/ Dr. N.J. Fiumara)

the hands, soles of the feet, face, and trunk [52]. Latent syphilis can manifest as either a re-occurrence of the generalized skin eruption seen in secondary syphilis or simply an absence of any symptoms. Finally, tertiary syphilis can present with gummas, which are rubbery painless tumors that can appear in any organ but most frequently are found on the skin, bones, and mucous membranes [52, 53].

Primary, secondary, or early latent syphilis is treated with a single intramuscular injection of benzathine penicillin G (2.4 million units) [54]. If an individual has late latent or tertiary syphilis, they will need multiple injections or intravenous penicillin G treatment [54]. Treatment with benzathine penicillin G will treat the *Treponema pallidum* spirochete, but will not reverse any physical damage done by the disease.

Of note, the emergence of clinically significant azithromycin resistance in *Treponema pallidum* species has led to treatment failures in patients who use macrolides, a second-line treatment for syphilis [55]. Macrolides are generally used for syphilis treatment when penicillin or doxycycline is not feasible, such as when patients are allergic to penicillin. Azithromycin resistance is due to point mutations in rRNA genes. Treponemal resistance to penicillin, however, is unlikely as it would require multistep mutational changes such as horizontal gene transfer, which is a mechanism that *Treponema pallidum* lacks [56].

Rickettsia spp.

Rickettsial diseases include epidemic typhus, murine typhus, Rocky Mountain spotted fever, and rickettsial pox, in addition to other spotted fevers [57]. Rickettsial diseases are caused by *Rickettsia* spp., obligate intracellular Gram-negative bacteria found in ticks, lice, fleas, mites, chiggers, and mammals [57]. The rickettsial diseases can disseminate through the blood and affect many organs in the body, including the skin [57].

Murine typhus is caused by the bacterium *Rickettsia typhi*, which is transmitted by fleas

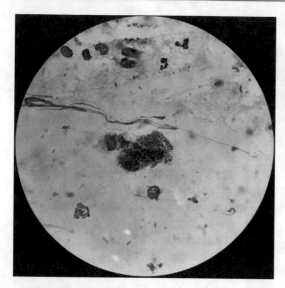

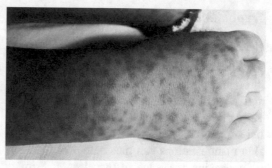

Fig. 3.6 Characteristic spotted rash of Rocky Mountain spotted fever, caused by *Rickettsia rickettsii*. (Source: CDC)

Fig. 3.5 Photomicrograph of a yolk sac culture, revealing numerous *Rickettsia typhi* bacteria at a magnification of 1000×. (Source: CDC/Armed Forces Institute of Pathology (AFIP))

from rodents to humans (Fig. 3.5). If a human host is infected, the symptoms include fever, chills, headache, myalgia, rash, cough, and relative bradycardia [58]. The rash associated with murine typhus appears as small erythematous papules on the extremities, which spread toward the trunk and abdomen [59]. Often, the face, palms, and soles are spared in murine typhus [59]. A black eschar may form at the site of the flea bite [58]. Murine typhus is endemic to tropical and coastal regions [60]. In the early 1900s, murine typhus was a significant problem for coastal areas, such as Galveston, TX. The implementation of an ectoparasite eradication program, involving the dispersion of the insecticide dichlorodiphenyltrichloroethane (DDT) to common paths that rats traversed, reduced the number of ectoparasites. Subsequently, the incidence of murine typhus in Galveston drastically decreased. However, recent climate change effects (most notably, flooding) in the area have led to increased number of cases in part due to poor vector control.

Rickettsia rickettsii, the causative organism of Rocky Mountain spotted fever (RMSF), can be transmitted to humans through the bite of an infected tick. The rash associated with RMSF appears as a generalized skin eruption with purpuric, blanching, or non-blanching macules and papules (Fig. 3.6) [61]. The rash is classically located on the extremities but can progress to involve the trunk. The palms and soles may be affected as well. The timing of the presentation of the rash can help a clinician ascertain if the condition might be related to a rickettsial disease. In general, patients with RMSF will develop a rash between the third and fifth day of illness, while in murine typhus, the rash will generally tend to appear at the end of the first week of illness.

RMSF can be a life-threatening condition, especially to those living in under-resourced settings [62]. The pathogenic mechanisms that have allowed for the re-emergence of RMSF in regions such as Arizona and Mexico have been attributed to large local infestations of the brown dog tick (*Rhipicephalus sanguineus* sensu lato) on domestic dogs that result in high rates of human exposure [63]. Children are especially at risk, since they may spend more time playing in tick-infested areas or playing with dogs. Poverty and lack of access to medical care are risk factors for more severe RMSF [63].

Because rickettsial disease can cause multisystem organ failure and death, timely treatment is essential [63]. Treatment is accomplished with doxycycline. A course of doxycycline for about 7 to 10 days is the most effective for the treatment of murine typhus, RMSF, and other rickettsial or tick-borne diseases [64].

Strategies for Mitigating Re-mergence

The principle of antibiotic stewardship, since conceptualized by two physicians at the Emory University School of Medicine in the mid-1990s [65], has evolved to become a critical healthcare philosophy that seeks to maximize the effective and efficient use of antibiotics in the treatment of illness while minimizing the potential consequences of antibiotic resistance. The Centers for Disease Control and Prevention (CDC), the Food and Drug Administration (FDA), and various advisory groups for the US government play essential roles in addressing the development of antibiotic resistance (Table 3.1). The CDC has established programs to maximize antibiotic stewardship and offer specific criteria for antibiotic use. For example, it advised medical facilities to assure that antibiotics are delivered for proper durations and at proper dosages while advocating that antibiotic "timeouts" be used after 48 to 72 hours to assess how well an antibiotic is functioning [66]. In addition, the CDC developed the standardized antimicrobial administration ratio (SAAR), a metric for comparing observed to predicted days of antimicrobial therapy based on nationally aggregated antimicrobial use data from about 200 hospitals as a benchmark for individual hospitals. However, the CDC's report on antibiotic resistance threats in 2013 grossly underreported the annual deaths from antibiotic-resistant infections [66, 67]. The recently released 2019 report shows that antibiotic-resistant bacteria and fungi caused more than 2.8 million infections and 35,000 deaths in the USA each year, nearly twice the annual deaths suggested by the 2013 report [68]. The report further indicated that prevention efforts have resulted in an 8% reduction in mortality from antibiotic-resistant infections.

To provide further data and guidance, the CDC's National Healthcare Safety Network (NHSN), an internet-based surveillance system responsible for integrating patient and healthcare personnel safety surveillance systems, created the Surveillance for Antimicrobial Use and

Table 3.1 US organizations that have contributed to the mitigation of antimicrobial resistance

Entity	Contribution
CDC National Healthcare Safety Network (NHSN)	Implements Surveillance for Antimicrobial Use and Antimicrobial Resistance Options Program to oversee national antibiotic use
FDA Center for Drug Evaluation and Research	Preserve effectiveness of currently available antibiotic drugs and reduce the emergence and spread of antibiotic-resistant bacteria
FDA Center for Biologics Evaluation and Research	
FDA Center for Veterinary Medicine	
FDA National Center for Toxicological Research	
FDA Office of the Chief Scientist	
Department of agriculture	Allows for "no antibiotics" food labeling to minimize the presence of antibiotic-fed animals in food supply nationally
Environmental Protection Agency (EPA)	Monitors data from antibiotic manufacturers and place limits on antibiotic usage
Centers for Medicare and Medicaid Services (CMS)	Regulates medical facilities and nursing homes as well as those managed/owned by the joint commission to implement antibiotic stewardship programs
Association for Professionals in Infection Control and Epidemiology (APIC)	Optimize antibiotic stewardship via epidemiological studies and the coordination of care between healthcare epidemiologists and infection specialists
Society for Healthcare Epidemiology of America (SHEA)	

Antimicrobial Resistance Options program, a national program that oversees antibiotic use. The program has established several resources for antibiotic stewardship, including three documents listed for January 2020 publication: the Antimicrobial Use and Resistance (AUR) Module, Identifying Healthcare-Associated Infections (HAI) for NHSN Surveillance, and Patient Safety Monthly Reporting Plan and Annual Surveys [69]. The AUR module provides a mechanism for individual healthcare facilities to report and analyze antimicrobial use and resistance data to inform benchmarking, reduce antimicrobial-resistant infections through antimicrobial stewardship, and interrupt transmission of resistant pathogens at individual facilities [70, 71]. The HAI module helps standardize the classification for data reporting to distinguish between infections present on admission or acquired within a healthcare facility [72]. The Patient Safety Monthly Reporting Plan and Annual Surveys help the CDC select data for creating national benchmarks by distinguishing whether the participating facility (hospital, long-term acute care, or inpatient rehabilitation facility) is using in-plan or off-plan surveillance [73]. The CDC also collects data on clinical outcomes of infections that vary with treatment plans, maintains an antibiotic resistance threat list, and determines trends and estimates of antibiotic-resistant infections and deaths over time [68]. Eighteen pathogens, including two new threats, drug-resistant *Candida auris* and carbapenem-resistant *Acinetobacter*, portend increasing resistance to antibiotics and are being closely monitored.

The Food and Drug Administration (FDA) is responsible for working with product sponsors and other government agencies to facilitate the efficient development of new antimicrobials, evaluating new antibiotic applications, and making recommendations concerning approval [67]. The agency promotes the appropriate and responsible use of antimicrobials and disseminates information that promotes interventions that help slow the development of resistance. This includes the ability to comment on the efficacy of antibiotics, to limit the patient population to whom the medication can be administered, and to discuss any discrepancies that exist between antibiotics on the market and those waiting to be released [74]. In addition, the FDA can determine the nature of data collected by institutions utilizing antimicrobials in addition to requiring ongoing data collection from companies in a post-approval process so that stakeholders can track, treat, and respond to antimicrobial resistance outbreaks. Several of the FDA Centers, including the Center for Drug Evaluation and Research, Center for Biologics Evaluation and Research, Center for Veterinary Medicine, National Center for Toxicological Research, and the Office of the Chief Scientist, play essential roles in helping to preserve the effectiveness of currently available antimicrobial drugs and reducing the emergence and spread of antimicrobial-resistant bacteria [67].

Additional government agencies may also play a role. The US Department of Agriculture has allowed for "antibiotic-free" food labeling in the hope of using market forces to minimize the presence of antibiotic-fed animals in our food supply. The presence of fewer antibiotic-fed animals may, in turn, slow the rise of antibiotic resistance. The US Environmental Protection Agency (EPA) can request data from antibiotic manufacturers and place limits on antibiotic usage. The EPA recently failed to limit the use of two medically important antibiotics to treat a disease affecting citrus production [75]. The Centers for Medicare and Medicaid Services (CMS) has mandated that antibiotic stewardship programs (ASPs) be implemented in medical facilities and nursing homes as well as in those managed or owned by the Joint Commission. Governmental agencies can play an important role in addressing the prevention of antibiotic resistance through the prevention of infection. Strategies such as immunization, safe and sanitary food preparation, and promoting handwashing are significant targets of prevention strategies [76] that would limit antibiotic use.

Elected official support in the fight against antibiotic resistance is also essential. The President of the USA can ask for the development of legislation and direct agencies to participate, and, in 2015, the White House created an action plan to fight antibiotic resistance, including funding state health departments to develop interventions and start antibiotic stewardship programs [74, 77]. In March of 2019, the Strategies to Address Antimicrobial Resistance (STAAR) Act was introduced to the US Senate. While the act remains stuck in Congress, it highlights the role government can play including the promotion of a partnership between the CDC and the government, the allocation of grants to healthcare facilities that study the development of antibiotics, the reauthorization of the Antimicrobial Resistance Task Force, the request of the National Institutes of Health to formulate a research plan, and the creation of an advisory board task force with the director from the Department of Health and Human Services [76]. Yet, many contend that the United States does not currently utilize programs to their maximum potential to help solve the problem of antibiotic resistance [76]. Barriers, including limited national and state personnel and financial resources, lack of program oversight, and the current antibiotic approval process lacking any antibiotic stewardship principles have been cited [76]. The irony is that instituting inappropriate regulations can contribute to the problem of antibiotic resistance rather than fixing it [78].

In 2012, the Association for Professionals in Infection Control and Epidemiology (APIC) and the Society for Healthcare Epidemiology of America (SHEA) recognized the essential role of epidemiologic studies in the optimizing antibiotic stewardship [79] and cooperation among infection preventionists and healthcare epidemiologists [76]. Epidemiologic studies provide an understanding of which specific resistant bacterial gene mutations are spreading and the morbidity and mortality associated with these mutations. Complicating epidemiologic studies is that they often study infection patterns among a population through molecular typing methods [80]. Evolving antibiotic resistance, with rapid mutation formation, can make tracking of antibiotic resistance using molecular typing techniques challenging [81]. Moreover, many feel that local hospital epidemiologists should be incentivized to provide higher levels of local leadership support, integrate education programs, share surveillance data and outbreak alerts, and bridge the gaps between antibiotic stewardship programs (ASPs) and microbiology departments [82].

Despite challenges, epidemiologic studies continue to reveal the details of antibiotic resistance that can assist clinicians in appropriate antibiotic stewardship. For instance, a recent study in inpatient facilities showed that even if a patient is treated with an antibiotic to which their bacterial infection is sensitive, it may result in a higher chance that the patient will host bacteria that are resistant to a different antibiotic [83]. The conclusion of the study found that the key to reducing the prevalence of antibiotic-resistant bacteria is to prevent bacterial transmission among patients in hospitals [83].

While healthcare organizations are complex entities with predominantly traditional structures of infection control, administration, and medical management [84], they do provide opportunities to ameliorate the potential for antibiotic resistance throughout the organization. Hospital administrators have the responsibility to promote safe antibiotic use by supporting the formation of multidisciplinary committees to turn local and national data into hospital and facility policy and best practices, join regional infection prevention efforts, and make sure that lab personnel, clinical prevention staff, and physicians are communicating [76]. They are also frequently either the barriers against or champions for hospital-based antibiotic stewardship programs. A study using data from the 2014 NHSN Annual Hospital Survey showed that 39% of 4184 US hospitals had a comprehensive antibiotic stewardship program and that hospitals with greater than 200 beds were more likely to have the program than hospitals with 50 beds or less (59% vs. 25%) [85]. Hospital leadership support and salary support for personnel were significantly associated with having a comprehensive ASP. The creation and implementation of antibiotic stewardship programs is a costly endeavor. Startup and management costs of ASPs in children's hospitals have been reported to range from $17,000 to $388,500 annually [86] The majority of the expense is due to the salaries of physicians and pharmacists who manage these programs. Making ASPs cost-effective is critical for adoption, and studies have suggested that savings from ASPs in both large and small hospitals can range from $200,000 to $900,000 annually [76]. A recent systematic review indicated that the mean cost savings varied by hospital size and region but, on average, was $732 per patient (range $2.50 to $2640) with the key cost savings resulting from a reduction in length of stay [87].

The CDC has highlighted cases in which proper antibiotic prescription and usage directly led to institutional cost savings. In one example, physicians prescribing cephalexin at a hospital in Brooklyn, NY, were required to receive approval from an infectious disease physician specialist. The hospital found that the costs due to the use of cephalexin decreased from $314,105 to $4166 over the year. In Jackson, MS, a teaching hospital restricted antibiotic use by requiring a pharmacist to approve all prescriptions. This practice decreased the usage of restricted antibiotics, usually the costliest ones, by 75%, and injectable antibiotic costs fell by almost $200,000 the following year. Pediatric programs with the financial ability to have an ASP show a clear reduction of antibiotic use [88].

Education and oversight of healthcare providers are critical in an ever-changing landscape of infections and antibiotic resistance in which it is vital that clinicians understand which infections are most prominent among their patients, understand how to prescribe antibiotics safely, and utilize a reassessment period every 48 to 72 hours [76]. De-escalation, where physicians prescribe antibiotics strictly based on culture results and thereby eliminate any unnecessary empiric therapies, is a technique that can also be used, especially in the ICU, where antibiotics are often prescribed quickly in a rapidly deteriorating patient. A two-step plan can also be implemented in the ICU where the first step includes identifying the infection and starting an appropriately dosed antibiotic. The second step encourages halting the therapy, or at least decreasing the dosage, and restricting the treatment to a maximum of 8 days [89]. Multiple avenues for education are available, including grand rounds, conferences, continuing medical education, and frequent emails, or other forms of communication. There is a push for publishers of scientific journals to view antibiotic resistance as a public health crisis and to incentivize the release of data even before publishing [74].

Oversight of programmatic failure in hospitals and outpatient centers is also an opportunity to optimize antibiotic stewardship. The data demonstrate that surgical patients are likely to receive more antibiotic courses and are less likely to have their antibiotic prescriptions reviewed regularly. In the ICU, the challenge lies in determining the appropriate timing of antibiotic therapy. While delaying a course of antibiotics for critically ill patients leads to increased mortality, a delay in the initiation of antibiotic therapy in stable patients actually lowers mortality [89]. In addition, patients that stay in the hospital for long periods often receive higher than necessary amounts of antibiotics [28]. Whether this is an association or causation requires further investigation. In the outpatient setting, research is especially alarming, where in one observed facility, it was determined that nearly 30% of prescribed antibiotics had no medical benefit, meaning the infection could have been treated without it [77].

Finally, education and management of expectations at the patient level are also important. Learned behaviors, most notably the expectation patients have of receiving antibiotics when ill, must be combated [78], and efforts to educate patients and prescribers are critical. Augmenting and encouraging new and established educational programs to accompany the prescription of antibiotics to the public, in collaboration with drug manufacturers, pharmacies, and hospitals, could be considered.

Interventions to ameliorate antibiotic resistance are centered on limiting the incidence of infections, improving antibiotic usage, developing new antibiotics, and encouraging efforts in education, surveillance, and feedback [66, 77, 84]. Critical antibiotic stewardship elements include leadership commitment, accountability, drug expertise, action, tracking, reporting, and education [66].

Funding Sources This article has no funding sources.

Conflict of Interest Disclosure The authors have no conflict of interest to declare.

This work has not been previously published or presented.

References

1. Emerging Infectious Diseases. World Health Organization; 1997. Available from: https://www.who.int/docstore/world-health-day/en/documents1997/whd01.pdf.

2. National Institutes of Health. Understanding emerging and re-emerging infectious diseases. In: NIH Curriculum Supplement Series: National Institutes of Health. Maryland: Bethesda; 2007.

3. World Health Organization. Global action plan on antimicrobial resistance. Switzerland: WHO Press; 2015.

4. Cosgrove SE. The relationship between antimicrobial resistance and patient outcomes: mortality, length of hospital stay, and health care costs. Clin Infect Dis. 2006;42(Suppl 2):S82–9.

5. Diaz Granados CA, Zimmer SM, Klein M, et al. Comparison of mortality associated with vancomycin-resistant and vancomyin-susceptible enterococcal bloodstream infections: a meta-analysis. Clin Infect Dis. 2005;41(3):327–33.

6. Sydnor ERM, Perl TM. Hospital epidemiology and infection control in acute-care settings. Clin Microbiol Rev. 2011;24(1):141–73.

7. Centers for Disease Control and Prevention. Antibiotic Resistance Threats in the United States, 2019. Atlanta: U.S. Department of Health and Human Resources, CDC; 2019.

8. Antimicrobial Resistance: Tackling a crisis for the future health and wealth of nations. Review of Antimicrobial Resistance; 2014.

9. Schweitzer V, Werkhoven CV, Baño JR, Bielicki J, Harbarth S, Hulscher M, et al. Optimizing design of research to evaluate antibiotic stewardship interventions: consensus recommendations of a multinational working group. Clin Microbiol Infect. 2019;26(1):41–50.

10. Burmeister AR. Horizontal gene transfer. Evol Med Public Health. 2015;2015(1):193–4.

11. Lim VK. Emerging and re-emerging infections. Med J Malaysia. 1999;54(2):287–91.

12. Griffiths AJF, Miller JH, Suzuki DT, et al. Bacterial transformation. In: An introduction to genetic analysis. 7th ed. New York: W. H. Freeman. p. 2000.

13. Thomas CM, Nielsen KM. Mechanisms of, and barriers to, horizontal gene transfer between bacteria. Nat Rev Microbiol. 2005;3(9):711–21.

14. Griffiths AJF, Miller JH, Suzuki DT, et al. Transduction. In: An introduction to genetic analysis. 7th ed. New York: W. H. Freeman. p. 2000.

15. Griffiths AJF, Miller JH, Suzuki DT, et al. Bacterial conjugation. In: An introduction to genetic analysis. 7th ed. New York: W. H. Freeman. p. 2000.

16. Munita JM, Arias CA. Mechanisms of antibiotic resistance. Microbiol Spectr. 2016;4(2):1–37.

17. Manson JM, Hancock LE, Gilmore MS. Mechanism of chromosomal transfer of Enterococcus faecalis pathogenicity island, capsule, antimicrobial resistance, and other traits. Proc Natl Acad Sci U S A. 2010;107(27):12269–74.

18. Blair JMA, Webber MA, Baylay AJ, Ogbolu DO, Piddock LJV. Molecular mechanisms of antibiotic resistance. Nat Rev Microbiol. 2015;13:42–51.

19. Ramirez MS, Tolmasky ME. Aminoglycoside modifying enzymes. Drug Resist Updat. 2010;13(6):151–71.

20. Bush K, Bradford PA. β-lactams and β-lactamase inhibitors: an overview. Cold Spring Harb Perspect Med. 2016;6(8):a025247.

21. Nikaido H. Molecular basis of bacterial outer membrane permeability revisited. Microbiol Mol Biol Rev. 2003;67(4):593–656.

22. Hancock RE, Brinkman FS. Function of pseudomonas porins in uptake and efflux. Annu Rev Microbiol. 2005;56:17–38.

23. Webber MA, Piddock LJV. The importance of efflux pumps in bacterial antibiotic resistance. J Antimicrob Chemother. 2003;51(1):9–11.

24. Poole K. Efflux-mediated antimicrobial resistance. J Antimicrob Chemother. 2005;56(1):20–51.

25. Portillo A, Ruiz-Larrea F, Zarazaga M, et al. Macrolide resistance genes in Enterococcus spp. Antimicrob Agents Chemother. 2000;44(4):967–71.

26. Leclercq R. Mechanisms of resistance to macrolides and lincosamides: nature of the resistance elements and their clinical implications. Clin Infect Dis. 2002;34(4):482–92.

27. Dönhöfer A, Franckenberg S, Wickles S, et al. Structural basis for TetM-mediated tetracycline resistance. Proc Natl Acad Sci U S A. 2012;109(42):16900–5.

28. Li W, Atkinson GC, Thakor NS, et al. Mechanism of tetracycline resistance by ribosomal protection protein Tet(O). Nat Commun. 2013;4:1477.

29. Rodríguez-Martínez JM, Cano ME, Velasco C, et al. Plasmid-mediated quinolone resistance: an update. J Infect Chemother. 2011;17(2):149–82.

30. Aldred KJ, Kerns RJ, Osheroff N. Mechanism of quinolone action and resistance. Biochemistry. 2014;53(10):1565–74.

31. Floss HG, Yu TW. Rifamycin-mode of action, resistance, and biosynthesis. Chem Rev. 2005;105(2):621–32.

32. Mendes RE, Deshpande LM, Jones RN. Linezolid update: stable in vitro activity following more than a decade of clinical use and summary of associated resistance mechanisms. Drug Resist Updat. 2014;17(1–2):1–12.

33. Weisblum B. Erythromycin resistance by ribosome modification. Antimicrob Agents Chemother. 1995;39(3):577–85.

34. Katz L, Ashley GW. Translation and protein synthesis: macrolides. Chem Rev. 2005;105(2):499–528.

35. Stapleton PD, Taylor P. Methicillin resistance in Staphylococcus aureus. Sci Prog. 2002;85(Pt 1):57–72.

36. Flensburg J, Sköld O. Massive overproduction of dihydrofolate reductase in bacteria as a response to the use of trimethoprim. Eur J Biochem. 1987;162(3):473–6.

37. Huovinen P. Resistance to trimethoprim sulfamethoxazole. Clin Infect Dis. 2001;32(11):1608–14.

38. Tran TT, Munita JM, Arias CA. Mechanisms of drug resistance: daptomycin resistance. Ann N Y Acad Sci. 2015;1354:32–53.

39. Munita JM, Tran TT, Diaz L, et al. A liaF codon deletion abolishes daptomycin bactericidal activity against vancomycin-resistant Enterococcus faecalis. Antimicrob Agents Chemother. 2013;57(6):2831–3.

40. Bayer AS, Schneider T, Sahl HG. Mechanisms of daptomycin resistance in Staphylococcus aureus: role of the cell membrane and cell wall. Ann N Y Acad Sci. 2013;1277:139–58.

41. Gardete S, Tomasz A. Mechanisms of vancomycin resistance in Staphylococcus aureus. J Clin Invest. 2014;124(7):2836–40.

42. Watanabe Y, Cui L, Katayama Y, et al. Impact of rpoB mutations on reduced vancomycin susceptibility in Staphylococcus aureus. J Clin Microbiol. 2011;49(7):2680–4.

43. Howden BP, Davies JK, Johnson PD, et al. Reduced vancomycin susceptibility in Staphylococcus aureus, including vancomycin-intermediate and heterogeneous vancomycin-intermediate strains: resistance mechanisms, laboratory detection, and clinical implications. Clin Microbiol Rev. 2010;23(1):99–139.

44. Institute of Medicine. Vector-borne disease emergence and resurgence. In: Vector-borne disease: understanding the environmental, human health, and ecological connections, workshop summary. Washington, DC: The National Academies Press; 2008. p. 16–64.

45. Drexler NA, Yaglom H, Casal M, et al. Fatal Rocky Mountain spotted fever along the United States–Mexico border, 2013–2016. Emerg Infect Dis. 2017;23(10):1621–6.

46. Stamm LV. Syphilis: re-emergence of an old foe. Microbial Cell. 2016;3(9):363–70. https://doi.org/10.15698/mic2016.09.523.

47. Lakhundi S, Zhang K. Methicillin-resistant Staphylococcus aureus: molecular characterization, evolution, and epidemiology. Clin Microbiol Rev. 2018;31(4):e00020–18.

48. Liu C, Bayer A, Cosgrove SE, et al. Clinical practice guidelines by the infectious diseases society of america for the treatment of methicillin-resistant Staphylococcus aureus infections in adults and children. Clin Infect Dis. 2011;52(3):e18–55.

49. O'Gara JP. Into the storm: chasing the opportunistic pathogen Staphylococcus aureus from skin colonisation to life-threatening infections. Environ Microbiol. 2017;19(10):3823–33.

50. Lowy FD. Staphylococcus aureus infections. N Engl J Med. 1998;339(8):520–32.

51. Hassoun A, Linden PK, Friedman B. Incidence, prevalence, and management of MRSA bacteremia across patient populations-a review of recent developments in MRSA management and treatment. Crit Care. 2017;21(1):211.

52. Ingram B. The many presentations of syphilis. J Dermatol Nurses Assoc. 2016;8(5):318–24. https://doi.org/10.1097/jdn.0000000000000252.

53. Cherniak W, Silverman M. Syphilitic Gumma. N Engl J Med. 2014;371(7):667. https://doi.org/10.1056/nejmicm1313142.

54. Workowski K, Bolan G. Sexually transmitted diseases guidelines 2015. MMWR. 2015;64(3):1–137.

55. Stamm LV. Syphilis: antibiotic treatment and resistance. Epidemiol Infect. 2014;143(8):1567–74. https://doi.org/10.1017/s0950268814002830.

56. Stamm LV. Global challenge of antibiotic-resistant *Treponema pallidum*. Antimicrob Agents Chemother. 2010;54:583–9.

57. Walker DH. Rickettsiae. In: Baron S, editor. Medical microbiology. 4th ed. Galveston: University of Texas Medical Branch at Galveston; 1996. Chapter 38. Available from: https://www.ncbi.nlm.nih.gov/books/NBK7624/.

58. Minahan N, Chao C-C, Tsai K-H. The reemergence and emergence of vector-borne rickettsioses in Taiwan. Trop Med Infect Dis. 2017;3(1):1. https://doi.org/10.3390/tropicalmed3010001.

59. Gorchynski JA, Langhorn C, Simmons M, Roberts D. What's hot, with spots and red all over? Murine Typhus West J Emerg Med. 2009;10(3):207. https://doi.org/10.1111/j.1442-2026.1998.tb00616.x.

60. Blanton LS, Vohra RF, Bouyer DH, Walker DH. Reemergence of murine typhus in Galveston, Texas, USA, 2013. Emerg Infect Dis. 2015;21(3):484–6. https://doi.org/10.3201/eid2103.140716.

61. Kao GF, Evancho CD, Ioffe O, Lowitt MH, Dumler JS. Cutaneous histopathology of Rocky Mountain spotted fever. J Cutan Pathol. 1997;24(10):604–10. https://doi.org/10.1111/j.1600-0560.1997.tb01091.x.

62. Alvarez-Hernandez G, Murillo-Benitez C, Candia-Plata MC, Moro M. Rocky Mountain Spotted Fever Reemergence in children from Sonora, Mexico. 2004–12. Int J Epidemiol. 2015;44(suppl_1):i243. https://doi.org/10.1093/ije/dyv096.440.

63. Straily A, Drexler N, Cruz-Loustaunau D, Paddock CD, Alvarez-Hernandez G. Notes from the field: community-based prevention of Rocky Mountain spotted fever — Sonora, Mexico, 2016. MMWR Morb Mortal Wkly Rep. 2016;65(46):1302–3. https://doi.org/10.15585/mmwr.mm6546a6.

64. Botelho-Nevers E, Socolovschi C, Raoult D, Parola P. Treatment of rickettsia spp. infections: a review. Expert Rev Anti-Infect Ther. 2012;10(12):1425–37. https://doi.org/10.1586/eri.12.139.

65. McGowan JE Jr, Gerding DN. Does antibiotic restriction prevent resistance? New Horizon. 1996;4(3):370–6.

66. Antibiotic resistance threats in the United States, 2013. Atlanta, GA: Centres for Disease Control and Prevention, U.S. Department of Health and Human Services; 2013.

67. Commissioner Of the. Antimicrobial Resistance Info [Internet]. U.S. Food and Drug Administration. FDA; [cited 2019Dec17]. Available from: https://www.fda.gov/emergency-preparedness-and-response/mcm-issues/antimicrobial-resistance-information-fda.

68. Biggest Threats and Data [Internet]. Centers for Disease Control and Prevention. Centers for Disease Control and Prevention; 2019 [cited 2019Dec17]. Available from: https://www.cdc.gov/drugresistance/biggest-threats.html.

69. ACH Surveillance for Antimicrobial Use and Antimicrobial Resistance Options [Internet]. Centers for Disease Control and Prevention. Centers for Disease Control and Prevention; 2019 [cited 2019 Dec 17]. Available from: https://www.cdc.gov/nhsn/acute-care-hospital/aur/index.html.

70. Dellit TH, Owens RC, McGowan JE, et al. Infectious Diseases Society of America and the Society for Healthcare Epidemiology of America guidelines for developing an institutional program to enhance Antimicrobial stewardship. Clin Infect Dis. 2007;44:159–77.

71. Antimicrobial Use and Resistance (AUR) Option [Internet]. [cited 2019 Dec 17]. Available from: https://www.cdc.gov/nhsn/pdfs/pscmanual/11pscaurcurrent.pdf.

72. Identifying Healthcare-associated Infections (HAI) for ... [Internet]. [cited 2019 Dec 17]. Available from: https://www.cdc.gov/nhsn/pdfs/pscmanual/2psc_identifyinghais_nhsncurrent.pdf.

73. Monthly Reporting Plan – Centers for Disease Control and ... [Internet]. [cited 2019 Dec 17]. Available from: https://www.cdc.gov/nhsn/pdfs/pscmanual/3psc_monthlyreportingplancurrent.pdf.

74. Metz M, Shlaes DM. Eight more ways to deal with antibiotic resistance. Antimicrob Agents Chemother. 2014;58(8):4253–6.

75. Dall C. Lawmakers urge EPA to rethink use of antibiotics on citrus trees [Internet]. CIDRAP. 2019 [cited 2019 Dec 17]. Available from: http://www.cidrap.umn.edu/news-perspective/2019/08/lawmakers-urge-epa-rethink-use-antibiotics-citrus-trees.

76. MacDonald JV. Antimicrobial Resistance: Stewardship and Strategies for Conquering a Global Threat [Internet]. Infection Control Today. 2018 [cited 2019 Dec 17]. Available from: https://www.infectioncontroltoday.com/antibiotics-antimicrobials/antimicrobial-resistance-stewardship-and-strategies-conquering-global.

77. Measuring Outpatient Antibiotic Prescribing [Internet]. Centers for Disease Control and Prevention. Centers for Disease Control and Prevention; 2019 [cited 2019 Dec 17]. Available from: https://www.cdc.gov/antibiotic-use/community/programs-measurement/measuring-antibiotic-prescribing.html?CDC_AA_refVal=https://www.cdc.gov/getsmart/community/programs-measurement/measuring-antibiotic-prescribing.html.

78. New Societal Approaches for Empowering Antibiotic Stewardship [Internet]. [cited 2019 Dec 17]. Available from: https://jamanetwork.com/journals/jama/fullarticle/2498636.

79. Manning ML, Septimus EJ, Ashley ESD, Cosgrove SE, Fakih MG, Schweon SJ, et al. Antimicrobial stewardship and infection prevention—leveraging the synergy: a position paper update. Am J Infect Control. 2018;46(4):364–8.

80. Stefani S, Agodi A. Molecular epidemiology of antibiotic resistance. Int J Antimicrob Agents. 2000;13(3):143–53.

81. Mcarthur AG, Wright GD. Bioinformatics of antimicrobial resistance in the age of molecular epidemiology. Curr Opin Microbiol. 2015;27:45–50.

82. Abbas S, Stevens MP. The role of the hospital epidemiologist in antibiotic stewardship. Med Clin North Am. 2018;102(5):873–82.

83. Lipsitch M, Bergstrom CT, Levin BR. The epidemiology of antibiotic resistance in hospitals: paradoxes and prescriptions. Proc Natl Acad Sci. 2000;97(4):1938–43.

84. Robb F, Seaton A. What are the principles and goals of antimicrobial stewardship? Oxford Medicine Online. 2016.

85. Pollack LA, van Santen KL, Weiner LM, Dudeck MA, Edwards JR, Srinivasan A. Antibiotic stewardship programs in U.S. acute care hospitals: findings from the 2014 National Healthcare Safety Network Annual Hospital Survey. Clin Infect Dis. 2016;63(4):443–9.

86. Zachariah P, Newland JG, Gerber JS, Saiman L, Goldman J, Hersh AL, The SHARPS Collaborative Project Group. Costs of Antimicrobial stewardship programs at U.S. Children's hospitals. Infect Control Hosp Epidemiol. 2016;37(7):852–4.

87. Nathwani D, Varhese D, Stephens J, Ansari W, Martin S, Charbonneau C. Value of hospital antimicrobial stewardship programs [ASPs]: a systematic review. Antimicrob Resist Infect Control. 2019;8:35.

88. Zachariah P, Newland JG, Gerber JS, Saiman L, Goldman JL, Hersh AL. Costs of Antimicrobial stewardship programs at US Children's hospitals. Infect Control Hospital Epidemiol. 2016;37(7):852–4.

89. Luyt C-E, Bréchot N, Trouillet J-L, Chastre J. Antibiotic stewardship in the intensive care unit. Crit Care. 2014;18(5)

90. Burmeister A. Horizontal Gene Transfer. Evolution, Medicine, and Public Health. 2015: 193–194. [Figure], Mechanisms of Bacterial Horizontal Gene Transfer; p. 193.

91. Public Health Image Library. MRSA Bacteria Photo 1 [Image on the Internet]. [Updated 2019, Jan 28; cited 2020 Mar 1]. Available from: available from: https://www.cdc.gov/mrsa/community/photos/photo-mrsa-1.html.

92. Moran G. MRSA Bacteria Photo 9 [Image on the Internet]. [Updated 2019, Jan 28; cited 2020 Mar 1]. Available from: Available from: https://www.cdc.gov/mrsa/community/photos/photo-mrsa-9.html.

Part II

Emerging Resistance to Antivirals

Mechanisms of Nonretroviral Resistance

4

Saira George and Ritu Swali

Abbreviations

AIDS	Acquired immunodeficiency syndrome
CMV	*Cytomegalovirus*
CRISPR	Clustered regularly interspaced short palindromic repeats
dCTP	Deoxycytidine triphosphate
dGTP	Deoxyguanosine triphosphate
dsDNA	Double-stranded DNA
EBV	Epstein-Barr Virus
FDA	Food and Drug Administration
GvHD	Graft-versus-host disease
HA	Hemagglutinin
HCT	Hematopoietic cell transplantation
HHV	Human herpes virus
HIV	Human immunodeficiency virus
HSCT	Hematopoietic stem cell transplantation
HSV	Herpes simplex virus
IV	Intravenous
NA	Neuraminidase
N-MCT	N-methanocarbathymidine
TFT	Trifluorothymidine
TK	Tyrosine kinase
VZV	Varicella zoster virus

S. George (✉)
MD Anderson Cancer Center, Department of Dermatology, Houston, TX, USA
e-mail: SJGeorge1@mdanderson.org

R. Swali
Department of Dermatology, University of Nebraska Medical Center, Omaha, TX, USA

Introduction

Most cutaneous findings related to viral infections are self-limited and do not require treatment. Skin findings such as the classic childhood viral exanthems are often due to the host's immune response to infection, rather than to the virus itself, and resolve as the infection clears. Several common viral infections such as orolabial herpes, genital herpes, chickenpox, and shingles are, however, the result of direct viral infection of the skin and can be associated with significant cutaneous and extracutaneous complications, especially among the immunocompromised. The effectiveness of antiviral drugs and degree of viral drug resistance is thus critical to the management of these infections. Other viruses, such as the influenza viruses, do not typically cause skin findings but are clinically relevant to all providers because of their far-reaching epidemics and viral mechanisms of drug resistance. The focus of this chapter is to understand the mechanisms and management of antiviral resistance in the treatment of HSV, VZV, and influenza.

© Springer Nature Switzerland AG 2021
S. K. Tyring et al. (eds.), *Overcoming Antimicrobial Resistance of the Skin*, Updates in Clinical Dermatology, https://doi.org/10.1007/978-3-030-68321-4_4

Herpesviridae Family and Antiviral Strategies

Herpesviridae is a large family of DNA viruses that includes eight human viruses: herpes simplex virus types 1 and 2 (HSV-1 and HSV-2), varicella zoster virus (VZV), human cytomegalovirus (CMV), human herpesviruses 6 and 7 (HHV-6 A/B and HHV-7), Epstein-Barr virus (EBV), and human herpes virus 8 (HHV-8). These ubiquitous viruses cause a range of pathologies that involve the skin. Members of the *Herpesviridae* family share the ability to establish latency after initial infection and then reactivate under certain circumstances.

Herpes virus family members are similar in structure and consist of dsDNA enclosed within an icosahedral capsid, protein tegument, and lipid envelope. To multiply, *Herpesviridae* use the host cell nucleus for DNA replication and transcription of gene products resulting in characteristic inclusions in the nucleus of infected cells [1].

FDA-approved drugs are currently available for the treatment of HSV-1, HSV-2, VZV, and CMV [2, 3] (Table 4.1). The ultimate target of all currently available antiviral drugs is the viral DNA polymerase (Fig. 4.1).

Antiviral therapy for Herpesviridae

Nucleoside Analogues: Acyclovir and Valacyclovir, Penciclovir and Famciclovir, Ganciclovir and Valganciclovir

Acyclovir, a deoxyguanosine analogue, is the prototypic selective inhibitor of HSV type 1 and 2 and VZV replication. Acyclovir is activated by a virally encoded thymidine kinase (TK) which converts it to a monophosphate derivative. This activation occurs only in infected cells [4]. Cellular kinases subsequently dephosphorylate and triphosphorylate the acyclovir monophosphate, resulting in high concentrations of acyclovir triphosphate within infected cells. Acyclovir triphosphate competes with deoxyguanosine triphosphate (dGTP) as a substrate for viral DNA polymerase; when incorporated into a replicating DNA strand by viral DNA polymerase, it results in strand termination [4, 5]. Valacyclovir, the L-valine ester of acyclovir, is an orally administered prodrug that was designed to overcome acyclovir's poor oral bioavailability [6]. It is well absorbed from the gastrointestinal tract and rapidly metabolized by the liver to yield acyclovir and L-valine, resulting in peak plasma acyclovir concentrations that are three to fivefold higher with oral valacyclovir than with oral acyclovir [7].

Table 4.1 Licensed drugs currently available for the treatment of HSV-1, HSV-2, VZV, and CMV

Antiherpesviral agents currently licensed for use			
Drug	Antiviral activity	Mechanism of action	Approved clinical indications
Acyclovir (valacyclovir)	All herpesviruses	Nucleoside analogue – polymerase inhibitor	Treatment and suppression of HSV and VZV infections
Penciclovir (famciclovir)	HSV VZV	Nucleoside analogue – polymerase inhibitor	Treatment of zoster and treatment and suppression of genital HSV[en]. Penciclovir topical for HSV labialis
Ganciclovir (valganciclovir)	All herpesviruses	Nucleoside analogue – polymerase inhibitor	Treatment and suppression of CMV infections
Foscarnet	All herpesviruses	Pyrophosphate analogue – polymerase inhibitor	Treatment of acyclovir- or ganciclovir-resistant HSV, VZV, and CMV infections
Cidofovir	All herpesviruses	Nucleotide analogue – polymerase inhibitor	Treatment of acyclovir-, ganciclovir-, and foscarnet-resistant HSV and CMV infections
Letermovir	CMV	Terminase complex inhibitor; inhibits cleavage of CMV genome units and viral particle packaging	Suppression of CMV infection posttransplantation

Reprinted with permission from Poole and James [100]. Copyright 2018 by Elsevier. No changes were made to the original content

CMV cytomegalovirus, *HSV* herpes simplex virus, *VZV* varicella zoster virus

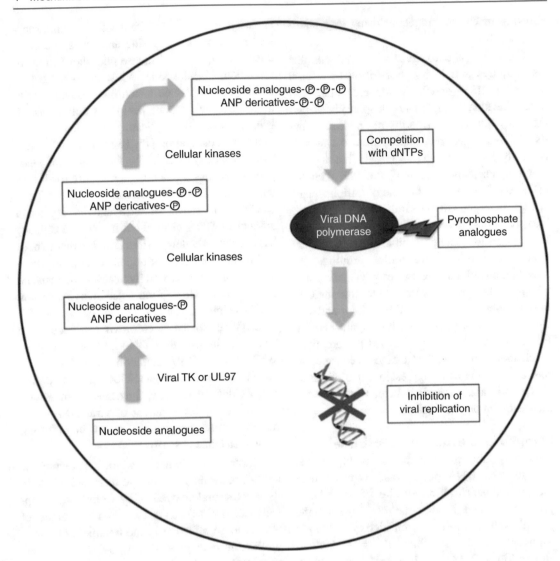

Fig. 4.1 Mechanism of action of different antiviral drugs. Nucleoside analogues such as acyclovir require an initial phosphorylation by viral thymidine kinase or UL97 and then two subsequent phosphorylations by cellular kinases to form a nucleoside analogue triphosphate. Cidofovir, an acyclic nucleoside phosphonate, requires only cellular kinases for phosphorylation to form an ANP derivate phosphate. Both the nucleoside analogue triphosphate and the ANP derivative phosphonate then compete with dNTPs to inhibit viral replication. Pyrophosphate analogues like foscarnet directly inhibit DNA polymerase. (Reprinted with permission from Pieret and Boivin [22]. Copyright 2014 by Wiley. No changes were made to the original content)

Penciclovir is a deoxyguanosine analogue that is very similar to acyclovir in structure, mechanism of action, and spectrum [8]. Like acyclovir, penciclovir must first be monophosphorylated in HSV- and VZV-infected cells by virally encoded TK and then further phosphorylated by cellular kinases. The triphosphate derivative then competitively inhibits viral DNA polymerase.

Just as acyclovir's poor bioavailability led to the development of valacyclovir, penciclovir's poor bioavailability is addressed by its prodrug famciclovir, which is well absorbed and has an oral bioavailability of 77%. Prompt first pass metabolism in the intestine and liver results in its conversion to penciclovir [7]. One key feature of penciclovir is its long intracellular half-life allowing much less frequent dosing than short-lived acyclovir.

Ganciclovir is deoxyguanosine analogue that also requires initial phosphorylation by a viral kinase. In HSV- and VZV-infected cells, viral thymidine kinase (TK) monophosphorylates ganciclovir [9]. CMV lacks a thymidine kinase, but its UL97-encoded phosphotransferase can successfully phosphorylate ganciclovir (but not acyclovir or penciclovir) making it the drug of choice in CMV infections [10]. Ganciclovir triphosphate is then incorporated by viral DNA polymerase into the elongating viral DNA where it slows DNA extension. The poor bioavailability of ganciclovir with oral administration prompted the development of its oral prodrug valganciclovir which exhibits an approximately tenfold increase in oral bioavailability [11]. Ganciclovir and acyclovir have similar in vitro activity against HSV1, HSV2, and VZV, but ganciclovir is preferentially much more active against CMV. Because of its risk of bone marrow suppression, use of ganciclovir and valganciclovir is primarily limited to the treatment of CMV infections.

Pyrophosphate Analogue: Foscarnet

Foscarnet is a pyrophosphate analogue that inhibits viral DNA polymerase. It binds near the pyrophosphate-binding site of viral DNA polymerase and blocks the cleavage of the pyrophosphate moiety from deoxynucleotide triphosphates (dNTPs) thus halting DNA chain elongation [12–14]. It has in vitro activity against HSV, VZV, CMV, EBV, and HHV 6. Clinically, it is used primarily for acyclovir-resistant HSV and VZV and as an alternative to ganciclovir for treatment of CMV. Because foscarnet does not require phosphorylation for activation, TK-deficient HSV and VZV isolates resistant to acyclovir and UL97-mutated CMV isolates resistant to ganciclovir should remain susceptible to foscarnet. Foscarnet must be administered intravenously due to its poor oral bioavailability.

Nucleotide Analogue: Cidofovir

Cidofovir, a nucleotide analogue of cytosine monophosphate, has potent antiviral activity against a broad range of DNA viruses. Unlike acyclovir and other nucleoside analogues, cidofovir does not require viral kinase phosphorylation for activation. Cellular kinases phosphorylate it to a diphosphate molecule which then competes with dCTP as a substrate for viral DNA polymerase. It is incorporated into replicating viral DNA and disrupts chain elongation [15, 16]. Cidofovir's selectivity is largely due to the fact that viral DNA polymerase has a much higher affinity for it than does cellular DNA polymerase.

Cidofovir shows in vitro activity against a number of DNA viruses but its clinical efficacy has been mostly demonstrated in the treatment of CMV. Since it does not require viral phosphorylation, it also retains activity in acyclovir-resistant TK-mutated HSV and ganciclovir-resistant UL97-mutated CMV [17].

CMV resistance to cidofovir can occur with mutations in the viral DNA polymerase gene. While CMV UL97 mutations that develop in patients on prolonged ganciclovir therapy do not affect cidofovir directly, they have been associated with the development of viral DNA polymerase mutations that do result in cidofovir cross-resistance [18, 19].

Cidofovir is only approved for intravenous use and is not available in an oral formulation due to its very low oral bioavailability. Compounded topical cidofovir has been documented in a number of reports to be effective in the treatment of warts, molluscum contagiosum, acyclovir-resistant herpes simplex, and trichodysplasia spinulosa. There are also a few reports of the successful use of intralesional cidofovir to treat warts.

Mechanisms of HSV/VZV Resistance

Mutations in Viral Thymidine Kinase

Acyclovir and its related nucleosides require activation by viral thymidine kinase. The vast majority (95%) of acyclovir-resistant strains of HSV and VZV harbor mutations in the genes encoding TK (UL23 in HSV and ORF 36 in VZV) that result in either the loss of all TK activity or significantly reduced TK activity [17, 20–22]. These acyclovir-resistant isolates are thus also resistant to valacyclovir, penciclovir, famciclovir, and ganciclovir - all of which also require viral TK phosphorylation for activation. A small percentage of TK mutants that demonstrate normal TK activity are able to phosphorylate thymidine but not acyclovir and/or penciclovir due to the expression of altered substrate specificity [23].

HSV TK is encoded by the UL23 gene. In acyclovir-resistant strains, mutation hotspots in UL23 have been identified in homopolymer stretches of guanines and cytosines [20, 24] where nucleotide deletions and substitutions result in frameshift reading and the introduction of termination codons leading to the expression of a truncated TK peptide.

Altered TK expression in acyclovir-resistant HSV may also arise from single amino acid substitutions that usually occur in one of six highly conserved domains that are important for TK enzyme activity such as the ATP-binding site, nucleoside-binding site, or cysteine at codon 336 which maintains the three-dimensional structure of the active site [20, 25–27].

Most acyclovir-resistant strains of HSV exhibit cross-resistance to penciclovir. Penciclovir resistance usually maps to mutations of UL-23 encoded TK as well. Some acyclovir- and foscarnet-resistant isolates that remain susceptible to penciclovir have been reported. These strains demonstrate altered thymidine kinase and DNA polymerase substrate specificity [25, 28].

Nucleoside analogue resistance has been reported to occur with VZV as well, but it appears to occur less commonly than with HSV. Since the first case was reported in a patient with AIDS in 1988, only approximately 35 cases of infections with acyclovir-resistant VZV strains have been described in the literature [29, 30]. As with HSV, acyclovir resistance in VZV is almost always associated with mutations in the gene that encodes viral TK (ORF 36) [31–35].

Mutations in Viral DNA Polymerase

All the antivirals discussed ultimately target viral DNA polymerase. Though uncommon, mutations in viral DNA polymerase that lead to acyclovir, foscarnet, and cidofovir resistance in HSV clinical isolates have been identified [17, 21, 22, 33]. Varying susceptibilities to acyclovir, foscarnet, and cidofovir may result depending on the type and location of the mutation in the DNA polymerase gene. For example, some foscarnet-resistant HSV isolates with single amino acid substitutions in certain conserved regions of the DNA polymerase remain fully or partly susceptible to acyclovir and cidofovir [36, 37], whereas isolates that harbor mutations in other conserved regions of the DNA polymerase gene may be resistant to both foscarnet and acyclovir [38]. Additionally, mutations in HSV DNA polymerase which confer cross-resistance to acyclovir and foscarnet as well as reduced susceptibility to cidofovir have been described [21, 22, 33].

Mutations in DNA polymerase (ORF 26) in VZV appear to be uncommon but have been identified in some acyclovir and/or foscarnet resistant VZV isolates [39–41].

Clinical Features of Drug-Resistant HSV and VZV

Resistant HSV can develop at a low rate spontaneously due to natural variability of the HSV population, as evidenced by the detection of acyclovir-resistant HSV in patients who had not been treated with acyclovir. But these resistant strains do not appear to lead to severe primary infection, reactivation, or increased person-to-person spread in immunocompetent hosts [42] . The low background prevalence of acyclovir-resistant HSV in healthy adults has been reported to be 0.1–0.7% in extensive surveys and has remained essentially constant since the introduction of acyclovir, despite its widespread use [42–46].

There is some evidence to suggest that antiviral-resistant HSV mutants may be less "fit" than the wild-type virus and that viral TK and DNA polymerase mutations may negatively affect viral pathogenicity [47]. It also appears to be very unusual for HSV strains in treated immunocompetent hosts to acquire acyclovir resistance. This is likely due to the fact that, in the normal immunocompetent host, both primary and recurrent herpes infections remain localized and are rapidly cleared by the immune response within a few days, leaving only a very limited time when selection of a resistant virus could occur during the treatment of active infection. The immune response to HSV occurs so efficiently among patients with normal immune function that persistent HSV infection, especially with an acyclovir-resistant strain, should raise suspicion for an unappreciated immune deficit.

Immunosuppressed patients with HSV tend to have recurrences that are more frequent and longer in duration than immunocompetent patients. They often present with chronic extensive mucocutaneous ulcerations that may be atypical in appearance. Neurologic complications of HSV such as aseptic meningitis, sacral radiculopathy, and transverse myelitis are rare but have been occasionally reported in severely immunocompromised patients such as transplant recipients and patients with advanced HIV [48].

The prevalence of acyclovir-resistant HSV isolates is much higher among immunocompromised patients. Reported ranges are as high as 3.5–7% in human immunodeficiency virus (HIV)-positive patients [45, 49], 2.5–10% in solid organ transplant recipients [44, 45], and 4.1–36% in hematopoietic stem cell transplant recipients [45, 50–52]. High levels of viral replication permitted by the lack of adequate antiviral immunity would allow for higher rates of spontaneous mutations that confer drug resistance. Selection pressure from prolonged antiviral therapy often required to manage immunosuppressed patients would also favor the emergence of drug-resistant strains.

Drug-resistant strains of HSV can present clinically like other HSV infections in immunocompromised patients, most often as chronic ulcerative mucocutaneous lesions without visceral or neurologic complications in immunocompromised patients. Clinically, most cases of ACV-resistant HSV involve HSV-2 [53]. Incidences of verrucous HSV in HIV (Fig. 4.2) have been noted in the literature [53, 54]. Disseminated infection can

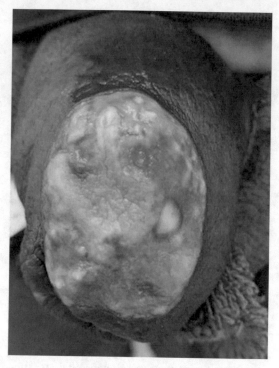

Fig. 4.2 Verrucous acyclovir-resistant HSV in AIDS

occur rarely; cases of acyclovir-resistant HSV causing fulminant hepatitis, pneumonia, meningoencephalitis, and lethal systemic disease have been reported [49, 55–58].

Acyclovir-resistant VZV isolates have not been reported in immunocompetent individuals [59, 60], but they have been reported in the severely immunosuppressed such as those with HIV, anticancer therapy, and transplant immunosuppression who developed treatment-resistant VZV reactivation [60]. The prevalence of acyclovir-resistant VZV cases in these different populations is unknown because most published reports are case reports. In a 2013 study, 27% of 87 patients, including HSCT patients, with persistent treatment-refractory infections were found to have strains with mutations that could confer resistance to acyclovir [60]. There are also scattered reports of VZV strains resistant to foscarnet in immunocompromised patients [32, 41].

Immunocompromised patients with VZV often develop prolonged infection with atypical cutaneous involvement (such as extra-dermatomal lesions or verrucous lesions) and have significant morbidity and mortality associated with visceral involvement and fulminant disseminated infection [61–65]. Infections with acyclovir-resistant VZV strains appear to present in a similar fashion [30]. Chronic verrucous skin lesions in acyclovir-resistant VZV infections have been reported [62, 66]. Disseminated infection with acyclovir-resistant, Oka vaccine strains has also been reported in two immunocompromised children being treated for zoster [62, 67].

Management of Drug-Resistant HSV Infections

Antiviral drug resistance should be suspected in patients with documented HSV who have minimal to no improvement, or an increase in lesion size, within 7 to 10 days of appropriately dosed antiviral therapy [17, 22, 68]. It is important to note that appropriately dosed antiviral therapy for immunocompromised patients is generally higher and of longer duration than for immunocompetent patients and should be ensured before consideration of viral resistance.

Patients with clinical treatment failure to nucleoside analogue therapy should undergo HSV antiviral susceptibility testing for acyclovir, foscarnet, and cidofovir [69, 70]. The most commonly used method for the evaluation of HSV antiviral susceptibility is the plaque reduction assay [17, 32]. In this assay, cells are incubated with the sample HSV strain in the presence of serial drug concentrations, and viral plaques are counted. The concentration of drug that reduces the viral plaque number by 50% is known as the IC_{50}. An IC50 $\geq$ 2 mcg/mL for acyclovir indicates that phenotypic resistance is present. The assay is commercially available and is preferred over other tests, as correlations between in vitro drug susceptibility levels and clinical response have been established. The downside of the test is that it takes approximately 15–17 days.

Genotypic testing for HSV acyclovir resistance can also be done in research labs. Since 95% of acyclovir-resistant strains have mutations in viral thymidine kinase and the remaining 5% have mutations in viral DNA polymerase, sequencing of these genes can be carried out. As more thymidine kinase polymorphisms and mutants associated with acyclovir drug resistance are identified, a commercially available molecular assay for HSV resistance testing may one day be available.

Since approximately 95% of acyclovir-resistant HSV isolates harbor a mutation in the TK enzyme, patients who have failed to respond to acyclovir or valacyclovir are unlikely to respond to famciclovir due to cross-resistance. No effective oral therapies are currently available for nucleoside-resistant HSV infections.

Intravenous Acyclovir

For patients with suspected acyclovir-resistant HSV who are being treated with oral antivirals, a trial of IV acyclovir for 7 days has been recommended as an initial step, while awaiting drug resistance testing. High-dose IV acyclovir (10 mg/kg IV every 8 hours, renally adjusted) achieves better serum concentrations than oral acyclovir and has a favorable safety profile [17].

Intravenous Foscarnet

If the lesions fail to improve or if they progress after 5–10 days of IV acyclovir, empiric treatment with foscarnet (40 mg/kg intravenously every 8 hours) should be started and continued for a minimum of 3 weeks or until healing of all mucocutaneous ulcers occurs. Patients on foscarnet require aggressive hydration to prevent nephrotoxicity and careful clinical and laboratory monitoring for toxicities including electrolyte abnormalities, renal dysfunction, and bone marrow suppression [22, 68].

The treatment of acyclovir-resistant HSV infections with foscarnet has been reported in AIDS patients [71–74] and BMT recipients [75].

Intravenous Cidofovir

In the rare cases of HSV resistance to foscarnet, intravenous cidofovir (5 mg/kg/week) has been used with some success, though the data on the efficacy of IV cidofovir in immunocompromised patients with acyclovir-resistant HSV treatment is limited [50, 76–79] and it is not approved for this indication. Intravenous cidofovir has been used more extensively in HIV-infected patients with cytomegalovirus retinitis. Treatment in these cases can be associated with severe toxicity, including neutropenia, nausea and vomiting, and nephrotoxicity. Cidofovir is co-administered with oral probenecid and aggressive intravenous hydration to minimize these toxicities.

Continuous High-Dose Acyclovir

Continuous high-dose acyclovir (30 to 45 mg/kg/day) has been successfully used for acyclovir-resistant or multidrug-resistant HSV infections in other immunocompromised patient populations (i.e., hematopoietic stem cell transplant recipients) [80, 81].

Thalidomide

Thalidomide has also been used as salvage therapy in severe cases of acyclovir-resistant herpes [82, 83].

Topical Therapy for Acyclovir-Resistant HSV

Topical therapies have been used with some success as either alternative or adjunct treatment of acyclovir-resistant HSV lesions that are refractory to foscarnet or in patients that cannot tolerate foscarnet.

1% foscarnet cream [84] and 2.4% foscarnet solution [85] were reported as effective therapies for mucocutaneous HSV lesions unresponsive to acyclovir.

A 1% topical solution of trifluorothymidine (TFT), a fluorinated nucleoside drug used in herpetic eye infections, has also been reported as potentially helpful in the treatment of acyclovir-resistant mucocutaneous HSV [86].

Application of 5% imiquimod, a commercially available immunomodulatory drug FDA approved for HPV, was effective in the treatment of recurrent and severe mucocutaneous lesions due to acyclovir and foscarnet-resistant HSV2 isolates in HIV-infected individuals [87].

There are a number of reports of topical cidofovir in the successful treatment of drug-resistant mucocutaneous HSV infections [78, 88–92]. In a double-blind clinical trial, 30 AIDS patients with acyclovir-resistant HSV infection (median of two lesions at baseline) were randomly assigned to topical cidofovir gel or placebo gel for 5 days [78]. Ten of 20 patients in the cidofovir treatment group achieved complete lesion resolution or 50 percent improvement in clinical symptoms compared with none of the patients receiving placebo. Topical cidofovir is not commercially available so requires compounding by the pharmacy and is costly but may be a valuable alternative or adjunct treatment for patients with acyclovir-resistant strains without the adverse effects associated with IV administrations of foscarnet and cidofovir. Although not approved by the Food and Drug Administration, cidofovir compounded in a 1% topical formulation is recommended by the Centers for Disease Control and Prevention for the therapy of acyclovir-resistant herpes simplex infections.

Long-Term Management of Acyclovir-Resistant HSV

Immunocompromised patients with acyclovir-resistant HSV should be initiated on standard prophylactic therapy once their acute infection resolves. While exposure to antivirals during the treatment of active HSV infection is thought to play a role in the emergence of acyclovir-resistant strains in immunocompromised patients, the same does not appear to be true for prophylactic antiviral therapy; unlike with other infections, daily suppressive antiviral therapy in these patients has been shown to reduce, rather than increase, the risk of developing acyclovir resistance [93]. It has also been shown that recurrent infection among immunosuppressed patients with a history of acyclovir-resistant HSV infection is most often with an acyclovir-sensitive strain [17].

Management of Drug-Resistant VZV Infections

The possibility of antiviral resistance should be considered in patients with documented VZV who have continued signs of active VZV infection despite 10–14 days of high-dose oral acyclovir [22].

With VZV, phenotypic testing for antiviral resistance using the plaque reduction assay can be done but is difficult because of the low rate of virus isolation from vesicle samples and its slow growth in cell culture [94].

Genotypic testing of the ORF36 gene that codes for the TK protein can also be performed on a biopsy of mucocutaneous lesions or from other infected tissue samples [95]. Unfortunately, only a limited number of mutations associated with drug resistance have been confirmed thus far, and genotypic analyses have failed to identify a cause for resistance in up to 50% of patients not responding to therapy [40].

Clinical experience with the treatment of acyclovir-resistant VZV is limited; in most cases, IV foscarnet is used. There are scattered reports documenting foscarnet's use in HIV-infected patients with ACV-resistant VZV [74, 96] and in some oncology patients [62, 66, 67]. The recommended intravenous dosage is 60 mg/kg every 8 h (adjusted for renal function) for at least 10 days or until complete lesion healing is observed.

Available data on cidofovir in the treatment of drug-resistant VZV diseases is also minimal [97, 98]. Brincidofovir, an experimental oral prodrug of cidofovir, was reported in the successful treatment of disseminated acyclovir and resistant VZV in an immunocompromised hematopoietic stem-cell transplant patient with chronic graft-versus-host disease who was intolerant to foscarnet [99].

Investigational Drugs and Future Directions for Treatment of Acyclovir-Resistant HSV and VZV

Treatment options for acyclovir-resistant HSV and VZV are limited, and new drugs with alternative mechanisms of action and acceptable safety profiles are needed, especially as the number of patients living with immunosuppression grows. Experimental drugs currently in clinical trials and drugs in early development may offer promise as potential future therapies [100].

Brincidofovir (CMX001) is a lipid acyclic nucleotide phosphonate that is the prodrug of cidofovir. It has demonstrated wide activity against a number of dsDNA viruses in in vitro studies and animal models. Brincidofovir's lipid side chain is cleaved in target cells to release cidofovir intracellularly. With brincidofovir, > 100-fold higher intracellular levels of the active substrate cidofovir phosphate and > 1000-fold antiviral activity against HSV, CMV, and VZV are achieved compared with cidofovir [97, 101, 102]. It also appears to be more potent than ganciclovir and foscarnet. Furthermore, brincidofivir is orally administered and does not appear to be nephrotoxic [101, 102]. Preclinical analyses of brincidofovir were promising, but its approval has been slowed by findings from a Phase III trial evaluating the prophylactic use of brincidofovir for the prevention of clinically significant CMV infection in seropositive alloHCT transplant recipients. Patients were randomized to receive brincidofovir or placebo until week 14 post-HCT and assessed through week 24 post-HCT. Although fewer brincidofovir recipients developed CMV viremia while receiving treatment through week 14 compared with placebo recipients, prophylaxis did not decrease clinically significant CMV infection through post-hematopoietic cell transplantation (HCT) week

24 compared with placebo. Serious adverse events were also ultimately more frequent among brincidofovir recipients, primarily due to a higher number of patients diagnosed with acute graft-versus-host disease (needing corticosteroid therapy) and higher incidence of diarrhea. Since the gastrointestinal toxicity in the brincidofovir treatment group could not be differentiated from acute gastrointestinal GvHD in the blinded study, this may have resulted in an excess diagnosis of acute GvHD and corticosteroid exposure in the treatment group, both of which are risk factors for "late" CMV infections after discontinuation of antivirals in HCT patients. Because of this study, all proposed future studies comparing oral brincidofovir for the prevention of CMV disease are currently suspended, although investigations into its utility in the treatment of other viral infections are ongoing. It may still hold therapeutic promise in the treatment of HSV and VZV infections; brincidofovir, obtained for compassionate use, has been already used successfully in the treatment of an immunocompromised hematopoietic stem cell transplant patient with chronic graft-versus-host disease and disseminated acyclovir- and foscarnet-resistant zoster who was unable to tolerate foscarnet [99].

N-Methanocarbathymidine (N-MCT) is a thymidine analogue that is phosphorylated by thymidine kinases and then host kinases to become an active triphosphate nucleoside analogue that competitively inhibits viral DNA polymerase. It has in vitro activity against HSV-1, HSV-2, EBV, and HHV-8, has shown superior efficacy to acyclovir in animal models, and is currently in a Phase I clinical trial [103].

Valomaciclovir, a carboxylic nucleoside analogue, has demonstrated potent activity against replicating forms of VZV and EBV. A Phase II trial with the drug for the treatment of zoster indicated that valomaciclovir is well tolerated in adults and is noninferior to valacyclovir [104]. Mutations in the TK gene that confer resistance to ACV also confer resistance to valomaciclovir as well.

FV-100, a bicyclic nucleoside analogue has highly specific antiviral activity against VZV. In Phase II trials for herpes zoster, it appears to be well tolerated and effective [105]. Although its precise mechanism of action is unclear, VZV thymidine kinase appears to play a key role as TK-negative mutants in vitro are resistant to the drug [105].

Since currently available antivirals for HSV and VZV target viral DNA polymerase, drugs with alternative targets such as the viral helicase-primase complex would be especially valuable therapeutic additions [106] (Fig. 4.3). The viral helicase unwinds the DNA double helix to create a replication fork with two strands of ssDNA; the primase synthesizes short RNA primers for initiation of replication. The helicase-primase inhibitor pritelivir has been shown to have potent in vitro activity against HSV-1 and HSV-2 isolates, including strains resistant to nucleoside analogues, and has also been shown to have efficacy in animal studies. A Phase II, randomized, double-blind, crossover clinical trial to compare the efficacy of pritelivir with valacyclovir for suppression of genital HSV-2 infection showed decreased viral shedding with pritelivir compared with valacyclovir among adults with frequently recurring genital HSV-2 [107]. An ongoing open-label trial is underway, comparing its efficacy and safety to foscarnet's in the treatment of acyclovir-resistant mucocutaneous HSV infections in immunocompromised patients. Amenamevir (ASP2151) is another helicase-primase inhibitor that is in development. It has potent activity against both HSV and VZV and was approved for the treatment of zoster in Japan in September 2017 after a trial there showed efficacy in the treatment of the disease. ASP2131 is not currently in clinical trials in the United States because of adverse events in a Phase I trial comparison study against valacyclovir in healthy patients but may be a future option for acyclovir-resistant HSV and VZV that warrants further investigation [100, 108].

A humanized monoclonal antibody has also been shown to be effective for immunotherapy of severe HSV infections, including those caused by multidrug-resistant isolates, in immunocompromised mice and warrants further investigation [109].

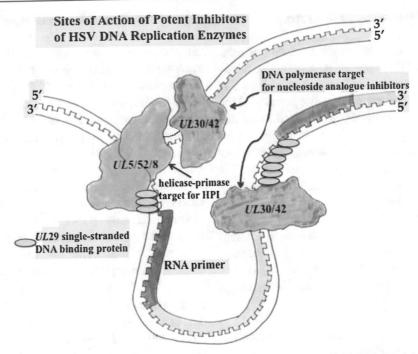

Fig. 4.3 Schematic diagram showing the site of action of nucleoside analogue triphos-phates (e.g. acyclovir or penciclovir) and helicase-primase inhibitors (e.g. BAY 57-1293, BILS 22 BS, or amenamevir). (Reprinted with permission from Field and Biswas [128]. Copyright 2011 by Elsevier. No changes were made to the original content)

Future methods of antiviral treatment may involve alterations of the genome of target viruses. Investigators have used CRISPR/Cas9-mediated genome editing to target genomic sites necessary for viral fitness in the genomes of three different herpesviruses (HSV1, CMV, and EBV) with the demonstration of complete inhibition. Because viral replication is not needed for this technique to work, it could potentially be used to address both active and latent herpesvirus infections, eradicating the virus from all infected cells. These applications could potentially revolutionize the management of viral infections in immunocompromised patients such as transplant recipients [110, 111].

Influenza: Antiviral Strategies and Resistance

Influenza viruses, though not classically known to cause cutaneous manifestations, are the epitome of re-emerging viral infections. RNA viruses such as influenza mutate at much faster rates than DNA viruses due to the inherently lower stability of RNA and the lack of proofreading during RNA replication. Influenza has a remarkable ability to rapidly evolve genetically; changes in its genome result in the periodic alterations of its key antigenic viral envelope glycoproteins, hemagglutinin (HA) and neuraminidase (NA) [112] . This allows the virus to evade the lasting immunity acquired through prior infection or vaccination and to circumvent the action of antiviral drugs.

Influenza type A and B viruses are responsible for the vast majority of influenza infections in humans. Seasonal outbreaks of influenza A and B are due to the steady accumulation of minor point mutations that result in gradual changes in the viruses' antigenic proteins known as "antigenic drift." Less frequently, abrupt and major changes in the circulating virus genome known as "antigenic shift" arise from reassortment of genetic material between viral subtypes or animal and human strains in influenza A and cause pandemics of influenza A [113–115].

Antiviral Therapy for Influenza

FDA-approved drugs for the treatment of influenza fall into three classes: neuraminidase inhibitors, adamantanes, and selective inhibitors of influenza cap-dependent endonuclease [116]. Since influenza is usually self-limited, symptomatic treatment is the mainstay of treatment, but infection can result in significant morbidity and mortality especially in high-risk individuals. The initiation of antiviral drugs, generally oseltamivir, as early as possible is currently recommended for any patient with confirmed or suspected influenza who is hospitalized, has severe, complicated, or progressive illness, or is at higher risk for complications (such as children <2 years of age, adults >65 years of age, and immunosuppressed individuals) [117].

Neuraminidase Inhibitors: Oseltamivir, Zanamivir, and Peramivir

Influenza's hemagglutinin (HA) and neuraminidase (NA) surface glycoproteins are key antigens in the host immune response to the virus, but they also play important roles in viral propagation. HA helps initiate viral infection by attaching the virus to the sialic acid residues of surface glycoproteins on human respiratory epithelial cells. NA releases progeny virions for more rounds of infection by cleaving their attachment to host cell glycoproteins at sialic acid residues. Oseltamivir, peramivir, and zanamivir are sialic acid analogues that competitively inhibit neuraminidase on the surface of both influenza A and B [118]. Oseltamivir is orally administered, peramivir is IV, and zanamivir is an inhaled powder.

Mutations that cause amino acid substitutions in the active site of the neuraminidase cause most cases of viral resistance to neuraminidase inhibitors. Although oseltamivir resistance has been observed rarely among influenza B viruses, most oseltamivir resistance has occurred in influenza A viruses. In influenza A, the H275Y neuraminidase mutation was responsible for the oseltamivir resistance that emerged during the seasonal outbreak of H1N1 in 2007 and became widespread among H1N1 viruses during the 2008 to 2009 influenza season, with resistant rates of >90% reported in several countries [118–121]. Due to their structural similarity, H275Y mutation confers cross-resistance to both oseltamivir and peramivir but not to zanamivir, making zanamivir the treatment of choice for H1N1 influenza A infections with H275Y mutations.

Since 2009's H1N1 influenza A pandemic, the oseltamivir-susceptible strain responsible for the pandemic has since replaced the oseltamivir-resistant seasonal H1N1 strain worldwide to become the predominant strain of H1N1 influenza; rates of oseltamivir resistance have subsequently remained low (i.e., below 1%) [121].

Adamantanes

Amantadine and rimantadine target the M2 protein of influenza A. The M2 protein forms an ion channel in the viral membrane that is essential for efficient viral replication. Single point mutations leading to changes in the transmembrane portion of the M2 protein result in resistance to amantadine and rimantadine and confer cross-resistance between agents [122].

Adamantane resistance can occur both spontaneously or as rapidly as 2–3 days following initiation of adamantane treatment and generally occurs more readily than to neuraminidase inhibitors [122]. Rates of resistance vary with the virus's strain but have generally increased over time. Widespread dissemination of adamantane-resistant influenza was first reported in 2003–2004 among H3N2 viruses, primarily in Asia. By the 2009–2010 influenza season in the United States, all H3N2 influenza A and 2009 pandemic H1N1 isolates tested were resistant to the adamantanes [123]. Because nearly all currently circulating influenza strains exhibit resistance to these agents, adamantanes are no longer recommended for treatment of seasonal influenza.

Baloxavir Marboxil

Baloxavir, a single-dose tablet by mouth with activity against both influenza A and B, is a new first-in-class influenza drug that was approved in the United States in October 2018. It inhibits the cap endonuclease of influenza's polymerase acidic protein, a subunit of viral RNA polymerase and an attractive target for antivirals because of both its critical role in viral replication and its high degree of conservation [124]. Unfortunately, the development of baloxavir-resistant virus due to polymerase acidic protein variants with I38T/M/F substitutions was seen following a single dose of the drug in up to 10 percent of adolescents and adults in trials and 24 percent of children, raising concerns about the long-term feasibility of this currently promising drug as monotherapy, especially with its widespread use [125–127].

Summary

Current antiviral drugs provide for the safe, effective treatment of a number of cutaneous viral infections such as those caused by HSV and VZV, but the emergence of drug-resistant strains challenges our ability to manage these common infections. This is particularly true for immunocompromised patients with HSV and VZV who are not only the most vulnerable to complications from infection but are also most likely to develop drug-resistant disease. The ability of viruses to develop resistance mechanism to overcome antiviral drug therapy is exemplified by the influenza viruses. The recognition and appropriate management of drug-resistant infections and the identification of new antiviral targets will be critical in our success against these common viral infections.

References

1. Roizman BKD, Whitley R. Herpes simplex viruses. Philadelphia: LWW; 2013.
2. Andrei G, De Clercq E, Snoeck R. Viral DNA polymerase inhibitors. In: Cameron CE, Matthias G, Raney K, editors. Viral genome replication. New York: Springer; 2009. p. 481–526.
3. De Clercq E, Li G. Approved antiviral drugs over the past 50 years. Clin Microbiol Rev. 2016;29(3):695–747.
4. Elion GB. Mechanism of action and selectivity of acyclovir. Am J Med. 1982;73(1a):7–13.
5. Reardon JE, Spector T. Acyclovir: mechanism of antiviral action and potentiation by ribonucleotide reductase inhibitors. Adv Pharmacol. 1991;22:1–27.
6. Vigil KJ, Chemaly RF. Valacyclovir: approved and off-label uses for the treatment of herpes virus infections in immunocompetent and immunocompromised adults. Expert Opin Pharmacother. 2010;11(11):1901–13.
7. Perry CM, Wagstaff AJ. Famciclovir. A review of its pharmacological properties and therapeutic efficacy in herpesvirus infections. Drugs. 1995;50(2):396–415.
8. Hodge RAV. Famciclovir and Penciclovir. The mode of action of Famciclovir including its conversion to Penciclovir. Antivir Chem Chemother. 1993;4(2):67–84.
9. Crumpacker CS. Ganciclovir. N Engl J Med. 1996;335(10):721–9.
10. Faulds D, Heel RC. Ganciclovir. A review of its antiviral activity, pharmacokinetic properties and therapeutic efficacy in cytomegalovirus infections. Drugs. 1990;39(4):597–638.
11. Pescovitz MD, Rabkin J, Merion RM, Paya CV, Pirsch J, Freeman RB, et al. Valganciclovir results in improved oral absorption of ganciclovir in liver transplant recipients. Antimicrob Agents Chemother. 2000;44(10):2811–5.
12. Crumpacker CS. Mechanism of action of foscarnet against viral polymerases. Am J Med. 1992;92(2a):3s–7s.
13. Oberg B. Antiviral effects of phosphonoformate (PFA, foscarnet sodium). Pharmacol Ther. 1989;40(2):213–85.
14. Wagstaff AJ, Bryson HM. Foscarnet. A reappraisal of its antiviral activity, pharmacokinetic properties and therapeutic use in immunocompromised patients with viral infections. Drugs. 1994;48(2):199–226.
15. Cihlar T, Chen MS. Identification of enzymes catalyzing two-step phosphorylation of cidofovir and the effect of cytomegalovirus infection on their activities in host cells. Mol Pharmacol. 1996;50(6):1502–10.
16. Xiong X, Smith JL, Chen MS. Effect of incorporation of cidofovir into DNA by human cytomegalovirus DNA polymerase on DNA elongation. Antimicrob Agents Chemother. 1997;41(3):594–9.
17. Piret J, Boivin G. Resistance of herpes simplex viruses to nucleoside analogues: mechanisms, prevalence, and management. Antimicrob Agents Chemother. 2011;55(2):459–72.
18. Chou S, Marousek G, Guentzel S, Follansbee SE, Poscher ME, Lalezari JP, et al. Evolution of mutations conferring multidrug resistance during prophylaxis and therapy for cytomegalovirus disease. J Infect Dis. 1997;176(3):786–9.

19. Lurain NS, Chou S. Antiviral drug resistance of human cytomegalovirus. Clin Microbiol Rev. 2010;23(4):689–712.

20. Gaudreau A, Hill E, Balfour HH Jr, Erice A, Boivin G. Phenotypic and genotypic characterization of acyclovir-resistant herpes simplex viruses from immunocompromised patients. J Infect Dis. 1998;178(2):297–303.

21. Morfin F, Thouvenot D. Herpes simplex virus resistance to antiviral drugs. J Clin Virol. 2003;26(1):29–37.

22. Piret J, Boivin G. Antiviral drug resistance in herpesviruses other than cytomegalovirus. Rev Med Virol. 2014;24(3):186–218.

23. Pottage JC Jr, Kessler HA. Herpes simplex virus resistance to acyclovir: clinical relevance. Infect Agents Dis. 1995;4(3):115–24.

24. Sasadeusz JJ, Tufaro F, Safrin S, Schubert K, Hubinette MM, Cheung PK, et al. Homopolymer mutational hot spots mediate herpes simplex virus resistance to acyclovir. J Virol. 1997;71(5):3872–8.

25. Burrel S, Deback C, Agut H, Boutolleau D. Genotypic characterization of UL23 thymidine kinase and UL30 DNA polymerase of clinical isolates of herpes simplex virus: natural polymorphism and mutations associated with resistance to antivirals. Antimicrob Agents Chemother. 2010;54(11):4833–42.

26. Chibo D, Druce J, Sasadeusz J, Birch C. Molecular analysis of clinical isolates of acyclovir resistant herpes simplex virus. Antivir Res. 2004;61(2):83–91.

27. Sauerbrei A, Bohn K, Heim A, Hofmann J, Weissbrich B, Schnitzler P, et al. Novel resistance-associated mutations of thymidine kinase and DNA polymerase genes of herpes simplex virus type 1 and type 2. Antivir Ther. 2011;16(8):1297–308.

28. Sarisky RT, Bacon TH, Boon RJ, Duffy KE, Esser KM, Leary J, et al. Profiling penciclovir susceptibility and prevalence of resistance of herpes simplex virus isolates across eleven clinical trials. Arch Virol. 2003;148(9):1757–69.

29. Pahwa S, Biron K, Lim W, Swenson P, Kaplan MH, Sadick N, et al. Continuous varicella-zoster infection associated with acyclovir resistance in a child with AIDS. JAMA. 1988;260(19):2879–82.

30. Saint-Leger E, Caumes E, Breton G, Douard D, Saiag P, Huraux JM, et al. Clinical and virologic characterization of acyclovir-resistant varicella-zoster viruses isolated from 11 patients with acquired immunodeficiency syndrome. Clin Infect Dis. 2001;33(12):2061–7.

31. Boivin G, Edelman CK, Pedneault L, Talarico CL, Biron KK, Balfour HH Jr. Phenotypic and genotypic characterization of acyclovir-resistant varicella-zoster viruses isolated from persons with AIDS. J Infect Dis. 1994;170(1):68–75.

32. Fillet AM, Dumont B, Caumes E, Visse B, Agut H, Bricaire F, et al. Acyclovir-resistant varicella-zoster virus: phenotypic and genetic characterization. J Med Virol. 1998;55(3):250–4.

33. Gilbert C, Bestman-Smith J, Boivin G. Resistance of herpesviruses to antiviral drugs: clinical impacts and molecular mechanisms. Drug Resist Updat. 2002;5(2):88–114.

34. Morfin F, Thouvenot D, De Turenne-Tessier M, Lina B, Aymard M, Ooka T. Phenotypic and genetic characterization of thymidine kinase from clinical strains of varicella-zoster virus resistant to acyclovir. Antimicrob Agents Chemother. 1999;43(10):2412–6.

35. Talarico CL, Phelps WC, Biron KK. Analysis of the thymidine kinase genes from acyclovir-resistant mutants of varicella-zoster virus isolated from patients with AIDS. J Virol. 1993;67(2):1024–33.

36. Bestman-Smith J, Boivin G. Herpes simplex virus isolates with reduced adefovir susceptibility selected in vivo by foscarnet therapy. J Med Virol. 2002;67(1):88–91.

37. Schmit I, Boivin G. Characterization of the DNA polymerase and thymidine kinase genes of herpes simplex virus isolates from AIDS patients in whom acyclovir and foscarnet therapy sequentially failed. J Infect Dis. 1999;180(2):487–90.

38. Bestman-Smith J, Boivin G. Drug resistance patterns of recombinant herpes simplex virus DNA polymerase mutants generated with a set of overlapping cosmids and plasmids. J Virol. 2003;77(14):7820–9.

39. Kamiyama T, Kurokawa M, Shiraki K. Characterization of the DNA polymerase gene of varicella-zoster viruses resistant to acyclovir. J Gen Virol. 2001;82(Pt 11):2761–5.

40. Sauerbrei A, Taut J, Zell R, Wutzler P. Resistance testing of clinical varicella-zoster virus strains. Antivir Res. 2011;90(3):242–7.

41. Visse B, Huraux JM, Fillet AM. Point mutations in the varicella-zoster virus DNA polymerase gene confers resistance to foscarnet and slow growth phenotype. J Med Virol. 1999;59(1):84–90.

42. Collins P, Ellis MN. Sensitivity monitoring of clinical isolates of herpes simplex virus to acyclovir. J Med Virol. 1993;Suppl 1:58–66.

43. Bacon TH, Levin MJ, Leary JJ, Sarisky RT, Sutton D. Herpes simplex virus resistance to acyclovir and penciclovir after two decades of antiviral therapy. Clin Microbiol Rev. 2003;16(1):114–28.

44. Christophers J, Clayton J, Craske J, Ward R, Collins P, Trowbridge M, et al. Survey of resistance of herpes simplex virus to acyclovir in Northwest England. Antimicrob Agents Chemother. 1998;42(4):868–72.

45. Danve-Szatanek C, Aymard M, Thouvenot D, Morfin F, Agius G, Bertin I, et al. Surveillance network for herpes simplex virus resistance to antiviral drugs: 3-year follow-up. J Clin Microbiol. 2004;42(1):242–9.

46. Stranska R, Schuurman R, Nienhuis E, Goedegebuure IW, Polman M, Weel JF, et al. Survey of acyclovir-resistant herpes simplex virus in the Netherlands: prevalence and characterization. J Clin Virol. 2005;32(1):7–18.

47. Chen SH, Pearson A, Coen DM, Chen SH. Failure of thymidine kinase-negative herpes simplex virus to reactivate from latency following efficient establishment. J Virol. 2004;78(1):520–3.

48. Marks GL, Nolan PE, Erlich KS, Ellis MN. Mucocutaneous dissemination of acyclovir-resistant herpes simplex virus in a patient with AIDS. Rev Infect Dis. 1989;11(3):474–6.

49. Levin MJ, Bacon TH, Leary JJ. Resistance of herpes simplex virus infections to nucleoside analogues in HIV-infected patients. Clin Infect Dis. 2004;39(Suppl 5):S248–57.

50. Chen Y, Scieux C, Garrait V, Socie G, Rocha V, Molina JM, et al. Resistant herpes simplex virus type 1 infection: an emerging concern after allogeneic stem cell transplantation. Clin Infect Dis. 2000;31(4):927–35.

51. Langston AA, Redei I, Caliendo AM, Somani J, Hutcherson D, Lonial S, et al. Development of drug-resistant herpes simplex virus infection after haploidentical hematopoietic progenitor cell transplantation. Blood. 2002;99(3):1085–8.

52. Wade JC, McLaren C, Meyers JD. Frequency and significance of acyclovir-resistant herpes simplex virus isolated from marrow transplant patients receiving multiple courses of treatment with acyclovir. J Infect Dis. 1983;148(6):1077–82.

53. Erlich KS, Mills J, Chatis P, Mertz GJ, Busch DF, Follansbee SE, et al. Acyclovir-resistant herpes simplex virus infections in patients with the acquired immunodeficiency syndrome. N Engl J Med. 1989;320(5):293–6.

54. Carrasco DA, Trizna Z, Colome-Grimmer M, Tyring SK. Verrucous herpes of the scrotum in a human immunodeficiency virus-positive man: case report and review of the literature. J Eur Acad Dermatol Venereol. 2002;16(5):511–5.

55. Czartoski T, Liu C, Koelle DM, Schmechel S, Kalus A, Wald A. Fulminant, acyclovir-resistant, herpes simplex virus type 2 hepatitis in an immunocompetent woman. J Clin Microbiol. 2006;44(4):1584–6.

56. Gateley A, Gander RM, Johnson PC, Kit S, Otsuka H, Kohl S. Herpes simplex virus type 2 meningo-encephalitis resistant to acyclovir in a patient with AIDS. J Infect Dis. 1990;161(4):711–5.

57. Ljungman P, Ellis MN, Hackman RC, Shepp DH, Meyers JD. Acyclovir-resistant herpes simplex virus causing pneumonia after marrow transplantation. J Infect Dis. 1990;162(1):244–8.

58. Shahani L. Fulminant hepatic failure secondary to acyclovir-resistant herpes simplex virus. BMJ Case Rep. 2016;2016:bcr2016216322. Published 2016 Oct 17. https://doi.org/10.1136/bcr-2016-216322.

59. Cole NL, Balfour HH Jr. Varicella-Zoster virus does not become more resistant to acyclovir during therapy. J Infect Dis. 1986;153(3):605–8.

60. van der Beek MT, Vermont CL, Bredius RG, Marijt EW, van der Blij-de Brouwer CS, Kroes AC, et al. Persistence and antiviral resistance of varicella zoster virus in hematological patients. Clin Infect Dis. 2013;56(3):335–43.

61. Ahmed AM, Brantley JS, Madkan V, Mendoza N, Tyring SK. Managing herpes zoster in immunocompromised patients. Herpes. 2007;14(2):32–6.

62. Bryan CJ, Prichard MN, Daily S, Jefferson G, Hartline C, Cassady KA, et al. Acyclovir-resistant chronic verrucous vaccine strain varicella in a patient with neuroblastoma. Pediatr Infect Dis J. 2008;27(10):946–8.

63. Glesby MJ, Moore RD, Chaisson RE. Clinical spectrum of herpes zoster in adults infected with human immunodeficiency virus. Clin Infect Dis. 1995;21(2):370–5.

64. Gnann JW Jr, Barton NH, Whitley RJ. Acyclovir: mechanism of action, pharmacokinetics, safety and clinical applications. Pharmacotherapy. 1983;3(5):275–83.

65. Rusthoven JJ, Ahlgren P, Elhakim T, Pinfold P, Reid J, Stewart L, et al. Varicella-zoster infection in adult cancer patients. A population study. Arch Intern Med. 1988;148(7):1561–6.

66. Crassard N, Souillet AL, Morfin F, Thouvenot D, Claudy A, Bertrand Y. Acyclovir-resistant varicella infection with atypical lesions in a non-HIV leukemic infant. Acta Paediatr. 2000;89(12):1497–9.

67. Levin MJ, Dahl KM, Weinberg A, Giller R, Patel A, Krause PR. Development of resistance to acyclovir during chronic infection with the Oka vaccine strain of varicella-zoster virus, in an immunosuppressed child. J Infect Dis. 2003;188(7):954–9.

68. Balfour HH Jr, Benson C, Braun J, Cassens B, Erice A, Friedman-Kien A, et al. Management of acyclovir-resistant herpes simplex and varicella-zoster virus infections. J Acquir Immune Defic Syndr. 1994;7(3):254–60.

69. Gupta R, Wald A. Genital herpes: antiviral therapy for symptom relief and prevention of transmission. Expert Opin Pharmacother. 2006;7(6):665–75.

70. Piret J, Drouot E, Boivin G. Antiviral drug resistance in herpesviruses. In: Handbook of antimicrobial resistance. New York: Springer; 2014. p. 87–122.

71. Alvarez-McLeod A, Havlik J, Drew KE. Foscarnet treatment of genital infection due to acyclovir-resistant herpes simplex virus type 2 in a pregnant patient with AIDS: case report. Clin Infect Dis. 1999;29(4):937–8.

72. Chatis PA, Miller CH, Schrager LE, Crumpacker CS. Successful treatment with foscarnet of an acyclovir-resistant mucocutaneous infection with herpes simplex virus in a patient with acquired immunodeficiency syndrome. N Engl J Med. 1989;320(5):297–300.

73. Erlich KS, Jacobson MA, Koehler JE, Follansbee SE, Drennan DP, Gooze L, et al. Foscarnet therapy for severe acyclovir-resistant herpes simplex virus type-2 infections in patients with the acquired immunodeficiency syndrome (AIDS). An uncontrolled trial. Ann Intern Med. 1989;110(9):710–3.

74. Safrin S, Berger TG, Gilson I, Wolfe PR, Wofsy CB, Mills J, et al. Foscarnet therapy in five patients with

AIDS and acyclovir-resistant varicella-zoster virus infection. Ann Intern Med. 1991;115(1):19–21.

75. Verdonck LF, Cornelissen JJ, Smit J, Lepoutre J, de Gast GC, Dekker AW, et al. Successful foscarnet therapy for acyclovir-resistant mucocutaneous infection with herpes simplex virus in a recipient of allogeneic BMT. Bone Marrow Transplant. 1993;11(2):177–9.

76. Andrei G, Fiten P, Goubau P, van Landuyt H, Gordts B, Selleslag D, et al. Dual infection with polyomavirus BK and acyclovir-resistant herpes simplex virus successfully treated with cidofovir in a bone marrow transplant recipient. Transpl Infect Dis. 2007;9(2):126–31.

77. Kopp T, Geusau A, Rieger A, Stingl G. Successful treatment of an aciclovir-resistant herpes simplex type 2 infection with cidofovir in an AIDS patient. Br J Dermatol. 2002;147(1):134–8.

78. Lalezari J, Schacker T, Feinberg J, Gathe J, Lee S, Cheung T, et al. A randomized, double-blind, placebo-controlled trial of cidofovir gel for the treatment of acyclovir-unresponsive mucocutaneous herpes simplex virus infection in patients with AIDS. J Infect Dis. 1997;176(4):892–8.

79. LoPresti AE, Levine JF, Munk GB, Tai CY, Mendel DB. Successful treatment of an acyclovir- and foscarnet-resistant herpes simplex virus type 1 lesion with intravenous cidofovir. Clin Infect Dis. 1998;26(2):512–3.

80. Engel JP, Englund JA, Fletcher CV, Hill EL. Treatment of resistant herpes simplex virus with continuous-infusion acyclovir. JAMA. 1990;263(12):1662–4.

81. Kim JH, Schaenman JM, Ho DY, Brown JM. Treatment of acyclovir-resistant herpes simplex virus with continuous infusion of high-dose acyclovir in hematopoietic cell transplant patients. Biol Blood Marrow Transplant. 2011;17(2):259–64.

82. Holmes A, McMenamin M, Mulcahy F, Bergin C. Thalidomide therapy for the treatment of hypertrophic herpes simplex virus-related genitalis in HIV-infected individuals. Clin Infect Dis. 2007;44(11):e96–9.

83. Verberkmoes A, Boer K, Wertheim PM, Bronkhorst CM, Lange JM. Thalidomide for genital ulcer in HIV-positive woman. Lancet. 1996;347(9006):974.

84. Javaly K, Wohlfeiler M, Kalayjian R, Klein T, Bryson Y, Grafford K, et al. Treatment of mucocutaneous herpes simplex virus infections unresponsive to acyclovir with topical foscarnet cream in AIDS patients: a phase I/II study. J Acquir Immune Defic Syndr. 1999;21(4):301–6.

85. Pechere M, Wunderli W, Trellu-Toutous L, Harms M, Saura JH, Krischer J. Treatment of acyclovir-resistant herpetic ulceration with topical foscarnet and antiviral sensitivity analysis. Dermatology. 1998;197(3):278–80.

86. Kessler HA, Hurwitz S, Farthing C, Benson CA, Feinberg J, Kuritzkes DR, et al. Pilot study of topical trifluridine for the treatment of acyclovir-resistant mucocutaneous herpes simplex disease in patients with AIDS (ACTG 172). AIDS Clinical Trials Group. J Acquir Immune Defic Syndr Hum Retrovirol. 1996;12(2):147–52.

87. Lascaux AS, Caumes E, Deback C, Melica G, Challine D, Agut H, et al. Successful treatment of aciclovir and foscarnet resistant Herpes simplex virus lesions with topical imiquimod in patients infected with human immunodeficiency virus type 1. J Med Virol. 2012;84(2):194–7.

88. Epstein JB, Gharapetian S, Rejali AR, Zabner R, Lill M, Tzachanis D. Complex management of resistant oral herpes simplex virus infection following hematopoietic stem cell transplantation: potential role of topical cidofovir. Support Care Cancer. 2016;24(8):3603–6.

89. Evans KG, Morrissey KA, Goldstein SC, Vittorio CC, Rook AH, Kim EJ. Chronic acyclovir-resistant HSV-2 ulcer in an immunosuppressed patient treated with topical cidofovir. Arch Dermatol. 2011;147(12):1462–3.

90. Lateef F, Don PC, Kaufmann M, White SM, Weinberg JM. Treatment of acyclovir-resistant, foscarnet-unresponsive HSV infection with topical cidofovir in a child with AIDS. Arch Dermatol. 1998;134(9):1169–70.

91. Muluneh B, Dean A, Armistead P, Khan T. Successful clearance of cutaneous acyclovir-resistant, foscarnet-refractory herpes virus lesions with topical cidofovir in an allogeneic hematopoietic stem cell transplant patient. J Oncol Pharm Pract. 2013;19(2):181–5.

92. Sacks SL, Shafran SD, Diaz-Mitoma F, Trottier S, Sibbald RG, Hughes A, et al. A multicenter phase I/II dose escalation study of single-dose cidofovir gel for treatment of recurrent genital herpes. Antimicrob Agents Chemother. 1998;42(11):2996–9.

93. Erard V, Wald A, Corey L, Leisenring WM, Boeckh M. Use of long-term suppressive acyclovir after hematopoietic stem-cell transplantation: impact on herpes simplex virus (HSV) disease and drug-resistant HSV disease. J Infect Dis. 2007;196(2):266–70.

94. Sauerbrei A, Eichhorn U, Schacke M, Wutzler P. Laboratory diagnosis of herpes zoster. J Clin Virol. 1999;14(1):31–6.

95. Brink AA, van Gelder M, Wolffs PF, Bruggeman CA, van Loo IH. Compartmentalization of acyclovir-resistant varicella zoster virus: implications for sampling in molecular diagnostics. Clin Infect Dis. 2011;52(8):982–7.

96. Breton G, Fillet AM, Katlama C, Bricaire F, Caumes E. Acyclovir-resistant herpes zoster in human immunodeficiency virus-infected patients: results of foscarnet therapy. Clin Infect Dis. 1998;27(6):1525–7.

97. Aldern KA, Ciesla SL, Winegarden KL, Hostetler KY. Increased antiviral activity of 1-O-hexadecyloxypropyl-[2-(14)C]cidofovir in MRC-5 human lung fibroblasts is explained by unique cellular uptake and metabolism. Mol Pharmacol. 2003;63(3):678–81.

98. Schliefer K, Gumbel HO, Rockstroh JK, Spengler U. Management of progressive outer retinal necrosis with cidofovir in a human immunodeficiency virus-infected patient. Clin Infect Dis. 1999;29(3):684–5.

99. Mullane KM, Nuss C, Ridgeway J, Prichard MN, Hartline CB, Theusch J, et al. Brincidofovir treatment of acyclovir-resistant disseminated varicella zoster virus infection in an immunocompromised host. Transpl Infect Dis. 2016;18(5):785–90.

100. Poole CL, James SH. Antiviral therapies for herpesviruses: current agents and new directions. Clin Ther. 2018;40(8):1282–98.

101. Ciesla SL, Trahan J, Wan WB, Beadle JR, Aldern KA, Painter GR, et al. Esterification of cidofovir with alkoxyalkanols increases oral bioavailability and diminishes drug accumulation in kidney. Antivir Res. 2003;59(3):163–71.

102. Painter W, Robertson A, Trost LC, Godkin S, Lampert B, Painter G. First pharmacokinetic and safety study in humans of the novel lipid antiviral conjugate CMX001, a broad-spectrum oral drug active against double-stranded DNA viruses. Antimicrob Agents Chemother. 2012;56(5):2726–34.

103. Bernstein DI, Bravo FJ, Clark JR, Earwood JD, Rahman A, Glazer R, et al. N-Methanocarbathymidine is more effective than acyclovir for treating neonatal herpes simplex virus infection in Guinea pigs. Antivir Res. 2011;92(2):386–8.

104. Tyring SK, Plunkett S, Scribner AR, Broker RE, Herrod JN, Handke LT, et al. Valomaciclovir versus valacyclovir for the treatment of acute herpes zoster in immunocompetent adults: a randomized, double-blind, active-controlled trial. J Med Virol. 2012;84(8):1224–32.

105. Andrei G, Topalis D, Fiten P, McGuigan C, Balzarini J, Opdenakker G, et al. In vitro-selected drug-resistant varicella-zoster virus mutants in the thymidine kinase and DNA polymerase genes yield novel phenotype-genotype associations and highlight differences between antiherpesvirus drugs. J Virol. 2012;86(5):2641–52.

106. Whitley RJ, Prichard M. A novel potential therapy for HSV. N Engl J Med. 2014;370(3):273–4.

107. Wald A, Timmler B, Magaret A, Warren T, Tyring S, Johnston C, et al. Effect of Pritelivir compared with Valacyclovir on genital HSV-2 shedding in patients with frequent recurrences: a randomized clinical trial. JAMA. 2016;316(23):2495–503.

108. Chono K, Katsumata K, Kontani T, Kobayashi M, Sudo K, Yokota T, et al. ASP2151, a novel helicase-primase inhibitor, possesses antiviral activity against varicella-zoster virus and herpes simplex virus types 1 and 2. J Antimicrob Chemother. 2010;65(8):1733–41.

109. Krawczyk A, Arndt MA, Grosse-Hovest L, Weichert W, Giebel B, Dittmer U, et al. Overcoming drug-resistant herpes simplex virus (HSV) infection by a humanized antibody. Proc Natl Acad Sci U S A. 2013;110(17):6760–5.

110. Lee C. CRISPR/Cas9-Based Antiviral Strategy: Current Status and the Potential Challenge. Molecules. 2019;24(7):1349. Published 2019 Apr 5. https://doi.org/10.3390/molecules24071349.

111. van Diemen FR, Lebbink RJ. CRISPR/Cas9, a powerful tool to target human herpesviruses. Cell Microbiol. 2017;19(2). https://doi.org/10.1111/cmi.12694. Epub 2016 Dec 23. PMID: 27860066.

112. CDC. How the Flu virus can change: "Drift" and "Shift". Centers for Disease Control and Prevention. https://www.cdc.gov/flu/about/viruses/change.htm. Published October 15, 2019. Accessed January 20, 2020.

113. CDC. 2009 H1N1 Pandemic (H1N1pdm09 virus). Centers for Disease Control and Prevention. https://www.cdc.gov/flu/pandemic-resources/2009-h1n1-pandemic.html. Published June 11, 2019. Accessed January 20, 2020.

114. CDC. 2019–2020 U.S. Flu Season: Preliminary Burden Estimates. Centers for Disease Control and Prevention. https://www.cdc.gov/flu/about/burden/preliminary-in-season-estimates.htm. Published January 10, 2020. Accessed January 19, 2020.

115. CDC. Flu Vaccination Coverage, United States, 2018–19 Influenza Season. Centers for Disease Control and Prevention. https://www.cdc.gov/flu/fluvaxview/coverage-1819estimates.htm. Published September 26, 2019. Accessed January 20, 2020.

116. Hayden FG, de Jong MD. Emerging influenza antiviral resistance threats. J Infect Dis 2011;203(1):6–10.

117. CDC. Influenza Antiviral Medications. Centers for Disease Control and Prevention. https://www.cdc.gov/flu/professionals/antivirals/. Accessed Jan 20, 2020. [updated July 10, 2019].

118. Gubareva LV. Molecular mechanisms of influenza virus resistance to neuraminidase inhibitors. Virus Res. 2004;103(1–2):199–203.

119. Hurt AC, Chotpitayasunondh T, Cox NJ, Daniels R, Fry AM, Gubareva LV, et al. Antiviral resistance during the 2009 influenza a H1N1 pandemic: public health, laboratory, and clinical perspectives. Lancet Infect Dis. 2012;12(3):240–8.

120. Tamura D, Sugaya N, Ozawa M, Takano R, Ichikawa M, Yamazaki M, et al. Frequency of drug-resistant viruses and virus shedding in pediatric influenza patients treated with neuraminidase inhibitors. Clin Infect Dis. 2011;52(4):432–7.

121. Organization WH. WHO/ECDC frequently asked questions for Oseltamivir Resistance https://www.who.int/influenza/patient_care/antivirals/oseltamivir_faqs/en/. Published February 15, 2008. Accessed Jan 20, 2020.

122. Belshe RB, Smith MH, Hall CB, Betts R, Hay AJ. Genetic basis of resistance to rimantadine emerging during treatment of influenza virus infection. J Virol. 1988;62(5):1508–12.

123. Bright RA, Medina MJ, Xu X, Perez-Oronoz G, Wallis TR, Davis XM, et al. Incidence of adamantane resistance among influenza A (H3N2) viruses isolated worldwide from 1994 to 2005: a cause for concern. Lancet. 2005;366(9492):1175–81.

124. Hayden FG, Sugaya N, Hirotsu N, Lee N, de Jong MD, Hurt AC, et al. Baloxavir Marboxil for uncomplicated Influenza in adults and adolescents. N Engl J Med. 2018;379(10):913–23.

125. Boivin G. Detection and management of antiviral resistance for influenza viruses. Influenza Other Respir Viruses. 2013;7(Suppl 3):18–23.

126. Hirotsu N, Sakaguchi H, Sato C, Ishibashi T, Baba K, Omoto S, et al. Baloxavir marboxil in Japanese pediatric patients with influenza: safety and clinical and virologic outcomes. Clin Infect Dis. 2019;71(4):971–81.

127. Uehara T, Hayden FG, Kawaguchi K, Omoto S, Hurt AC, De Jong MD, et al. Treatment-emergent Influenza variant viruses with reduced Baloxavir susceptibility: impact on clinical and Virologic outcomes in uncomplicated Influenza. J Infect Dis. 2020;221(3):346–55.

128. Biswas S, Field HJ. Herpes simplex virus helicase-primase inhibitors: recent findings from the study of drug resistance mutations. Antivir Chem Chemother. 2008;19(1):1–6. https://doi.org/10.1177/095632020801900101. PMID: 18610552.

Mechanisms of Retroviral Resistance

5

Alfredo Siller Jr., Joseph Jebain, Chetan Jinadatha, and Stephen K. Tyring

Abbreviations

ARV	Antiretroviral
CCR5	CC chemokine receptor 5
CXCR4	CXC chemokine receptor 4
DHHS	Department of Health and Human Services
DRT	Drug resistance testing
FDA	Food and Drug Administration
HIV	Human immunodeficiency virus
HR1	First heptad repeat
HTLV	Human T-cell lymphotropic virus
INSTI	Integrase strand transfer inhibitor
NNRTI	Non-nucleoside reverse transcriptase inhibitors
NRTI	Nucleoside/nucleotide reverse transcriptase inhibitors
PI	Protease inhibitor
PrEP	Pre-exposure prophylaxis
RT	Reverse transcriptase
TAM	Thymidine analog mutation
TDF	Tenofovir disoproxil fumarate

A. Siller Jr. (✉)
Baylor Scott and White Medical Center, Department of Internal Medicine, Temple, TX, USA

J. Jebain
Center for Clinical Studies, Houston, TX, USA

C. Jinadatha
Infectious Diseases Section, Central Texas Veterans Health Care System, Department of Internal Medicine, Temple, TX, USA
e-mail: Chetan.Jinadatha@va.gov

S. K. Tyring
Department of Dermatology, University of Texas Health Science Center, Houston, TX, USA

Center for Clinical Studies, Houston, TX, USA
e-mail: styring@ccstexas.com

Introduction

Retroviruses are enveloped, icosahedral RNA-based viruses that arise from the family *Retroviridae* [1]. These viruses revolutionized the central dogma of molecular biology with their unique ability to store and replicate genetic information. Retroviruses contain reverse transcriptase, an enzyme that functions as an RNA-dependent DNA polymerase for the transcription of RNA into DNA. Once converted to DNA, the viral genetic material is integrated into the host cell genome by an integrase enzyme and then transcribed and translated by the host's cellular machinery to produce new copies of the virus. Only two genera of retroviruses cause infection in humans – the *Deltaretrovirus*, which gives rise to the human T-cell lymphotropic virus (HTLV) subtypes (I-IV), and the *Lentivirus*, which gives rise to human immunodeficiency virus (HIV) [2]. The advent of antiretroviral (ARV) drug therapy, particularly for HIV, has resulted in a significant reduction in the morbidity and mor-

© Springer Nature Switzerland AG 2021
S. K. Tyring et al. (eds.), *Overcoming Antimicrobial Resistance of the Skin*, Updates in Clinical Dermatology, https://doi.org/10.1007/978-3-030-68321-4_5

tality associated with infection; however, the efficacy of these agents continues to be threatened by the rise in ARV resistance [3].

Antiretrovirals

ARVs are divided into seven distinct drug classes, each with a unique mechanism of action. These include (1) nucleoside/nucleotide analog reverse transcriptase inhibitors (NRTIs), (2) nonnucleoside reverse transcriptase inhibitors (NNRTIs), (3) integrase inhibitors, (4) protease inhibitors (PIs), (5) fusion inhibitors, (6) CCR5 co-receptor antagonists, and (7) CD4-directed post-attachment inhibitors [4]. The virologic efficacy of these ARV agents is dependent on several factors, including the inherent resistance to treatment of a virus, also known as the genetic barrier to resistance, or the number of mutations required before the development of resistance to an ARV occurs, and the regimen of ARVs used. Inadequate ARV efficacy leads to virologic failure, defined as the inability to suppress persistently a viral load below 200 copies/ml. The application of genotypic resistance testing has provided valuable insight in determining the causes of virologic failure and continues to be a useful tool in guiding therapy for both ARV-naïve and ARV-resistant individuals. Even so, the most common reasons for virologic failure of ARV agents are nonadherence, pharmacokinetic factors, and co-infection with a resistant minority variant [5] (Fig. 5.1).

General Overview of Retroviral Mechanisms of Resistance

Human retroviruses have been shown to express low fidelity during DNA replication. This results in a high mutation rate and a rapid turnover rate for HIV that results in innumerable viral variants referred to as quasi-species. The ability to rapidly produce new quasi-species allows retroviruses to elude the immune system and generate mutations that decrease their susceptibility to ARV agents [5, 6]. Still, naturally occurring drug-resistant viruses are rare, with the majority of drug-resistant strains acquired through drug selection pressures or person-to-person transmission. ARV resistance mutations can be classified into two categories – primary mutations, which directly reduce the susceptibility of a virus to an ARV agent, or accessory mutations, which enhances viral fitness and further decreases susceptibility when combined with a major mutation. Although cross-resistance is common among strains with high-level resistance to ARV agents within the same class, cross-resistance between classes is extremely uncommon [5].

NRTIs (Nucleoside and Nucleotide Reverse Transcriptase Inhibitors)

NRTIs are nucleoside or nucleotide analogs that are incorporated into a growing DNA chain by a reverse transcriptase (RT) protein and lead to chain termination during the DNA replication cycle. To accomplish this task, NRTIs must enter the cell and become phosphorylated in order to act as a synthetic substrate for the active site of RT during DNA polymerization. The most commonly utilized NRTIs include zidovudine, lamivudine, abacavir, emtricitabine, and tenofovir (disoproxil fumarate or alafenamide). Other agents, such as zalcitabine, didanosine, and stavudine, are rarely used. Although this class of antiretrovirals helps prevent the infection of susceptible cells, they demonstrate no effect on cells already infected with a virus [3].

Retroviral resistance to NRTIs occurs through two different mechanisms. The first mechanism of resistance requires a discriminatory mutation of a residue on or proximal to the catalytic site of RT, resulting in the inability of an NRTI to be incorporated into the growing DNA chain. Most commonly, discriminatory mutations involve the following numeric positions and amino acid letter codes: M184V/I, K65R, K70E/G, L74V, Y115F, and the Q151M complex [5]. A mutation on M184V/I results in high-level resistance to analogs lamivudine (cytidine) and emtricitabine (cytosine) with low-level cross-resistance to abacavir (guanosine) and, to lesser extent, didano-

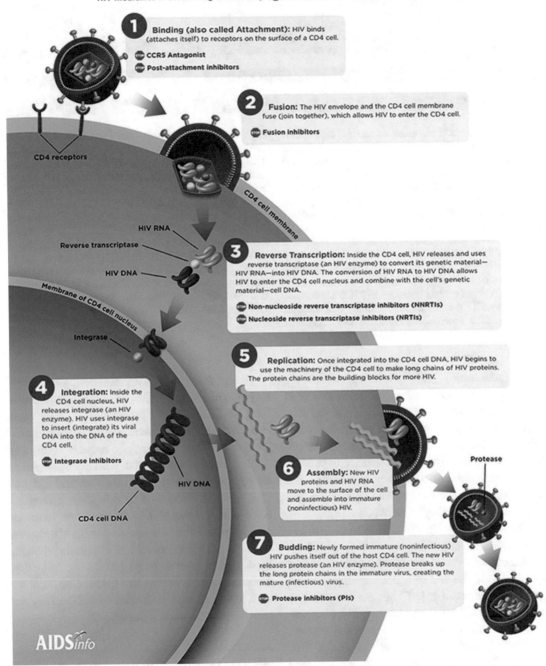

Fig. 5.1 The HIV lifecycle and sites of action for major antiretroviral drug classes. (Reference: US Department of Health and Human Services. https://hivinfo.nih.gov/ understanding-hiv/fact-sheets/hiv-life-cycle.   Accessed October 12, 2019)

	Major Nucleoside RT Inhibitor (NRTI) Resistance Mutations											
	Non-TAMs					TAMS						MDR	
	184	65	70	74	115	41	67	70	210	215	219	69	151
Cons	M	K	K	L	Y	M	D	K	L	T	K	T	Q
3TC	**VI**	R										INS	M
FTC	**VI**	R										INS	M
ABC	VI	R	E	**VI**	**F**	L			W	FY		INS	M
TFV	***	**R**	E		F	L	R		W	FY		INS	M
ZDV	***	***	*	*		L	N	R	W	FY	QE	INS	M

Fig. 5.2 Major NRTI resistance mutations. *Bold underline*: High-level reduced susceptibility or virological response. *Bold*: Reduced susceptibility or virological response. Plain text: Reduced susceptibility in combination with other NRTI resistance mutations. Asterisk: Increased susceptibility. *TAMs*: Thymidine analog mutations. Selected by AZT and d4T; facilitate primer unblocking. Non-TAMs prevent NRTI incorporation. *MDR*: Multidrug resistance mutations. T69 insertions occur with TAMs. Q151M occurs with non-TAMs and the accessory mutations A62V, V75I, F77L, and F116Y. *M184VI*: Although they cause high-level in vitro resistance to 3TC/FTC, they are not contraindications to 3TC/FTC because they increase TFV and AZT susceptibility and decrease viral replication fitness. *TFV, TDF, and TAF*: Tenofovir (TFV) disoproxil fumarate (TDF) and TFV alafenamide (TAF) are TFV triphosphate prodrugs. Although TDF and TAF have similar resistance profiles, TAF attains higher intracellular levels. *Additional mutations*: K65N similar but weaker than K65R. K70GQNT similar to K70E. T69D and V75MT reduce susceptibility to d4T and ddI, which are not shown because they are no longer recommended for HIV treatment. T215SCDEIVALN (T215 revertants) emerge from T215YF in the absence of NRTIs. E40F, E44DA, D67GE, V118I, and K219NR are accessory TAMs. D67, T69, K70 deletions have not been well studied. They usually occur in combination with K65R and/or Q151M. (*References*: Reproduced with permission from hivdb.stanford.edu/s/nrtinotes)

sine (adenosine) [3]. However, M184V/I mutations have also been shown to reduce viral fitness and to increase susceptibility to the analogs tenofovir (adenosine) and zidovudine (thymidine). The next most significant mutation, K65R, confers intermediate resistance to lamivudine, emtricitabine, tenofovir, abacavir, and didanosine, low-level resistance to stavudine, and increased vulnerability to zidovudine [5].

The second mechanism of resistance involves a thymidine analog mutation (TAM) of RT for enhanced removal of an NRTI from its site of attachment at the end of a DNA chain via phosphorolytic excision [3]. TAMs are classified as either type I or type II and have overlapping patterns that mainly affect the thymidine analogs zidovudine and stavudine at M41L, D67N, K70R, L210W, T215F/Y, and K219Q/E. Type I TAMs (M41L, L210W, and T215Y) demonstrate higher levels of clinical resistance and cross-resistance to the drugs abacavir, didanosine, and tenofovir compared to type II TAMs (D67N, K70R, T215F, and K219Q/E) [5].

Except for the M184V/I mutation, discriminatory mutations and TAMs arise through two distinct and divergent pathways. It has been demonstrated that retroviruses expressing multiple TAMs are more likely to acquire additional TAMs, even when treated with non-thymidine analogs such as tenofovir, abacavir, and didanosine, and to induce discriminatory mutations K65R or L74V [7–9]. Furthermore, viruses expressing as much as four to five TAMs plus an M184V mutation are highly associated with high-level resistance to all NRTIs. Additionally, while mutations T69ins and Q151M also confer high levels of cross-resistance to NRTIs, they are relatively uncommon [5] (Fig. 5.2).

NNRTIs (Nonnucleoside Reverse Transcriptase Inhibitors)

Despite functioning similarly to NRTIs, NNRTIs are not nucleoside/nucleotide analogs but inhibit viral DNA replication without incorporation into the DNA chain [3]. Instead, these agents allosterically bind to a position adjacent to the catalytic site of reverse transcriptase (RT), leading to a conformational change that alters the enzyme's ability to polymerize DNA [4]. The five commonly utilized drugs in this class include nevirapine, efavirenz, etravirine, rilpivirine, and doravirine. Delavirdine is rarely used due to its low efficacy and inconvenient dosing. Due to their mechanism of action, NNRTIs have a low genetic barrier to resistance, so rapidly develop mutations that prohibits function [5]. Virtually all NNRTI resistance mutations occur adjacent to the NNRTI-binding pocket on RT; therefore, resistance to one agent confers high levels of cross-resistance to other agents of the same class. Consequently, NNRTIs are never used as monotherapy for the treatment of retroviral infections [3].

Most NNRTIs develop high-level resistance with as few as one to two mutations, with nevirapine, rilpivirine, efavirenz, etravirine, and doravirine, respectively, listed in order of increasing genetic barrier of resistance [10–13]. The most common mutations involve L100I, K101EP, K103NS, V106AM, Y181CIV, Y188L, G190ASE, and M230L [4, 5]. All these mutations induce high-level resistance to nevirapine, except for L100I, and intermediate to high-level resistance to efavirenz, with the exception of V106A and Y181CIV [10]. Decreased susceptibility to etravirine and rilpivirine has also been demonstrated in all the above mutations, excluding K103NS and V106AM [5].

In patients who develop virologic failure while receiving rilpivirine, close to 50% acquire an E138K mutation, which is known to confer a degree of cross-resistance to all other NNRTIs. Interestingly, when rilpivirine is used in combination with tenofovir and emtricitabine, virologic failure is more likely to occur as a result of "cross-talk" between NRTI and NNRTI combination mutations (E138K and M184I) rather than from the more common M184V mutation. Y188L is another mutation that causes high-level resistance to rilpivirine, nevirapine, and efavirenz; however, it causes only low-level resistance to

etravirine. K103N and Y181C are the most common mutations selected by efavirenz and nevirapine, respectively. In those on nevirapine, the development of Y181C mutations often confers partial cross-resistance to etravirine; in contrast, those on efavirenz with K103N mutations are less likely to develop cross-resistance to etravirine. Due to the variability of etravirine's responsiveness in the presence of the above NNRTI mutations, a genotypic susceptibility score has been developed to better predict etravirine susceptibility [5]. In 2018, a novel NNRTI agent, doravirine, was approved for use in combination therapy for treatment-naïve patients. Overall, the prevalence of resistance mutations was found to be higher in all other NNRTIs compared to doravirine, making it an excellent first-line therapeutic in treatment-naïve patients [13] (Fig. 5.3).

PIs (Protease Inhibitors)

Gag and Gag/pol are viral protein precursors required for the maturation of HIV particles into fully functional and infectious viruses. PIs prevent the proteolytic cleavage of viral proteins (Gag and Gag/pol) by competitively inhibiting the active site of the HIV-1 protease enzyme [5]. To date, ten PIs (saquinavir, indinavir, lopinavir, amprenavir, fosamprenavir, atazanavir, tipranavir, darunavir, nelfinavir, and ritonavir) have been approved by the Food and Drug Administration (FDA) for the treatment of HIV [4]. In recent years, the agents indinavir, nelfinavir, amprenavir, fosamprenavir, and saquinavir have fallen out favor and are rarely used due to their poor efficacy, toxicity, or discontinuation in the USA. Atazanavir, darunavir, lopinavir, and ritonavir are most commonly utilized with tipranavir reserved for salvage therapy. Ritonavir and cobicistat, a pharmacokinetic enhancer, have the unique ability to inhibit cytochrome P450 (CYP3A) and are often combined at smaller doses with other protease and integrase inhibitors (e.g., atazanavir/r, darunavir/r, elvitegravir/cobicistat, etc.) in order to boost their plasma

Major Non-Nucleoside RT Inhibitor (NNRTI) Resistance Mutations

	100	101	103	106	181	188	190	272	230
Cons	L	K	K	V	Y	Y	G	F	M
DOR	I	EP		AM	CIV	**L**	SE	**LC**	**L**
EFV	*I*	E**P**	**NS**	AM	CIV	**L**	A**S**E	LC	**L**
ETR	*I*	E**P**		.	**CIV**	L	ASE	C	L
RPV	*I*	E**P**			**CIV**	L	ASE	**LC**	**L**
NVP	I	EP	**NS**	**AM**	**CIV**	L	**ASE**	**LC**	**L**

Fig. 5.3 Major NNRTI resistance mutations. *Bold underline*: High-level reduced susceptibility or virological response. *Bold*: Reduced susceptibility or virological response. Plain text: Reduced susceptibility in combination with other NNRTI resistance mutations. *Abbreviations*: Doravirine (DOR), efavirenz (EFV), etravirine (ETR), rilpivirine (RPV), nevirapine (NVP). *Additional Mutations*: A98G (DOR, EFV, ETR, NVP, RPV) and E138GQKR are nonpolymorphic mutations associated with intermediate-/high-level RPV resistance. E138A is a polymorphic mutation associated with low-level RPV resistance. Y188CH are associated with intermediate-/high-level resistance to EFV and potential low-level DOR resistance; G190Q is a rare mutation which may have an effect similar to G190E; P225H (DOR, EFV); L234I (DOR), Y318F (DOR, NVP). *Synergistic combinations*: V179D + K103R reduce NVP and EFV susceptibility >tenfold. Y181C + V179F causes high-level ETR and RPV resistance. *DOR and ETR often require multiple mutations*: DOR – high level with Y188L, V106A, F227L/C, M230L, or any combination of V106 and F227 mutations. ETR: L100I, K101P, Y181C/I/V, M230L. But multiple non-DOR mutations at common positions such as Y181 and G190 can reduce susceptibility. (*References*: Reproduced with permission from hivdb. stanford.edu/s/nnrtinotes)

concentrations and lower their side effect profile [5]. Resistance to the aforementioned PI develops as a result of amino acid mutations near or on the catalytic binding site of the drug; however, PIs are known for having a much higher genetic barrier to resistance compared to other drug classes [3].

PI resistance mutations are numerous and can be classified into two categories – major and accessory mutations. Major mutations function to reduce the susceptibility to one or more agents, while accessory mutations work synergistically with one or more major mutations to further reduce the efficacy of PIs. Additionally, the majority of viruses that carry PI resistance mutations must also carry a compensatory cleavage site mutation on the Gag protein for resistance to confer [14, 15]. The index of major PI mutations includes the positions D30N, V32I, L33, M46IL, G48VM, I50VL, I54VTALM, L76V, V82ATFS, I84V, N88S, and L90M. All of these mutations confer resistance to two or more

PI's except for D30N and I50L, which specifically target nelfinavir and atazanavir, respectively, for high-level resistance. Resistance mutations at identical amino acid positions have been noted to produce markedly variable effects on PI susceptibility. This, coupled with the large number of PI resistance mutations, makes the ability to identify and predict PI cross-resistance, especially for mutations at the 50, 54, and 82 positions, a complex process [5]. Despite this, ritonavir-boosted PIs have a particularly high genetic barrier to resistance, requiring at least one or more combined major and accessory mutations, including a cleavage site mutation on the Gag protein, for resistance to occur [14, 15]. Of the PI-ritonavir combinations, lopinavir/r and darunavir/r possess the highest genetic barrier to resistance. Lopinavir/r requires at least three to four mutations, and darunavir/r requires even more mutations than lopinavir/r for high-level resistance to occur [16, 17].

Major Protease Inhibitor (PI) Resistance Mutations										
	32	46	47	48	50	54	76	82	84	88	90
Cons	V	M	I	G	I	I		L	V	I	N	L
ATV/r	I	IL	V	**VM**	**L**	VTALM		AFTS	**V**	**S**	**M**
DRV/r	**I**		VA	V		**LM**	V	F	**V**		
LPV/r	**I**	IL	**VA**	**VM**	V	VTALM	V	**AFTS**	V		M

Fig. 5.4 Major PI resistance mutations. *Bold underline*: High-level reduced susceptibility or virological response. *Bold*: Reduced susceptibility or virological response. Plain text: Reduced susceptibility in combination with other PI resistance mutations. *Abbreviations*: atazanavir (ATV), darunavir (DRV), lopinavir (LPV), '/r' (ritonavir). *Additional mutations*: L10F, V11I, K20TV, L23I, L33F, K43T, F53L, Q58E, A71IL, G73STCA, T74P, N83D, and L89V are common nonpolymorphic accessory resistance mutations. L10F, V11IL, L33F, T74P, and L89V are accessory resistance mutations associated with reduced DRV/r susceptibility. D30N and N88D are nonpolymorphic resistance mutations selected by NFV. L10RY, V11L, L24F, M46V, G48ASTLQ, F53Y, I54S, V82CM, I84AC, and N88TG are rare nonpolymorphic variants. *Hypersusceptibility*: I50L (each PI except ATV); L76V (ATV). (*References*: Reproduced with permission from hivdb.stanford.edu/s/pinotes)

According to the DHHS guidelines, darunavir/r and atazanavir/r are considered first-line recommended agents, while lopinavir/r is considered an acceptable alternative. As such, in patients receiving first-line therapy boosted by ritonavir, PI resistance mutations have rarely been recorded, suggesting that virologic failure of these agents may stem from decreased adherence or other unidentified variables. Tipranavir is not recommended for first-line therapy but is utilized as a salvage agent for lopinavir/r- and occasionally darunavir/r-resistant viruses. Its genetic barrier to resistance is poorly understood, but it is hypothesized that resistance mutations to lopinavir/r and darunavir/r confer increased susceptibility to tipranavir [5] (Fig. 5.4).

Integrase Inhibitors (INSTI)

Integrase is an enzyme produced by retroviruses that catalyzes the incorporation of retroviral DNA into host DNA. After the production of double-stranded viral DNA by reverse transcriptase, retroviral integrase catalyzes two chemical reactions: a 3′-processing reaction and the strand transfer reaction, for the successful integration of retroviral DNA into the host genome. Integrase inhibitors function by binding to integrase when it is already bound to viral DNA during the strand transfer reaction. INSTIs disrupt the correct positioning of viral DNA on the integrase enzyme by binding close to its active site and altering its interaction with two essential magnesium ions [4]. The most commonly utilized INSTIs are raltegravir, elvitegravir, dolutegravir, and bictegravir. First-generation antiretroviral agents (raltegravir and elvitegravir) have a modest genetic barrier to resistance compared to second-generation INSTIs (dolutegravir and bictegravir), and all but raltegravir are available in fixed drug combinations [5, 18].

The archetypical integrase inhibitor, raltegravir, was the first in its class and quickly became approved for first-line and salvage antiretroviral therapy. It was followed by elvitegravir, dolutegravir, and bictegravir in 2012, 2013, and 2018, respectively. The index of major INSTI mutations includes T66AIK, E92Q, G118R, E138KAT, G140SAC, Y143RCH, S147G, Q148HRK, N155H, and R263K. Resistance mutations to raltegravir occur through three main and sometimes overlapping pathways. These mutations occur in the positions N155H, E92Q, Q148HRK + G140SA, and Y143CR + T97A and are often coupled with other accessory mutations [19, 20]. The individual mutations N155H, Q148R, and Y1433R appear to impede raltegravir's ability to bind integrase and the essential magnesium ions and have been shown to lower the susceptibility of raltegravir by as much as tenfold. Moreover, retroviruses with many combinations of these mutations lead to a decrease in susceptibility of raltegravir by more than 100-fold. In addition to the mutations shared by raltegravir, elvitegravir harbors major resistance mutations at the positions T66I/A/K and S147G [5].

All raltegravir resistance mutations, except for Y143CR, confer cross-resistance to elvitegravir and vice versa [5, 21]. This suggests these agents have a low genetic barrier to resistance compared to the second-generation INSTIs bictegravir and dolutegravir, which have no reported resistance when used as part of a triple therapy regimen and often require at least three resistance mutations to confer cross-resistance [18]. Despite this, maintenance monotherapy with dolutegravir for 24 weeks may breach this high genetic barrier to resistance with a high rate of virologic failure [22]. Lastly, a new INSTI, cabotegravir, is currently undergoing Phase III trials and is projected to have a similar profile for resistance as bictegravir and dolutegravir [18] (Fig. 5.5).

Chemokine Receptor 5 (CCR5) Antagonists

In order for HIV to infect CD4+ T cells, the virus must first attach itself to receptors on the cell's surface to gain entry. This process is accomplished via attachment of the R5 HIV-1 glycoprotein (gp120) to the CD4+ T cell receptor, which results in a conformational change in gp120, allowing it to bind to the CCR5 protein and precipitate the glycoprotein 41-mediated fusion of the viral envelope with the host cell membrane. This step in viral entry is inhibited by the CCR5 co-receptor antagonists maraviroc, aplaviroc, and vicriviroc, which are hypothesized to allosterically disrupt the CCR5 receptor by locking it in a conformation, hindering its co-receptor function [23]. Currently, maraviroc is the only FDA-approved CCR5 antagonist available for use; however, a new agent, leronlimab, a monoclonal antibody that functions by competitively inhibiting CCR5, should be released in 2020. Maraviroc is often combined with two NRTI's as an alternative regimen for first-line therapy and is used in salvage therapy for patients infected with CCR5-tropic viruses [5].

Major Integrase Inhibitor (INST) Resistance Mutations										
	66	92	118	138	140	143	147	148	155	263
Cons	T	E	G	E	G	Y	S	Q	N	R
BIC	K	Q	**R**	KAT	SAC	-		**HRK**	H	K
DTG	**K**	Q	**R**	KAT	SAC			**HRK**	H	K
EVG	AI**K**	**Q**	**R**	**KAT**	**SAC**		**G**	**HRK**	**H**	K
RAL	AI**K**	**Q**	**R**	**KAT**	**SAC**	**RC**		**HRK**	**H**	K

Fig. 5.5 Major INSTI resistance mutations. *Bold underline*: High-level reduced susceptibility or virological response. *Bold*: Low-level reduced susceptibility or reduced susceptibility or virological response. Plain text: Reduced susceptibility in combination with other INSTI resistance mutations. *Abbreviations*: Bictegravir (BIC), dolutegravir (DTG), elvitegravir (EVG), raltegravir (RAL). *Additional mutations*: L74MI, T97A, V151I, E157Q, and G163KR are common polymorphic accessory DRMs. H51Y, F121Y, S153YF, and S230R are additional nonpolymorphic mutations associated with reduced susceptibility to one or more INSTIs. E92GV, Y143HKSGA, P145S, Q146P, Q148N, V151AL, and N155ST are rare nonpolymorphic IN mutations that reduce RAL and/or EVG susceptibility. Mutations outside of IN in the polypurine tract have also rarely been reported to reduce INSTI susceptibility. *Cabotegravir (CAB)*: CAB has a resistance profile similar to DTG/BIC; however, mutations associated with these INSTIs cause greater reductions in CAB susceptibility. G140R is a novel mutation that emerges under CAB selection pressure and reduces CAB susceptibility. (*References*: Reproduced with permission from hivdb.stanford.edu/s/instnotes)

CCR5 antagonists are limited to use in patients infected with viruses that use the CCR5 receptor for viral entry. CXC chemokine receptor 4 tropic viruses (CXCR4) and viruses that use both CCR5 and CXCR4 receptors for viral entry do not respond to CCR5 antagonist therapy. In fact, the most common reason for virologic failure with the use of maraviroc is co-infection with a minority CXCR4 tropic virus at levels below the limit of assay detection [18]. It is estimated that 80% of patients infected with HIV are solely infected with CCR5 tropic viruses. However, nearly 50% of patients chronically infected with HIV will eventually become co-infected with a CXCR4 tropic minority variant [5]. Although it is possible for resistance mutations that allow HIV-1 gp120 to bind a CCR5 receptor that is already bound to a CCR5 inhibitor to emerge from the V3 loop region of HIV (the major determinant of viral tropism), such reports have only been documented in a small number of viruses in vitro [18, 23]. No consensus currently exists on specific signature resistance mutations for CCR5 antagonists [18].

Fusion Inhibitors

Fusion inhibitors, also known as entry inhibitors, are a class of antiretrovirals that work by inhibiting the envelope of HIV from merging with the host cell membrane of CD4+ T cells. Enfuvirtide is the only FDA-approved fusion inhibitor on the market. It functions by binding the first heptad repeat (HR1) on the glycoprotein 41 (gp41) subunit and preventing the conformational change required for the fusion of viral and cellular membranes [24]. The index of resistance mutations to enfuvirtide occurs at the gp41 codons 36–45, which code for HR1, and includes G36DEV, V38EA, Q40H, N42T, and N43D. Any of the above resistance mutations can decrease susceptibility for enfuvirtide tenfold; however, combination mutations can reduce susceptibility 100-fold. Despite its unique mechanism of action, enfuvirtide has a low genetic barrier

for resistance. As such, its use has virtually been displaced by such agents as maraviroc, efavirenz, lopinavir/r, and raltegravir, with a similar level of activity and an easier route of administration [5].

Novel Post-Attachment Inhibitors: CD4-Directed (Ibalizumab) and gp120 Attachment Inhibitor (Fostemsavir)

In 2018, the FDA approved ibalizumab, a humanized IgG4 monoclonal antibody, for the treatment of HIV-1 infection. Ibalizumab works by blocking HIV from binding the CCR5 and CXCR4 co-receptors after HIV has already bound the CD4 receptor. This CD4-directed post-attachment inhibitor prevents the entry of HIV into CD4+ T cells while preserving the CD4+ T cell's normal immunologic function. Ibalizumab is reserved for patients who are treatment refractory and are experiencing virologic failure with their current ARV regimen due to multidrug-resistant strains [25].

Most recently, fostemsavir, the first-in-class gp120 attachment inhibitor received FDA approval on July 2, 2020. Fostemsavir is the oral prodrug form of temsavir which functions by attaching to the gp120 protein on the outer surface of HIV-1, thereby blocking HIV from entering and infecting CD4+ T cells. Preliminary studies have demonstrated a unique resistance profile with no in vitro cross-resistance to other classes of ARV drugs. Other advantages to the use of fostemsavir include a favorable drug-drug interaction profile and potent antiviral activity irrespective of HIV-1 tropism. Four amino acid substitutions at positions in gp120 (S375H/I/N/M/T, M426L/P, M434I/K, and M475I) have been shown to affect the susceptibility of HIV-1 to temsavir. Much like the novel CD4-directed post-attachment inhibitor, ibalizumab, fostemsavir is reserved for individuals with multidrug-resistant HIV-1 infection and limited therapeutic options [26] (Fig. 5.6).

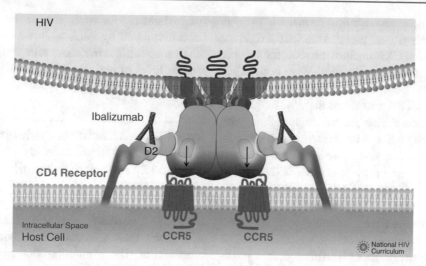

Fig. 5.6 Mechanism of action of CD4 post-attachment inhibitors. The CD4 post-attachment inhibitor ibalizumab is a humanized monoclonal antibody that binds to the domain 2 region of the human CD4 cell receptor. This binding does not prevent attachment of HIV gp120 with the host CD4 receptor, but, through steric hindrance, it prevents normal post-binding conformational changes in gp120 that are required for gp120-coreeptor binding. (From National HIV Curriculum, illustration by David H. Spach, MD, Retrieved from: www.hiv.uw.edu. Accessed October 7th, 2019)

First-in-Class HIV Capsid Inhibitor

Late-breaking Phase I clinical trials on GS-6207, lenacapavir, have shown great promise in the efficacy and safety profile of this investigational drug for the treatment of HIV-1 [27]. Lenacapavir was developed as a first-in-class HIV capsid inhibitor that targets several functions of the HIV capsid in the viral cycle, including viral particle assembly, capsid formation, and nuclear entry [28]. Data from the two Phase I studies has demonstrated that lenacapavir not only has potent antiviral activity with high synergy and no cross-resistance with approved antiretroviral drugs but is also very long-acting and amenable to dosing intervals of 6 months, given its low in vivo systemic clearance and slow-release kinetics [27]. Both studies showed that lenacapavir was overall well tolerated without any serious adverse effects reported by participants [29]. In vitro genotypic analysis has demonstrated an absence of naturally occurring resistance mutations [28] nor the emergence of resistance mutations in in vivo analysis of individuals with multidrug-resistant HIV-1 mutations, making lenacapavir an ideal therapy for heavily treatment-experienced individuals living with HIV. Further clinical trials are underway to assess lenacapavir in combination with other antiretrovirals [29] (Fig. 5.7).

HTLV ARV Resistance

Although HTLV originates from the same family as HIV, shares similar tropism, and utilizes similar structural proteins, antiretroviral therapy has been reported to be highly inefficient for the treatment of HTLV infections, possibly because of differences in how these two viruses are transmitted and replicated. HTLV is transmitted through cell-to-cell contact, while HIV is transmitted via cell-free viral particles. Unlike HIV, HTLV does not normally replicate via reverse transcription but instead through clonal expansion. It is thought that these attributes confer

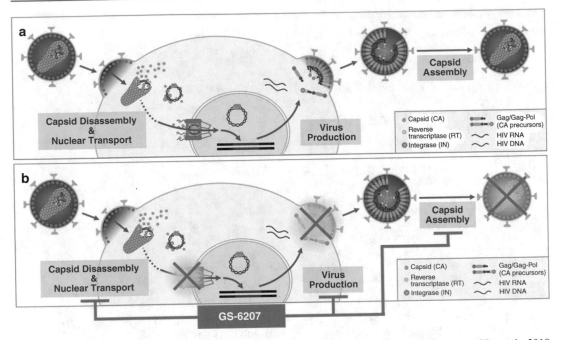

Fig. 5.7 HIV capsid inhibitor mechanism of action. (**a**) HIV capsid is essential at multiple stages in the viral life cycle. (**b**) GS-6207 inhibits multiple processes essential for viral replication; GS-6207 modulates the stability and/ or transport of capsid complexes. (Yang SR, et al., 2019 CROI Conference, Seattle, WA. Poster 480 – "GS-6270, a potent and selective first-in-class long-acting HIV-1 capsid inhibitor". © Gilead Sciences 2020)

inherent drug resistance to NRTIs, NNRTIs, integrase inhibitors, and protease inhibitors, which have been shown to demonstrate no significant decrease in HTLV proviral load [30, 31].

DHHS Guidelines for First-Line ARV Therapy

The initial regimen for first-line ARV therapy in treatment-naïve patients typically consists of two NRTIs, often abacavir/lamivudine or tenofovir alafenamide/emtricitabine, administered in combination with an INSTI, NNRTI, or a boosted PI. Selecting the appropriate drug and treatment regimen should be an individualized process based on resistance testing, predicted virologic efficacy, potential adverse effects, childbearing potential and use of effective contraception, pill burden, dosing frequency, drug-drug interaction potential, comorbid conditions, and cost [32]. Newer data support the use of two-drug regimens such as abacavir/lamivudine, tenofovir alafenamide/emtricitabine, tenofovir disoproxil fumarate (TDF)/lamivudine, or TDF/emtricitabine. In cases where abacavir, TDF, or tenofovir alafenamide cannot be used, or use is suboptimal, dolutegravir plus lamivudine is recommended [33].

Please see Tables 5.1 and 5.2 for more details on first-line ARV therapy [32].

Strategies to Overcome Retroviral Resistance

Strategies to improve response to treatment and combat ARV resistance, especially for those infected with HIV, requires a multifaceted approach with targeted intervention at multiple levels. First and foremost, drug resistance testing (DRT) is highly recommended for guidance in

Table 5.1 First-line antiretroviral agents

Recommended initial regimens for most people with HIV
Recommended regimens are those with demonstrated durable virologic efficacy, favorable tolerability and toxicity profiles, and ease of use

INSTI plus two NRTIs
Note: For individuals of childbearing potential, see Table 6b before prescribing one of these regimens.
   BIC/TAF/FTC (**AI**)
   DTG/ABC/3TC (**AI**)—**If HLA-B*5701 negative**
   DTG plus (TAF or TDF)[a] plus (FTC or 3TC) (**AI**)
   RAL plus (TAF or TDF)[a] plus (FTC or 3TC) (**BI** for TDF/[FTC or 3TC], **BII** for TAF/FTC)

INSTI plus one NRTI
   DTG/3TC (**AI**), except for individuals with HIV RNA >500,000 copies/mL, HBV coinfection, or in whom ART is to be started before the results of HIV genotypic resistance testing for reverse transcriptase or HBV testing are available

Rating of recommendations: *A, strong; B, moderate; C, optional*
Rating of evidence: *I, data from randomized controlled trials; II, data from well-designed nonrandomized trials, observational cohort studies with long-term clinical outcomes, relative bioavailability/bioequivalence studies, or regimen comparisons from randomized switch studies; III, expert opinion*

[a]TAF and TDF are two forms of TFV approved by FDA. TAF has fewer bone and kidney toxicities than TDF, while TDF is associated with lower lipid levels. Safety, cost, and access are among the factors to consider when choosing between these drugs.

Note: The following are available as coformulated drugs: ABC/3TC, ATV/c, BIC/TAF/FTC, DOR/TDF/3TC, DRV/c, DRV/c/TAF/FTC, DTG/3TC, DTG/ABC/3TC, EFV (400 mg or 600 mg)/TDF/3TC, EFV/TDF/FTC, EVG/c/TAF/FTC, EVG/c/TDF/FTC, RPV/TAF/FTC, RPV/ TDF/FTC, TAF/FTC, TDF/3TC, and TDF/FTC.

Key: *3TC* lamivudine, *ABC* abacavir, *ART* antiretroviral therapy, *ARV* antiretroviral, *ATV* atazanavir, *ATV/c* atazanavir/cobicistat, *ATV/r* atazanavir/ritonavir, *BIC* bictegravir, *CD4* CD4 T lymphocyte, *DOR* doravirine, *DRV* darunavir, *DRV/c* darunavir/cobicistat, *DRV/r* darunavir/ritonavir, *DTG* dolutegravir, *EFV* efavirenz, *EVG* elvitegravir, *EVG/c* elvitegravir/cobicistat, *FDA* Food and Drug Administration, *FTC* emtricitabine, *HLA* human leukocyte antigen, *INSTI* integrase strand transfer inhibitor, *NNRTI* nonnucleoside reverse transcriptase inhibitor, *NRTI* nucleoside reverse transcriptase inhibitor, *PI* protease inhibitor, *RAL* raltegravir, *RPV* rilpivirine, *STR* single-tablet regimen, *TAF* tenofovir alafenamide, *TFV* tenofovir, *TDF* tenofovir disoproxil fumarate

Source: Panel on Antiretroviral Guidelines for Adults and Adolescents. Guidelines for the Use of Antiretroviral Agents in Adults and Adolescents with HIV. Department of Health and Human Services. What to start: initial combination regimens for the antiretroviral-naive patient. Accessed November 7th, 2019. https://clinicalinfo.hiv.gov/sites/default/files/inline-files/AdultandAdolescentGL.pdf

Table 5.2 Considerations before initiating dolutegravir and other integrase strand transfer inhibitors as initial therapy for persons of childbearing potential

Background:
Preliminary data from a study in Botswana suggested that there is an increased risk of NTDs (0.9%) in infants born to women who were receiving DTG at the time of conception [5, 9]. Updated results have shown that the prevalence of NTDs in infants who were exposed to DTG at the time of conception is lower (0.3%) than reported in the preliminary data, but still higher than in infants who were exposed to ART that did not contain DTG (0.1%) [6, 7]

It is not yet known whether use of other INSTIs around the time of conception also poses a risk of NTDs (i.e., a class effect)

There are insufficient data to determine whether use of BIC around the time of conception and during pregnancy is safe

There is limited data on RAL use around the time of conception. Thus far, based on data collected from the antiretroviral pregnancy registry, the drug manufacturer, and in a cohort study from the United States and other countries, no case of NTD has been reported [10–12]. Among those receiving RAL during pregnancy, the rate of fetal malformations is within the expected range for pregnancy outcomes in the United States [10–12]

Before initiating an INSTI-containing regimen in a person of childbearing potential

A pregnancy test should be performed (**AIII**)

To enable individuals of childbearing potential to make informed decisions, providers should discuss the benefits and risks of using DTG around the time of conception, including the low risk of NTDs and the relative lack of information on the safety of using other commonly prescribed ARV drugs, including other INSTIs, around the time of conception (**AIII**)

For individuals who are trying to conceive, the panel recommends initiating one of the following regimens, which are designated as *Preferred* regimens during pregnancy in the perinatal guidelines: RAL, ATV/r or DRV/r plus TDF/FTC, TDF/3TC, or ABC/3TC. DTG would be an *Alternative*, rather than a *Preferred*, option (**BII**)

For individuals who are not planning to conceive but who are sexually active and not using contraception, consider a regimen's effectiveness and tolerability, the available data on potential teratogenicity, and the person's preferences (e.g., low pill burden) when choosing among regimens recommended for initial therapy. In this situation, DTG would be an *Alternative*, rather than *Preferred*, option (**BII**). If the person becomes pregnant, changes to the ARV regimen may be warranted. Clinicians should refer to the perinatal guidelines for recommendations

For individuals who are using effective contraception, a DTG-based regimen is one of the recommended options; however, clinicians should discuss the risks and benefits of using DTG with patients to allow them to make an informed decision (**AIII**)

An approach similar to that outlined for DTG should be considered for BIC-containing ART (**AIII**)

EVG/c *should not be used during pregnancy* because of inadequate drug concentrations in the second and third trimesters (**AII**).

Clinicians should refer to the perinatal guidelines when prescribing ART for a pregnant person with HIV

Rating of recommendations: *A, strong; B, moderate; C, optional*

Rating of evidence: *I, data from randomized controlled trials; II, data from well-designed nonrandomized trials, observational cohort studies with long-term clinical outcomes, relative bioavailability/bioequivalence studies, or regimen comparisons from randomized switch studies; III, expert opinion*

Key: *3TC* lamivudine, *ABC* abacavir, *ART* antiretroviral therapy, *ATV/r* atazanavir/ritonavir, *BIC* bictegravir, *DRV/r* darunavir/ritonavir, *DTG* dolutegravir, *EVG/c* elvitegravir/cobicistat, *FTC* emtricitabine, *INSTI* integrase strand transfer inhibitor, *NTD* neural tube defect, *RAL* raltegravir, *TDF* tenofovir disoproxil fumarate

Source: Panel on Antiretroviral Guidelines for Adults and Adolescents. Guidelines for the Use of Antiretroviral Agents in Adults and Adolescents with HIV. Department of Health and Human Services. What to start: initial combination regimens for the antiretroviral-naive patient. Accessed November 7th, 2019. https://clinicalinfo.hiv.gov/sites/default/files/inline-files/AdultandAdolescentGL.pdf

the selection of initial therapy in ARV-naïve individuals newly diagnosed with HIV. Genotypic resistance testing looks for mutations in the genetic code for reverse transcriptase, protease, and integrase enzymes. This initial step is paramount in optimizing virologic efficacy and preventing further transmission of the virus. For individuals who defer therapy, repeat testing should be considered upon initiation of ARV therapy at a later date. In patients who are experiencing virologic failure or have a suboptimal viral load (HIV RNA >500 copies/mL) while already on ARV therapy, repeat drug resistance testing should be performed to aid in the selection of new active ARV agents [34]. Those experiencing virologic failure on an INSTI based therapy should have INSTI genotypic testing before switching to another drug in the same class [35]. DRT should be performed while patients are actively on their ARV regimen. If this is not possible, optimal testing should occur within 4 weeks following discontinuation of therapy. When complex drug resistance mutations are known or suspected, the application of both phenotypic and genotypic resistance testing is often preferred and is beneficial in the selection of salvage therapy [32].

A patient commencing a new ARV regimen should receive at least two, if not three, fully active agents. In general, patients on at least three active ARV agents experience higher and more sustained virologic response compared to those receiving fewer agents; however, newer data suggest a similar response may be achieved with two agents if combination therapy is INSTI-based [36]. A thorough review of a patient's drug resistance profile and prior ARV history is key in determining which ARV agents are likely to be therapeutic. Additionally, when considering the use of a CCR5 antagonist, tropism testing is necessary for the identification of minority variant retroviruses that may interfere with response to treatment [37]. It is important to note that certain mutations may necessitate an adjustment to a twice-daily dose, as is the case for darunavir/ritonavir- or lopinavir/ritonavir-based therapies in the presence of specific dolutegravir resistance mutations. Adding a single ARV to a failing regimen is not recommended due to an increased risk of developing resistance to all the drugs in that regimen. Instead, DRT should be used to help guide what drug substitutions are likely to result in an increased virologic response [32].

For those patients who are ARV-experienced and have extensive drug resistance and are experiencing virologic failure, the goal of treatment should be to reestablish virologic suppression. The implementation of a salvage regimen can be complicated, and it often requires the use of multiple ARVs with partial residual activity and compromised genetic barriers to resistance to achieve acceptable virologic suppression. In some cases, maximal virologic suppression may not be possible, but ARV therapy should still be continued with a regimen designed to preserve CD4 cell counts, minimize drug toxicity, and ultimately delay clinical progression [38]. Furthermore, these patients should be enrolled in a clinical trial of investigational agents or connected with a manufacturer drug program designed to provide patients with investigational agents not currently on the market for the treatment of multidrug-resistant viruses [32].

Pre-exposure Prophylaxis with Truvada

In 2012, the FDA approved the landmark use of Truvada (TDF/emtricitabine) for pre-exposure prophylaxis (PrEP) in individuals considered at substantial risk for HIV infection [39]. Although PrEP markedly reduces the risk of HIV infection, those who become acutely infected with HIV, while on Truvada, are at increased risk for drug resistance. It is estimated that 0.1% of PrEP users will develop emtricitabine or tenofovir resistance mutations due to an unrecognized HIV infection prior to the initiation of therapy [40–43]. However, for every case of emtricitabine resistance attributed to PrEP, 8–50 HIV infections are prevented. The most commonly reported PrEP-associated resistance mutations for emtricitabine and TDF are the M184/I and K65R mutations, respectively. While the incidence of resistance mutations associated with PrEP is very low, this risk may increase as PrEP is more widely implemented; however, this can be mitigated through frequent laboratory testing for unrecognized HIV infections prior to the initiation of PrEP therapy [40–43].

Post-Exposure Prophylaxis

The recommended post-exposure prophylaxis for HIV is typically a three-drug regimen (e.g.. a nucleoside/tide combination plus an integrase inhibitor), but the regimen should take into account the known or anticipated drug resistance profile of the source virus [44]. If the source HIV strain is known to be resistant or has a high probability of resistance to ARV agents, post-exposure prophylaxis regimens should include dolutegravir or boosted darunavir (if not otherwise contraindicated), and the regimens can be further tailored to the specific resistance pattern of the source strain once genotype testing has resulted [44]. Although the true efficacy of ARV agents as post-exposure prophylaxis for HIV in humans is unknown, data from animal models have displayed that zidovudine is effective in preventing viral transmission when used as post-exposure prophylaxis and administered soon after exposure [45, 46]. It is thus recommended that ARV be initiated within 72 hours after exposure to HIV [44].

Conclusion

Although tremendous progress has been made in the development of new drugs with high ARV activity, increasing global resistance to ARV therapy continues to threaten the virologic efficacy, transmissibility, incidence, prevalence, morbidity, and mortality associated with HIV infection. ARV drug resistance is complex and multifactorial; however, lack of adherence and access remains the strongest contributors to the failure of ARV therapy. The recent development of drug combinations that are less toxic, with improved dosing and high genetic barriers to resistance, may prevent inadequate drug adherence and virologic failure. Continuous adherence support is essential in patients with possible adverse side effects or difficulty accessing their medications to prevent viral transmission, ARV resistance, and development of acquired immune deficiency syndrome.

References

1. Ryu W-S. Molecular virology of human pathogenic viruses. London, UK/San Diego, CA, USA/Cambridge, MA, USA/Oxford, UK: Academic Press; 2016.
2. Longo DL, Fauci AS. The human retroviruses. In: Kasper D, Fauci A, Hauser S, Longo D, Jameson J, Loscalzo J, editors. Harrison's principles of internal medicine, 19e. New York: McGraw-Hill; 2014. Accessed September 07, 2019.
3. Zdanowicz MM. The pharmacology of HIV drug resistance. Am J Pharm Educ. 2006;70(5):100.
4. Arts EJ, Hazuda DJ. HIV-1 antiretroviral drug therapy. Cold Spring Harb Perspect Med. 2012;2(4):a007161.
5. Tang MW, Shafer RW. HIV-1 antiretroviral resistance. Drugs. 2012;72(9):e1–e25.
6. Sharma R. Antiretroviral resistance: mechanisms, detection and clinical implications. J Pharm Pract. 2000;13(6):442–56.
7. Boucher S, et al. HIV-1 reverse transcriptase (RT) genotypic patterns and treatment characteristics associated with the K65R RT mutation. HIV Med. 2006;7(5):294–8.
8. Parikh UM, et al. The K65R mutation in human immunodeficiency virus type 1 reverse transcriptase exhibits bidirectional phenotypic antagonism with thymidine analog mutations. J Virol. 2006;80(10):4971–7.
9. Rhee S-Y, et al. HIV-1 subtype B protease and reverse transcriptase amino acid covariation. PLoS Comput Biol. 2007;3(5):e87.
10. Melikian GL, et al. Non-nucleoside reverse transcriptase inhibitor (NNRTI) cross-resistance: implications for preclinical evaluation of novel NNRTIs and clinical genotypic resistance testing. J Antimicrob Chemother. 2013;69(1):12–20.
11. Sluis-Cremer N, Tachedjian G. Mechanisms of inhibition of HIV replication by non-nucleoside reverse transcriptase inhibitors. Virus Res. 2008;134(1–2):147–56.
12. Vingerhoets J, et al. Resistance profile of etravirine: combined analysis of baseline genotypic and phenotypic data from the randomized, controlled Phase III clinical studies. AIDS. 2010;24(4):503–14.
13. Soulie C, et al. Rare occurrence of doravirine resistance-associated mutations in HIV-1-infected treatment-naive patients. J Antimicrob Chemother. 2018;74(3):614–7.
14. Foulkes-Murzycki JE, Scott WRP, Schiffer CA. Hydrophobic sliding: a possible mechanism for drug resistance in human immunodeficiency virus type 1 protease. Structure. 2007;15(2):225–33.
15. Fun A, et al. Human Immunodeficiency Virus Gag and protease: partners in resistance. Retrovirology. 2012;9(1):63.
16. De Meyer S, et al. Resistance profile of darunavir: combined 24-week results from the POWER trials. AIDS Res Hum Retrovir. 2008;24(3):379–88.
17. King MS, et al. Predictive genotypic algorithm for virologic response to lopinavir-ritonavir in protease inhibitor-experienced patients. Antimicrob Agents Chemother. 2007;51(9):3067–74.
18. Wensing AM, et al. 2019 Update of the Drug Resistance Mutations in HIV-1. Resistance Mutations Update 27(3) July/August 2019. https://www.iasusa.org/wp-content/uploads/2019/07/2019-drug-resistance-mutations-figures.pdf.
19. Blanco J-L, et al. HIV-1 integrase inhibitor resistance and its clinical implications. J Infect Dis. 2011;203(9):1204–14.
20. Geretti AM, Armenia D, Ceccherini-Silberstein F. Emerging patterns and implications of HIV-1 integrase inhibitor resistance. Curr Opin Infect Dis. 2012;25(6):677–86.
21. Abram ME, et al. Impact of primary elvitegravir resistance-associated mutations in HIV-1 integrase on drug susceptibility and viral replication fitness. Antimicrob Agents Chemother. 2013;57(6):2654–63.
22. Wijting I, et al. Dolutegravir as maintenance monotherapy for HIV (DOMONO): a phase 2, randomised non-inferiority trial. Lancet HIV. 2017;4(12):e547–54.
23. Tsibris A. Update on CCR5 inhibitors: scientific rationale, clinical evidence, and anticipated uses. PRN Notebook. 2007;12
24. Reeves JD, et al. Enfuvirtide resistance mutations: impact on human immunodeficiency virus envelope function, entry inhibitor sensitivity, and virus neutralization. J Virol. 2005;79(8):4991–9.
25. Markham A. Ibalizumab: first global approval. Drugs. 2018;78(7):781–5.

26. Kozal M, et al. Fostemsavir in adults with multidrug-resistant HIV-1 infection. N Engl J Med. 2020;382(13):1232–43.
27. Link JO, et al. Clinical targeting of HIV capsid protein with a long-acting small molecule. Nature. 2020;584:614–18.
28. Marcelin A-G, et al. Frequency of capsid substitutions associated with GS-6207 in vitro resistance in HIV-1 from antiretroviral-naive and-experienced patients. J Antimicrob Chemother. 2020;75(6):1588–90.
29. Rana AI, et al. Advances in long-acting agents for the treatment of HIV infection. Drugs. 2020;80;535–45.
30. Pasquier A, et al. How to control HTLV-1-associated diseases: preventing de novo cellular infection using antiviral therapy. Front Microbiol. 2018;9:278.
31. Soltani A, et al. Molecular targeting for treatment of human T-lymphotropic virus type 1 infection. Biomed Pharmacother. 2019;109:770–8.
32. Adolescents, P.o.A.G.f.A.a., Guidelines for the use of antiretroviral agents in adults and adolescents living with HIV. 2018, Department of Health and Human Services Washington, DC.
33. Gallant J, et al. Bictegravir, emtricitabine, and tenofovir alafenamide versus dolutegravir, abacavir, and lamivudine for initial treatment of HIV-1 infection (GS-US-380-1489): a double-blind, multicentre, phase 3, randomised controlled non-inferiority trial. Lancet. 2017;390(10107):2063–72.
34. Clutter DS, et al. HIV-1 drug resistance and resistance testing. Infect Genet Evol. 2016;46:292–307.
35. Paredes R, et al. Collaborative update of a rule-based expert system for HIV-1 genotypic resistance test interpretation. PLoS One. 2017;12(7):e0181357.
36. Lalezari JP, et al. Enfuvirtide, an HIV-1 fusion inhibitor, for drug-resistant HIV infection in North and South America. N Engl J Med. 2003;348(22):2175–85.
37. Westby M, et al. Emergence of CXCR4-using human immunodeficiency virus type 1 (HIV-1) variants in a minority of HIV-1-infected patients following treatment with the CCR5 antagonist maraviroc is from a pretreatment CXCR4-using virus reservoir. J Virol. 2006;80(10):4909–20.
38. Negredo E, et al. Compromised immunologic recovery in treatment-experienced patients with HIV infection receiving both tenofovir disoproxil fumarate and didanosine in the TORO studies. Clin Infect Dis. 2005;41(6):901–5.
39. Organization, W.H., Guideline on when to start antiretroviral therapy and on pre-exposure prophylaxis for HIV. World Health Organization; 2015.
40. Baeten JM, et al. Antiretroviral prophylaxis for HIV prevention in heterosexual men and women. N Engl J Med. 2012;367(5):399–410.
41. Fonner VA, et al. Effectiveness and safety of oral HIV preexposure prophylaxis for all populations. AIDS (London, England). 2016;30(12):1973.
42. Liegler T, et al. HIV-1 drug resistance in the iPrEx preexposure prophylaxis trial. J Infect Dis. 2014;210(8):1217–27.
43. Thigpen MC, et al. Antiretroviral preexposure prophylaxis for heterosexual HIV transmission in Botswana. N Engl J Med. 2012;367(5):423–34.
44. Kuhar DT, et al. Updated US Public Health Service guidelines for the management of occupational exposures to human immunodeficiency virus and recommendations for postexposure prophylaxis. Infect Control Hospital Epidemiol. 2013;34(9):875–92.
45. Martin LN, et al. Effects of initiation of 3′-azido, 3′-deoxythymidine (zidovudine) treatment at different times after infection of rhesus monkeys with simian immunodeficiency virus. J Infect Dis. 1993;168(4):825–35.
46. Shih C-C, et al. Postexposure prophylaxis with zidovudine suppresses human immunodeficiency virus type 1 infection in SCID-hu mice in a time-dependent manner. J Infect Dis. 1991;163(3):625–7.

Emerging Viral Infections

Eleanor Johnson, Shravya Reddy Pothula, and Julie H. Wu

Abbreviations

COVID-19	Coronavirus disease 2019
HFMD	Hand-foot-and-mouth disease
HLA	Human leukocyte antigen
HPyV	Human polyomavirus
HPyV6	Human polyomavirus 6
HPyV7	Human polyomavirus 7
HSV-1	Human simplex virus type 1
HSV-2	Human simplex virus type 2
IFN	Interferon
LT	Large tumor
MCC	Merkel cell carcinoma
MCPyV	Merkel cell polyomavirus
MHC	Major histocompatibility complex
MMR	Measles, mumps, and rubella
mT	Middle tumor
PD-1	Programmed cell death protein 1
PD-L1	Programmed cell death ligand-1
PHN	Post-herpetic neuralgia
prM	Precursor membrane protein
SARS-CoV-2	Severe acute respiratory syndrome coronavirus 2
sT	Small tumor
TLR	Toll-like receptors
TS	Trichodysplasia spinulosa
TSPyV	Trichodysplasia spinulosa-associated polyomavirus
VZV	Varicella zoster virus

Introduction

Emerging viral infections are viruses that have recently appeared within the human population or those whose incidence has increased rapidly in recent decades. Given the increasing trend in immigration, international travel, and intercontinental mobility, viral infections that were initially uncommon are being detected at higher frequency around the world. Emerging viral infections are considered to be a major public health concern, and a number of factors such as viral evolution, resistance to antiviral therapy, environmental factors, and changes in vaccination patterns have contributed to the rise of new viral infections. Many of these diseases present with cutaneous manifestations, which can serve as an aid to prompt diagnosis and identification of appropriate therapies. In this chapter, we review the cutaneous manifestations, epidemiol-

E. Johnson · S. R. Pothula
School of Medicine, Baylor College of Medicine, Houston, TX, USA

J. H. Wu (✉)
New York University School of Medicine, Department of Dermatology, New York, NY, USA

© Springer Nature Switzerland AG 2021
S. K. Tyring et al. (eds.), *Overcoming Antimicrobial Resistance of the Skin*, Updates in Clinical Dermatology, https://doi.org/10.1007/978-3-030-68321-4_6

ogy, and pathogenesis of these infections and evaluate the current diagnostic methods and therapeutic options.

Mechanisms of Viral Emergence

Host genetics, viral evolution, environmental factors, and decreasing herd immunity are several known mechanisms that contribute to viral re-emergence. The human immune system elicits a type I interferon (IFN) response to combat a viral infection. Mutations affecting this pathway can lead to more severe disease. Mutations in viral recognition receptors, such as Toll-like receptors (TLR) and immunoglobulin heavy chain receptors, also decrease the immune response. Human leukocyte antigen (HLA) alleles also affect an individual's susceptibility. HLA alleles encode the major histocompatibility complex (MHC) proteins of the adaptive immune system which is crucial for a robust T-cell response [1].

Viruses can evolve via point mutations, recombination, and reassortment. An organism's mutation rate is generally inversely proportional to its genome size. Thus, viral mutation rates are exponentially greater than bacterial or eukaryotic. Between viruses, those with a single-stranded RNA genome have the fastest rate of mutation, followed by double-stranded RNA, single-stranded DNA, and, finally, double-stranded DNA viruses. On average, each daughter cell's viral genome will contain one or two new mutations following the replication process [2]. Recombination occurs when there is an exchange of genetic material between two chromosomes by crossing over within regions of significant base sequence homology. This creates a more considerable change in the genome than point mutations and is a possible source for evolution. Reassortment can only occur in viruses with segmented genomes (bunyavirus, orthomyxovirus, arenavirus, and rotavirus). Genetic material is exchanged between two different strains causing an antigenic shift. This mechanism is a known cause of pandemics, particularly in influenza A [3].

Environmental factors include travel and migration, ecologic cycles, and increasing human population density [1]. Travel allows for the spread of microbe-infected persons and arthropod and rodent vectors. For example, *Aedes* mosquito eggs likely were brought to the Americas by water containers on slave ships. This allowed for the spread of many arboviruses [4]. Mosquitos require only small amounts of standing water to lay eggs, and thus arbovirus outbreaks often occurred after periods of substantial rainfall [5]. Rapid urbanization increases human-to-human transmission of viruses spread via fecal-oral, aerosolization, or droplet contact [6].

Vaccination practices date back as far as 1000 AD but did not have a global impact until the invention of the smallpox vaccine by Edward Jenner in 1796. The wonders of vaccines were realized when vaccination became compulsory in Europe and the United States in the 1800s, and smallpox was eventually eradicated. In 1974, the WHO set a goal to establish and strengthen routine immunization programs in developing countries via the Expanded Programme on Immunization (EPI). By 1990, it is estimated that nearly 80% of the children worldwide were vaccinated. This rate was not sustained due to lack of funding and internal instability, and some countries fell below 50%. As a result, other eradication efforts have been unsuccessful, and many viruses have recently re-emerged [7]. Currently, the CDC vaccination schedule protects against hepatitis B, rotavirus, diphtheria, tetanus, pertussis, Hib (*Haemophilus influenzae* type b), pneumococcal, polio, influenza, measles, mumps, and rubella, varicella, hepatitis A, and meningococcal [8]. According to the most recent publication by the CDC on vaccination coverage, rates have been relatively stable at above 90% for polio, MMR, hepatitis B, and varicella from 2011–2017. Factors associated with lower rates of vaccination are low socioeconomic status, living in a rural area, and being uninsured [9].

Herpes Simplex Viruses

Human simplex virus type 1 (HSV-1) and human simplex virus type 2 (HSV-2) are two linear double-stranded DNA viruses with icosahedral capsules that are part of the *Herpesviridae* family. HSV-1 and HSV-2 are spread primarily via bodily fluids transmitted across mucous membranes or contamination of skin abrasions. During the acute phase of HSV infection, the virus attaches to and enters dermal keratinocytes and epithelial cells via HSV surface glycoproteins [10]. The virus actively replicates at the initial contact site but then travels to sensory ganglia neurons through retrograde axonal transport. HSV establishes chronic latent infection in the dorsal root ganglion, and reactivation of the virus involves anterograde transport of the virus to epithelial cells of the skin and mucosa, where it actively replicates and can manifest clinically as dermatological lesions [11].

HSV-1

HSV-1 is highly prevalent in the human population with approximately 90% of individuals in Latin America and 48% of adults in the United States testing seropositive [12–14, 15]. HSV-1 infections are frequently asymptomatic. Approximately 25% of patients who are seropositive for the virus report a history of clinically significant oral or genital herpes [16]. Transmission of HSV-1 can occur through a number of modalities, including oral-oral, ora-genital, genital-genital contact, or infection of skin abrasions [17]. Accordingly, the most common dermatologic presentation is an orolabial rash (Fig. 6.1). In symptomatic HSV-1 primary infections, clinical symptoms typically occur

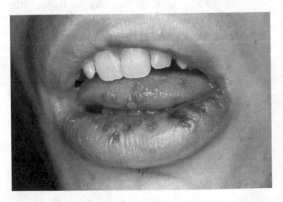

Fig. 6.1 Orolabial herpes caused by HSV-1. (Source: CDC/Robert E. Sumpter; https://phil.cdc.gov/Details.aspx?pid=12616)

2–12 days following initial exposure and are associated with pharyngitis herpetic gingivostomatitis. Oral lesions are classically described as vesiculopustular lesions on an erythematous base. Lymphadenopathy and flu-like symptoms including fever and headache may also occur [18]. If left untreated, lesions typically take 7–18 days to resolve [19]. Recurrent or secondary infection of the perioral region occurs in approximately 20–40% of infected individuals and infrequently manifests with systemic symptoms. Prodromal symptoms, which include pruritus and burning, typically occur 24 hours prior to reappearance of vesicular perioral lesions, which blister and crust in 5–8 days without antiviral treatment. Recurrent HSV infections are often less severe and shorter in duration in comparison to the primary infection. Immunosuppression is a major risk factor for HSV reactivation. Treatment of orolabial infection includes oral or topical antiviral therapy in combination with proper hygiene of the infected blisters [20].

HSV-1 infection can also manifest dermatologically as vesiculopustular lesions located on the neck and arms. This presentation of HSV-1 infection is classically referred to as herpes gladiatorum and occurs commonly in wrestlers or those who have close skin-to-skin contact. While mild cases do not require therapy, severe or extensive disease can be treated with antiviral therapy [21].

Eczema herpiticum is a result of the infection spreading to an area of skin with pre-existing damage. Patients with atopic dermatitis are at high risk for this condition, especially those who require immunosuppressive therapies. The compromised skin barrier allows HSV-1 infection to spread and establish itself within the skin's layers. Eczema herpiticum is described as small punched-out lesions with hemorrhagic crusting, and given that eczema herpiticum can spread rapidly, prompt antiviral therapy is encouraged, and intravenous acyclovir is recommended in severe presentations [22].

Herpetic whitlow occurs more frequently in individuals with HSV-2 infection although it can present in those with HSV-1 as well. Infection is primarily spread through an open wound or broken skin. Though herpetic whitlow can present in all age groups, it is most prevalent in children given that infection of the finger can occur via oral inoculation of the virus [23]. However, adults who are in contact with oral mucosa such as dentists, physicians, and dental hygienists are also at high risk. The dermatologic findings of herpetic whitlow first appear 1–20 days following inoculation and lesions progress and heal over 2–3 weeks. Similar to other forms of HSV-1 infection, herpetic whitlow can become recurrent [24]. Herpetic whitlow presents as a single vesicle or a cluster of vesicles erythematous base and become purulent and coalesce into large bullae that can spread below the nail bed. These lesions are associated with pain out of proportion to clinical presentation. Flu-like symptoms including body aches, headache, and fever are also common. Herpetic whitlow is frequently confused with bacterial infections, although the distinction is important given that antibiotic therapy will not be effective for herpetic whitlow. Although herpetic whitlow is self-limited, patients can be given antivirals to reduce the severity of symptoms and shorten the course of infection [25].

For mucosal or cutaneous disease, culture of the virus or DNA detection through polymerase chain reaction (PCR) is the mainstay of the diagnostic workup. The specimen for PCR or viral culture should be obtained once the vesicle has been unroofed. Other diagnostic tests, such as the Tzanck smear or fluorescent antibody testing, are also available, although these alternatives have a lower sensitivity and specificity [26].

HSV-2

HSV-2 is spread primarily through oral, vaginal, or anal sex, although the infection can also be spread from mother to child during childbirth [27].

Similar to HSV-1, HSV-2 infection is often asymptomatic and can establish primary and recurrent infections. In symptomatic disease, the most common dermatologic complication of HSV-2 is genital herpes. Primary infection is characterized by bilateral painful vesiculopustular genital lesions and can be accompanied by dysuria and systemic flu-like symptoms in 63% and 67% of patients, respectively. Moreover, tender lymphadenopathy is present in 80% of patients [28]. Primary infections generally resolve in 19 days on average, and infections are typically more severe in women [29]. Disease recurrence occurs with reactivation of latent HSV infection and is typically shorter in duration and less severe in comparison to primary infection. Recurrent genital herpes tend to be unilateral and resolve in 10 days [30]. While genital herpes is one of the most common sexually transmitted diseases, routine surveillance for HSV in asymptomatic adults is generally not recommended. Reactivation of genital herpes is common and can be triggered by menstrual cycles and urethritis among many other factors. Fortunately, genital herpes is treatable with oral antivirals such as acyclovir, although previous antiviral treatment has no impact on rates of recurrent infection [31]. Chronic suppressive therapy can be considered for those with frequent or severe infections that hinder quality of life and for patients who wish to decrease the risk of transmitting the virus to their sexual partners [32].

Infants who contract HSV-2 in utero or though vaginal delivery can develop neonatal skin-eye-mouth disease (SEM). Notably, SEM can also be caused by HSV-1, albeit less frequently. Parenteral administration of antiviral therapy is imperative in pregnant mother with known genital herpes infections, and a caesarean section is the preferred method of delivery in those with active infections. SEM disease with the absence of disseminated and CNS involvement generally has a good prognosis [33]. Infants with SEM should be treated with acyclovir for a minimum of 14 days. However, approximately 2% of infants may have developmental delay despite acyclovir therapy, and infants with more than three recurrent skin infections prior to the age of 6 months are at higher risk for adverse outcomes [34]. Notably, CNS involvement or disseminated disease that is not confined to the skin, eyes, and mouth is associated with high mortality and morbidity [35].

There is significant overlap between dermatological presentations of HSV-1 and HSV2. It is important to note that HSV-2 can also cause herpetic whitlow and orolabial herpes, which were previously described. Moreover, HSV-1 is becoming an increasingly common cause of genital herpes, especially in younger female patients and men who have sex with men [36, 37]. Type 1- versus type 2-induced genital herpes cannot be differentiated based on clinical features alone.

Acyclovir is considered to be the gold standard therapy for the majority of dermatologic HSV infections in immunocompetent patients [38, 39]. Famciclovir and valacyclovir can be used as alternatives for those who do not respond to acyclovir, although there are currently no randomized control trials that evaluate the efficacy of ganciclovir or valacyclovir for primary HSV-induced gingivostomatitis. Notably, valacyclovir is currently only approved for adult usage. HSV thymidine kinase plays a key role in selectively activating these medications in virus-infected cells, thus inhibiting viral DNA polymerase and impeding viral replication. HSV resistance to acyclovir is driven by mutations in the thymidine kinase (TK) enzyme, thus preventing antiviral activation [40]. Studies have demonstrated that mutation-induced acyclovir resistance occurs in approximately 0.3% of HSV strains, and resistance is more common in immunocompromised patients [41]. Antiviral therapies targeting DNA helicase or primase enzymes have been explored, although further research needs to be completed to assess the benefits and effectiveness of these approaches [42].

VZV

Varicella zoster virus (VZV) is a double-stranded, linear DNA virus that is third member of the *Herpesviridae* family. Much like other *Herpesviridae* described previously, VZV presents with two forms: primary infection in the form of varicella (chickenpox) and secondary infection in the form of herpes zoster [43]. VZV is primarily transmitted through airborne droplets and infects lymphoid tissue of the nasopharynx,

subsequently traveling throughout the body via T-cells and resulting in viremia [44]. VZV can be detected in blood 6–8 days prior to onset of dermatologic symptoms [45]. The virus is then thought to travel through retrograde transport from nerve endings in the skin to regional sensory ganglia, where it remains latent. VZZ infection is propagated through viral mechanisms that evade immune response, such as inhibition of interferon and MHC class I gene expression [44].

VZV infections are notable for their widespread involvement of the skin. The incubation period of the virus is 10–21 days, and the virus is thought to be highly infectious 48 hours prior to the onset of skin lesions [46]. Primary VZV infection occurs frequently during childhood, and varicella is self-limited in most immunocompetent individuals. However, severity of illness increases with age, and severe disease has been reported in adolescents and adults. Dermatological manifestations include a generalized pruritic vesicular rash that arises in successive crops and progresses over approximately 4 days and crust within 6 days (Fig. 6.2) [46]. Dermatologic symptoms are often preceded by a prodrome of fever, malaise, and/or pharyngitis. Superimposed bacterial skin infections are the most common reasons for hospitalization in young patients under the age of 15 [47]. Although infrequent, some patients may develop more serious extracutaneous neurologic complications such as encephalitis, aseptic meningitis, and transverse myelitis [43]. Introduced in 1995, the varicella

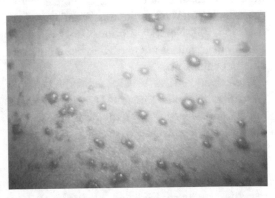

Fig. 6.2 Rash due to the varicella zoster virus (VZV). (Source: CDC/Joe Miller; https://phil.cdc.gov/Details. aspx?pid=5409)

vaccine is widespread in developed countries. Vaccinated individuals may have nonclassic dermatologic symptoms such as a maculopapular rash. Although 20% of children who receive one dose of the vaccine may acquire the infection, illness is typically more mild in nature with fewer extracutaneous complications [48].

Reactivation of latent VZV results in herpes zoster, which is characterized by a hallmark unilateral dermatomal vesicular rash that starts as erythematous papules and progresses to vesicles and bullae. The rash typically becomes pustular over 3–4 days of onset and crust within 7–10 days in immunocompetent hosts, although scarring and depigmentation may be a long-term complication that persists for months to years. Lesions can be hemorrhagic in patients with compromised immune systems. Viral reaction typically results in inflammation and hemorrhagic necrosis of sensory ganglion nerve cells, causing acute neuropathic pain. Prodromal pain precedes appearance of the rash in the majority (75%) of cases. Unlike primary VZV infection, only 20% of patients experience systemic flu-like symptoms [49]. Vaccination with the live-attenuated herpes zoster vaccine is safe and effective for patients over the age of 50, although certain contraindications, such as immunosuppression, must be considered [50]. A recombinant zoster vaccine has also been approved [51]. Although no randomized clinical trials have directly compared the live-attenuated versus recombinant zoster vaccines, meta-analytic studies have shown that the recombinant zoster vaccine is more effective for reducing rates of herpes zoster and complications [52, 53]. Notably, a prior history of herpes zoster or varicella is not needed to determine vaccination eligibility.

Reactivation of VZV in the second division of the fifth cranial nerve manifests as herpes zoster ophthalmicus, which, if untreated, can lead to blindness. The presence of classic herpes zoster skin findings on the medial nose is a pathognomonic feature referred to Hutchinson's sign. In addition to rash, other symptoms can include keratitis, conjunctivitis, and uveitis [54]. The infection can further spread to the geniculate ganglion, which can result in Ramsay Hunt syndrome. The geniculate ganglion includes cranial nerve seven and eight, resulting in impairment of ipsilateral facial muscles and hearing and partial loss of sensation and function of the tongue [55].

Post-herpetic neuralgia (PHN) is the most common complication of herpes zoster and occurs in 10–15% of patients with herpes zoster. Incidence rises with age, and immunocompromised individuals are at particularly high risk. PHN is characterized by acute pain that continues for at least 90 days following rash onset and can be accompanied by numbness, pruritis, and dysesthesias [56]. Studies have indicated that the live attenuated herpes zoster vaccine can reduce incidence of PHN [57].

Acyclovir is the gold standard treatment for VZV infections, although prolonged acyclovir treatment has led to a rise in antiviral-resistant strains of VZV infections. Similar to acyclovir-resistant HSV, antiviral resistance in VZV is caused by mutation of thymidylate kinase, which prevents acyclovir activation in virus-infected cells. Acyclovir-resistant strains of VZV can be fatal in immunocompromised patients, and patients with cancer, organ transplantation, and HIV are particularly susceptible [58]. Acyclovir-resistant VZV should be treated with alternative antiviral medications such as foscarnet, and treatment is generally recommended for at 10 days [59].

Coxsackievirus A6

Coxsackievirus belongs to the *Picornaviridae* family, which are naked viruses with a single-stranded, linear, positive-sense RNA genome and icosahedral capsid. Within the *Picornaviridae* family, coxsackievirus is subclassified as an enteroviral species virus and has two major groups, A and B [60]. Group B cause aseptic meningitis, pleurodynia, and myopericarditis [61, 62]. This section will focus on Group A coxsackievirus, which is a major pathogen associated with hand-foot-and-mouth disease (HFMD).

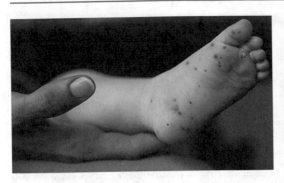

Fig. 6.3 Hand, foot, and Mouth disease (Source: CDC; https://www.cdc.gov/hand-foot-mouth/index.html)

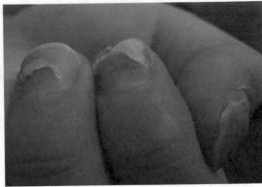

Fig. 6.4 Onychomadesis. (*Courtesy, Stephen Tyring, MD, PhD, MBA*)

HFMD causes a papulovesicular rash on the palms, souls, and oral cavity (Fig. 6.3). Outbreaks occur primarily from spring to fall in children less than 5 years old [63]. Treatment is supportive, as most cases resolve within 1 week [63]. In the United States, coxsackievirus A16 and enterovirus A71 are the major pathogens associated with HFMD. It is important to keep in mind that other serotypes within these classes can cause this disease [64]. Coxsackievirus A6 is a newly evolved strain that was first described in Finland in 2008 and has since been documented in the United Kingdom, the United States, and Asia [65]. This strain causes an atypical HFMD that caused widespread cutaneous manifestations at sites of atopic dermatitis or on the face, scalp, proximal extremities, lips, perianal region, groin, and dorsal aspects of feet and hands. Onychomadesis is a late dermatologic complication that arises 4–6 weeks after disease onset (Fig. 6.4) [66]. It also can present during winter and can affect adults [63, 67]. It is believed to have been circulating for 2 years before becoming a dominant pathogen, which is similar to the emergence of enterovirus A71 [64].

Viral transmission primarily occurs via fecal-oral transmission. The virus replicates in the oropharynx and lower GI tract [60]. It is thought that children play a larger role in local transmission, but that asymptomatic adults are more likely to have caused global spread [64]. Genetic analysis of the new Coxsackievirus A6 strand has shown that recombination with other HFMD-causing enteroviruses may have led to the pathogenicity of this strand, specifically in the P2-P3 region. Point mutations are key factors in creating viral population diversity because many of the isolated strains did not have evidence of recombination [68].

Arboviruses

Arbovirus refers to a group of viruses transmitted by arthropod (mosquito) vectors. Most arboviruses belong to one of the following families: bunyavirus, flavivirus, reovirus, and togavirus. This section will focus specifically on the chikungunya, dengue, and zika viruses. All three of these infections are transmitted by the *Aedes* mosquito, most commonly the *Aedes aegypti*. The *Aedes aegypti* has evolved to inhabit urban environments of the tropical and subtropical regions of the world, including the United States [4]. Because of this, rates of coinfection with multiple of these viruses are increasing. More research is needed to determine the clinical effects of coinfection. Each of these infections presents with fever, malaise, rash, headache, and arthralgias and thus can be difficult to distinguish. The emergence of these pathogens in new regions and re-emergence in endemic locations is highly dependent on environmental factors such as urbanization, increased travel, and climate change [69]. Unique symptoms and viral mutations are discussed below.

Chikungunya Fever

Chikungunya virus belongs to the *Togaviridae* family, which are enveloped viruses with a single-stranded, linear, positive-sense RNA genome and icosahedral capsid. Unlike dengue and zika, most chikungunya infections are symptomatic. The most distinguishing feature of chikungunya infection is the severe, often disabling polyarthralgia that is usually symmetrical and involves both the large and small joints of the upper and lower limbs. About half of infections result in persistent arthralgia for several months to years [4]. Treatment is mainly supportive. Chloroquine has been studied as a preventative measure for chronic arthralgias, but results were inconclusive. The most common dermatologic manifestation is a mildly pruritic, erythematous, maculopapular rash, usually with truncal involvement, with occasional spread to the face, extremities, palms, and soles. Other dermatologic manifestations are hyperpigmented macules, genital or oral ulcers, and rarely a vesiculobullous eruption seen only in children [70]. Neurological complications of infection, such as Guillain-Barre, encephalitis, and seizures, have been reported in 15–25% of cases. Death can occur due to infection, although rare and associated with multiple comorbidities, elderly, and neonatal infection. Due to the limited antigenic diversity, previous infection with any of the genotypes provides immunity to all Chikungunya infections. Vaccination would theoretically be effective, but due to the unpredictable nature of outbreaks and lack of financial incentive, none have progressed past phase 1 of development [4].

Over the past 15 years, there have been sporadic outbreaks of this disease in Africa, Asia, the Indian Ocean, and, most recently, in the Caribbean and the Americas. This, in part, is due to genetic adaptation of the chikungunya virus that allowed it to replicate in the *Aedes albopictus*, a mosquito with a wider distribution. This adaptation occurred during an outbreak in the Indian Ocean when a strain acquired a mutation in the envelope glycoprotein (the E1-A226V mutation) [71]. Host genetics also play a role in chikungunya susceptibility. Mutations associated with increased disease susceptibility are SNPs that affect TLR-7 and TLR-8 [72].

Dengue Hemorrhagic Fever

Dengue virus belongs to the flavivirus family, which are enveloped viruses with a single-stranded, linear, positive-sense RNA genome and icosahedral capsid. Dengue incidence has increased 30-fold over the last 50 years according to the WHO and of the three arboviruses discussed has the greatest risk of mortality [73]. There are four distinct serotypes of dengue virus, DENV-1–DENV-4. Serotypes DENV-1 and DENV-2 have been associated with severe disease [4], although the majority of infections (80%) are asymptomatic. In 2009, the WHO reclassified dengue infections into three categories: dengue without warning signs, dengue with warning signs, and severe dengue. To have the diagnosis of dengue without warning signs, the patient must have two of the following: nausea/vomiting, rash, headache, eye pain, muscle ache, or joint pain, leukopenia, or positive tourniquet test. If the patient also has abdominal pain or tenderness, persistent vomiting, ascites, or pleural effusion, mucosal bleeding, lethargy or restlessness, or hepatomegaly, then they are classified as having dengue with warning signs. Severe dengue occurs if the patient is in shock and respiratory distress having severe bleeding or organ failure [73].

Several vaccines have been created to help control the dengue virus. CYD-TDV is licensed in many countries, and TAK-003 is advanced clinical development. All vaccines include immunity to all four strains [74]. This is crucial because secondary infection with another strain of dengue increases the risk of severe dengue infection [75]. Treatment is again supportive. Fevers must be treated with acetaminophen instead of NSAIDs to avoid any potential bleeding risk. If the patient progresses to shock or massive hemorrhage, intravenous fluids or blood products are administered as needed [73].

Like other arboviruses, the increase in dengue virus epidemics and global spread is strongly linked to increased travel, increased population density, and inadequate mosquito control [1]. Studies done in Thailand and Taiwan have recognized a SNP that is important for dendritic cell functioning. This mutation is associated with the development of severe dengue [76, 77]. The HLA-A*24 allele is associated with an increased risk of developing severe dengue in children [78, 79].

Zika

Zika virus also belongs to the *Flavivirus* family. The virus was first discovered in the early 1940s. Originally, the illness was only reported on the African continent but by the 1960s was spread to Asian countries like Malaysia, Indonesia, the Philippines, Thailand, Maldives, Pakistan, and India. Most recently, the virus has spread to the Pacific Islands, South America, and southernmost states in the United States [80]. Like dengue, the majority of infections are asymptomatic. Symptomatic infection, which occurs in approximately 20% of cases, has the distinguishing feature of conjunctivitis, which affects half of patients. The most common symptom is a pruritic, maculopapular rash that starts on the trunk and extremities and then spreads to affect the face [70].

Transmission is primarily via mosquito bites but can occur by direct contact via sexual intercourse. Vertical transmission from mother to fetus is a major concern and can result in microcephaly or loss of the pregnancy [81, 82]. This was not noted until 2015 when health authorities noted increased rates of these conditions in Brazil [83]. A mutation in the viral precursor membrane protein (prM) may be the cause of this new consequence [84]. Zika virus enters cells via the cell surface protein AXL protein. AXL is highly expressed in the human fetal cortex, cutaneous fibroblasts, and epidermal keratinocyte [85]. The mutant seems to increase infectivity in these cells and induces apoptosis [84].

Zika virus also can cause several neurological complications. A study done in Columbia found that 97% of patients with Guillain-Barre syndrome (GBS) had symptoms of Zika virus infection within 1 month prior to the onset of GBS [86]. Other neurological complications associated with Zika virus include encephalitis, transverse myelitis, and chronic inflammatory demyelinating polyneuropathy [87].

Measles

Measles belongs to the paramyxovirus family, which are enveloped viruses with a single-stranded, linear, negative-sense RNA genome and helical capsid. The virus is highly contagious, with a reproductive rate of 12 to 17. It is spread via aerosolized respiratory droplets or by direct contact with infected secretions [88]. Classically, this infection presents 10–12 days after initial exposure with a prodrome of fever, cough, coryza, and conjunctivitis and followed 1–2 days later by a maculopapular rash that starts at the head and neck and spreads downward (Fig. 6.5). Rash usually resolved within a week. Koplik spots, bright red spots with blue-white center on the buccal mucosa, are a highly specific finding seen in 50–70% of patients [88].

Measles is still endemic to most of the world and remains the leading cause of death globally in young children [88]. Infection can cause serious sequelae that can affect many different organ systems. Croup, diarrhea, and malnutrition are the greatest contributors to mortality. The most common severe complication is pneumonia. Risk factors for complications include age < 5 years or > 30 years, malnutrition, immunosuppression, and vitamin A deficiency [7]. Treatment for measles is mainly supportive therapy. In severe infection, vitamin A can be given orally for 2 days. This treatment is associated with reduced risk of mortality and pneumonia-specific mortality in children less than 2 years old [89].

Primary infection control is prevention with vaccination. The measles vaccine was first licensed in the United States in 1963, which lead to an initial drastic decline in cases. Today, the measles vaccine is a live attenuated vaccine given in combination with mumps and rubella vaccines, known as MMR. It is a two-dose series that

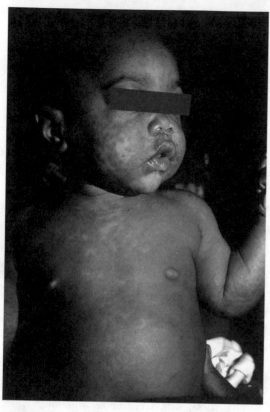

Fig. 6.5 The head, neck, and chest of an infant displaying the characteristic measles rash. (Source: CDC/ Betty G. Partin; https://phil.cdc.gov/Details.aspx?pid=17639)

begins at 12 months and can be given through 6 years. The second dose may be given as early as 4 weeks after the second dose [90]. There have been several resurgences of measles infections. From 1989 to 1991, there a reported 50,000 cases [91]. The incidence of measles declined again, to the point that in 2000 the United States declared that transmission of the measles virus was eliminated [88]. Around this time, a case series suggested that the MMR vaccine might cause autism, which has since gained much public attention. Such association has been rejected, and the paper has been formally retracted but has led to decreased vaccine compliance in the United States and Central and Western Europe [92]. According to the CDC, there were 1282 reported cases in the United States in 2019, which is the greatest number of cases since 1992. Similar trends are also being reported in Europe, especially Central and Western [93].

Polyomaviruses

Human polyomaviruses (HPyVs) are nonenveloped, double-stranded DNA viruses that were first described in 1971. Since then, 14 polyomavirus species have been identified, although only 4 have been definitively associated with cutaneous pathologies: Merkel cell polyomavirus (MCPyV), trichodysplasia spinulosa-associated polyomavirus (TSPyV), human polyomavirus 6 (HPyV6), and human polyomavirus 7 (HPyV7). Epidemiologic studies have indicated that polyomavirus infection occurs frequently during childhood with rates of seropositivity increasing sharply with age. For example, the prevalence of MCPyV seropositivity is 9% for children 1–4 years of age and increases to 35% for children 4–13 years of age and 88% for adults [94, 95]. Similar patterns have been observed in TSPyV, HPyV6, and HPyV7 [96]. Cutaneous HPyVs are continuously shed from the skin and are thought to be transmitted through skin-to-skin contact, although the route of transmission has not been definitively determined despite considerable research [97].

Cutaneous polyomaviruses contain genomes of approximately 5000 base pairs that are subdivided into early, late, and noncoding control regions (NCCR). The early transcription region is the first to be expressed during infection and encodes for the large tumor (LT) and small tumor (sT) antigens, which have been shown to play an integral part in polyomavirus pathogenesis. Notably, LT antigens of all human polyomaviruses contain highly conserved binding domains for retinoblastoma (pRb) family proteins, and polyomavirus association with pRb has been shown to inhibit tumor suppressor activity. Moreover, polyomavirus LT antigens possess Zinc-binding motifs and helicase domains that facilitate LT binding to viral DNA, thus mediating recruitment of host cell replication factors and promoting viral DNA replication. The small T antigen shares some sequence homology with LT antigen and is generated through alternative splicing. The C terminal end of sT contains characteristic binding motifs for protein phosphatase 2A (PP2A), and in vitro studies have demonstrated that sT-PP2A interaction dysregulates cellular pathways in all polyomaviruses implicated in cutaneous disease. While sT antigen of MCPyV is capable of inducing cell transformation, the transforming potential of other cutaneous HPyV sT antigens requires further investigation.

MCPyV

MCPyV sheds from the skin in 61.5% of healthy individuals and is considered to be part of the normal skin microbiome [97]. In healthy individuals, MCPyV infection is not typically associated with illness, although it is known to cause Merkel cell carcinoma in a subset of patients [98, 99]. Currently, MCPyV is the only HPyV definitively associated with tumorigenesis and has been incriminated as the causative agent for 80% of MCCs [97, 100, 101]. The oncogenic events that lead to MCC development are dependent upon mutation of the virus that enables clonal integration of MCPyV into the host cell genome and subsequent expression of viral oncoproteins, namely, LT and sT antigens [102]. Notably, a second mutation that truncates the LT antigen is required for oncogenesis and results in deletion of domains responsible for viral replication but preservation of pRB binding sites [103]. MCPyV sT antigen, in particular, is thought to drive Merkel cell carcinogenesis and facilitate clonal expansion of tumor cells through dysregulation of cap-dependent protein translation via hyperphosphorylation of 4E-binding protein 1 [104]. Interestingly, antibodies to sT and LT antigen are detected at high levels in MCC patients and in less than 1% of healthy individuals [105].

MCC is a highly aggressive cancer affecting neuroendocrine cells of the skin (Fig. 6.6). Although rare with an incidence of 0.79 cases per 100,000 people, the disease-associated mortality of MCC is 46% [106, 107]. Typically, MCC presents on sun-exposed skin and initially appears as a solitary, painless, flesh-colored, or bluish-red nodule that expands rapidly. Crusting and ulceration may be present, although appear infrequently [108]. 97% of cases are diagnosed in

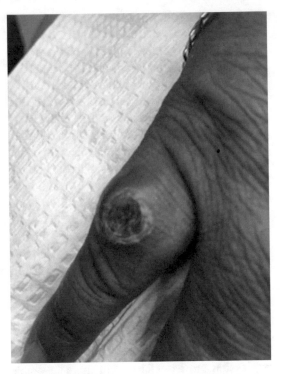

Fig. 6.6 Merkel cell carcinoma. (*Courtesy, Stephen Tyring, MD, PhD, MBA*)

patients over the age of 50, and MCC most commonly affects individuals of Caucasian ethnicity [108, 109]. Immunosuppression represents a significant risk factor for MCC, and studies have demonstrated that HIV-positive patients have a relative risk of 13.4 in comparison to those who are HIV-negative [98]. Moreover, spontaneous partial regression of MCC has been noted in organ-transplant recipients following withdrawal of immunosuppressive therapies [110].

MCC is diagnosed histologically by hematoxylin and eosin as well as immunohistochemical staining. Histologically, MCC is characterized by strands or nests of round, blue cells with large basophilic nuclei and scant cytoplasm [111]. Ultrastructurally, MCC cells, like other neuroendocrine cells, possess paranuclear dense core neurosecretory granules. Three histologic patterns have been identified: intermediate type (most common), small cell type, and trabecular type (least common) [111]. Currently, the therapeutic and prognostic implications of these histologic patterns require further investigation, although some studies have demonstrated that intermediate and small cell-type MCCs behave more aggressive clinically [112]. On immunohistochemistry, MCC is consistently immunoreactive to low-molecular-weight cytokeratin 20 (CK20), and paranuclear expression of CK20 has been shown to be a sensitive and specific marker for MCC [113]. Moreover, MCCs have been shown to express other neuroendocrine markers such as chromogranin, synaptophysin, somatostatin receptor, and calcitonin in addition to epithelial markers including Ber-EP4, pancytokeratin, CAM 5.2, and AE1/AE3 [114]. LT antigen expression can be detected, although immunohistochemical confirmation of LT presence is not required for diagnosis of MCC [113].

MCC has an exceedingly poor prognosis with overall 5-year survival rates of 51%, 35%, and 14% for local, nodal, and distant metastatic disease, respectively [109]. For unclear reasons, MCPyV positivity and presence of LT antigen expression are associated with more favorable prognosis [115]. Management of MCC is dependent upon the clinical stage of disease, and treatment guidelines for MCC are fully reviewed in the National Cancer Center Network (NCCN) Clinical Practice Guidelines. The mainstay treatment for local disease without evidence of metastasis or lymph node involvement is wide local excision. Radiation therapy to the primary tumor site may be used as an alternative in patients who are poor surgical candidates [116]. In patients with biopsy-confirmed lymph node involvement, careful workup for metastatic disease is indicated. Lymph node excision with radiation to affected nodes has shown promising results in patients without metastatic disease. For patients with high risk of recurrence, nodal radiation and radiation to the primary tumor bed can be considered [117, 118]. Treatment guidelines for Merkel cell carcinoma are rapidly evolving, and recent research has identified immunotherapy as the preferred intervention for metastatic disease [119]. Avelumab is a humanized monoclonal antibody directed against PD-L1, and a multicenter, phase II clinical trial has demonstrated an overall response rate of 33% and a 2-year progression-free survival rate of 26% [119–121]. Moreover, complete response was achieved in 11% of patients, and preliminary data has shown that treatment response is higher in patients who have not previously received chemotherapy [122]. Directed therapies against programmed cell death protein 1 (PD-1), such as pembrolizumab and nivolumab, are also currently being investigated in phase I and phase II clinical trials [123].

TSPyV

TSPyV is the eighth member of the polyomavirus family found to infect human hosts and is associated with *Trichodysplasia spinulosa* (TS), a hyperproliferative and disfiguring skin disease that primarily occurs in immunosupressed patients (Fig. 6.7) [124]. Similar to other HPyVs, TSPyV is ubiquitous and infects 65–80% of adults [125]. The virus is known to drive pathogenesis through the expression of sT and middle tumor (mT) antigens. TSPyV sT antigen mediated binding to protein phosphatase 2A and upregulation of MAPK pathway activity has been identified as mechanisms of particular importance in TS pathogenesis [126, 127]. Moreover, TSPyV mT has been shown to act through parallel mechanisms to modulate cell proliferation and inflammatory pathways [128].

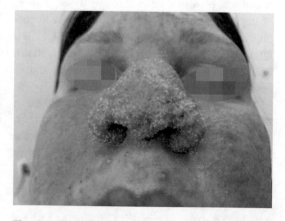

Fig. 6.7 Trichodysplasia spinulosa. (*Courtesy, Stephen Tyring, MD, PhD, MBA*)

Clinically, TS presents as flesh colored or erythematous folliculocentric papules with protrusion of keratin spines [129]. Lesions are located primarily on the central face. Alopecia of the eyebrows and scalp and deformity of leonine facies due to distortion of facial contours is often present [130]. One third of patients describe these lesions as pruritic [131]. TSPyV is thought to actively replicate within inner root sheath cells of hair follicles, and histopathologic analysis of TS lesions typically reveals dystrophy of inner root sheath cells and presence of eosinophilic, trichohyalin granules [124]. Treatment options for TS remain limited, and a gold standard regimen has yet to be established. Topical cidofovir (1–3%) cream appears to be the most effective, although oral valganciclovir has also shown promising results and is more widely available [132–135]. Acyclovir has been used in a limited number of case reports with mixed results [132, 136].

HPyV6 and HPyV7

Similar to other cutaneous polyomaviruses, HPyV6 and HPyV7 establish subclinical infection of the skin, and skin swabs from healthy adults are positive for HPyV6 and HPyV7 in 14–28% and 11–13% of samples, respectively [97, 137]. HPyV6 and HPy7 share 68% sequence homology and have both been linked to pruritic skin eruptions demonstrating "peacock plumage" histology in immunocompromised patients [138, 139]. HPyV7 in particular has been detected at high levels in pruritic parakeratotic and dyskeratotic dermatoses [139, 140]. Moreover, HPyV6 is detected in the majority of BRAF inhibitor-induced cutaneous squamous cell carcinomas, and a carcinogenic role for HPyV6 has been suggested given that HPyV6 sT antigen induces activation of MAPK pathway proteins [141, 142]. The clinical management of HPyV6- and HPyV7-associated cutaneous disease has not been clearly defined, and the possibility of using antivirals for the treatment of these lesions has not been studied.

Coronavirus Disease 2019

Coronavirus disease 2019 (COVID-19) is caused by severe acute respiratory syndrome coronavirus 2 (SARS-CoV-2), a positive-sense single-stranded RNA virus [143]. The virus was first identified in Wuhan, China, in late 2019 and subsequently spread rapidly around the world. Understanding of SARS-CoV-2 and COVID-19 are rapidly evolving. SARS-CoV-2 is thought to be transmitted primarily by direct person-to-person contact via respiratory droplets released by sneezing, coughing, and talking [144]. The virus is thought to infect human hosts through contact with mucous membranes and gains entry into cells using the angiotensin-converting enzyme 2 (ACE2) receptor [145]. However, airborne transmission of the SARS-CoV-2 through particles smaller than respiratory droplets remains controversial as long-range airborne transmission of the virus has not been clearly determined [146]. While SARS-CoV-2 has also been detected in blood and stool, the possible role of bloodborne or fecal-oral transmission in the spread of COVID-19 remains unknown, and there is currently no evidence to suggest the virus can be transmitted through skin-to-skin contact.

While COVID-19 is primarily a respiratory illness, a wide range of dermatologic presentations have been reported including exanthematous rash, urticaria, vesicular-pustular eruptions, pernio (chilblain)-like lesions, livedo reticularis, and retiform purpura (Fig. 6.8) [147, 148]. A morbilliform exanthem is the most common cutaneous manifestation of COVID-19 and presents in approximately 36% of patients either at disease onset or after recovery [148–150]. A varicella-like vesicular-pustular eruption has been described as the second most common cutaneous presentation and typically occurs 4–30 days following onset of respiratory symptoms (Fig. 6.9) [150–152]. Lesions resolve within 10 days, and PCR studies of vesicular lesions have been negative for SARS-CoV-2 [152].

Painful chilblain-like acral lesions have been reported in COVID-19 patients of all age groups, although they are more frequently detected in

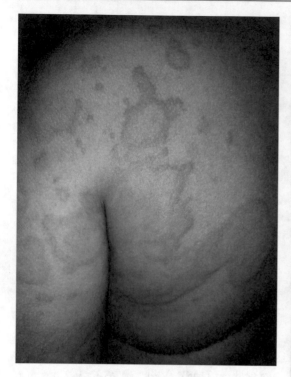

Fig. 6.8 Urticarial lesions due to COVID-19

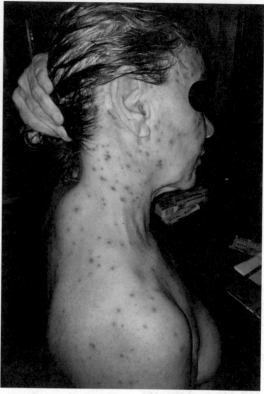

Fig. 6.9 Outbreak of varicella-like lesions in COVID-19 patient

young, healthy patients with few medical comorbidities and have mild symptoms of COVID-19 rather than severe disease (Fig. 6.10) [147, 153, 154]. The median time to resolution is 2 weeks, although lesions may be present for as long as 8 weeks. The pathogenesis of these lesions is thought to be attributed to an inflammatory response against viral infection [147]. Whether chilblain-like acral lesions in asymptomatic patients can signify underlying COVID-19 infection remains controversial [153, 155]. A limited number of studies have indicated that patients with chilblain-like acral lesions without a reasonable alternative cause may benefit from SARS-CoV-2 testing depending on regional availability of testing materials [153].

Necrotic vascular lesions are less common, although significant cutaneous presentation of COVID-19 has been described in patients with severe pulmonary symptoms [156]. Biopsy and histopathologic analysis of these necrotic lesions demonstrate complement-mediated vascular injury and thrombosis with deposition of C5b-9 and C4d co-localized with COVID-19 glycoproteins in both lesional and normal skin [156–158]. Interestingly, systemic coagulopathy appears to be a hallmark sign of severe COVID-19 disease; abnormal coagulation markers are often detectable early during hospitalization [159, 160]. Notably, treatment of these patients with low-molecular-weight heparin or other anticoagulants has been shown to lower mortality rates, and prompt recognition of cutaneous manifestations of COVID-19 indicative microvascular or thrombogenic disease can aid in the identification of proper therapies [160].

Conclusion

As patterns of infectious disease transmission continue to evolve, the threat of emerging and re-emerging viral infections will persist as an important public health concern. Given the high rates of immunosuppression and increasing international

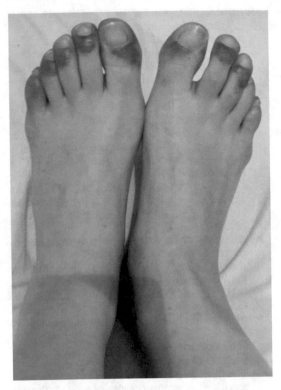

Fig. 6.10 Chilblain-like lesions on the toes due to COVID-19

travel, the incidence of these viral infections is expected to rise in the future. Delays in appropriate diagnosis and treatment of these infections are associated with increased patient morbidity and mortality. Thus, increased recognition of these viruses and their cutaneous manifestations is important to improve patient outcomes. Technological advancements have increased our ability to identify emerging viruses, and continued study of their pathogenesis is further needed to improve treatment options for patients.

References

1. Ketkar H, Herman D, Wang P. Genetic determinants of the re-emergence of Arboviral Diseases. Viruses. 2019;11(2):150.
2. Sanjuán R, Nebot MR, Chirico N, Mansky LM, Belshaw R. Viral mutation rates. J Virol. 2010;84(19):9733–48.
3. Manrubia SC, Lázaro E. Viral evolution. Phys Life Rev. 2006;3(2):65–92.
4. Fong IW. Emerging Zoonoses a worldwide perspective. 1st ed. Cham: Springer International Publishing; 2017.
5. Vu DM, Jungkind D, Angelle Desiree L. Chikungunya Virus. Clin Lab Med. 2017;37(2):371–82.
6. Lim VK. Emerging and re-emerging infections. Med J Malaysia. 1999;54(2):287–91. quiz 92
7. Mass Vaccination: Global aspects – Progress and obstacles. 1st ed. Plotkin SA, editor. Berlin, Heidelberg: Springer Berlin Heidelberg; 2006.
8. CDC Immunization Schedules [20 March 2020]. Available from: https://www.cdc.gov/vaccines/schedules/hcp/imz/child-adolescent.html.
9. Hill HA, Singleton JA, Yankey D, Elam-Evans LD, Pingali SC, Kang Y. Vaccination coverage by age 24 months among children born in 2015 and 2016 - National Immunization Survey-Child, United States, 2016-2018. MMWR Morb Mortal Wkly Rep. 2019;68(41):913–8.
10. Campadelli-Fiume G, Cocchi F, Menotti L, Lopez M. The novel receptors that mediate the entry of herpes simplex viruses and animal alphaherpesviruses into cells. Rev Med Virol. 2000;10(5):305–19.
11. van Velzen M, Jing L, Osterhaus AD, Sette A, Koelle DM, Verjans GM. Local CD4 and CD8 T-cell reactivity to HSV-1 antigens documents broad viral protein expression and immune competence in latently infected human trigeminal ganglia. PLoS Pathog. 2013;9(8):e1003547.
12. Looker KJ, Magaret AS, May MT, Turner KM, Vickerman P, Gottlieb SL, et al. Global and regional estimates of prevalent and incident herpes simplex virus type 1 infections in 2012. PLoS One. 2015;10(10):e0140765.
13. Sukik L, Alyafei M, Harfouche M, Abu-Raddad LJ. Herpes simplex virus type 1 epidemiology in Latin America and the Caribbean: systematic review and meta-analytics. PLoS One. 2019;14(4):e0215487.
14. McQuillan G, Kruszon-Moran D, Flagg EW, Paulose-Ram R. Prevalence of Herpes Simplex Virus Type 1 and Type 2 in Persons Aged 14–49: United States, 2015–2016. NCHS Data Brief. 2018;304:1–8.
15. Bradley H, Markowitz LE, Gibson T, McQuillan GM. Seroprevalence of herpes simplex virus types 1 and 2–United States, 1999–2010. J Infect Dis. 2014;209(3):325–33.
16. Oliver L, Wald A, Kim M, Zeh J, Selke S, Ashley R, et al. Seroprevalence of herpes simplex virus infections in a family medicine clinic. Arch Fam Med. 1995;4(3):228–32.
17. Douglas RG Jr, Couch RB. A prospective study of chronic herpes simplex virus infection and recurrent herpes labialis in humans. J Immunol. 1970;104(2):289–95.
18. Amir J. Clinical aspects and antiviral therapy in primary herpetic gingivostomatitis. Paediatr Drugs. 2001;3(8):593–7.

19. Amir J, Harel L, Smetana Z, Varsano I. The natural history of primary herpes simplex type 1 gingivostomatitis in children. Pediatr Dermatol. 1999;16(4):259–63.

20. Whitley R, Kimberlin DW, Prober CG. Pathogenesis and disease. In: Arvin A, Campadelli-Fiume G, Mocarski E, Moore PS, Roizman B, Whitley R, Yamanishi K, editors. Human Herpesviruses: Biology, Therapy, and Immunoprophylaxis. Cambridge: Cambridge University Press; 2007. Chapter 32. PMID: 21348130.

21. Anderson BJ. The epidemiology and clinical analysis of several outbreaks of herpes gladiatorum. Med Sci Sports Exerc. 2003;35(11):1809–14.

22. Wollenberg A, Wetzel S, Burgdorf WH, Haas J. Viral infections in atopic dermatitis: pathogenic aspects and clinical management. J Allergy Clin Immunol. 2003;112(4):667–74.

23. Rubright JH, Shafritz AB. The herpetic whitlow. J Hand Surg Am. 2011;36(2):340–2.

24. Walker LG, Simmons BP, Lovallo JL. Pediatric herpetic hand infections. J Hand Surg Am. 1990;15(1):176–80.

25. Saleh D, Yarrarapu SNS, Sharma S. Herpes Simplex Type 1. [Updated 2020 Nov 21]. In: StatPearls [Internet]. Treasure Island (FL): StatPearls Publishing; 2020. Available from: https://www.ncbi.nlm.nih.gov/books/NBK482197/.

26. Corey L. Laboratory diagnosis of herpes simplex virus infections. Principles guiding the development of rapid diagnostic tests. Diagn Microbiol Infect Dis. 1986;4(3 Suppl):111S–9S.

27. Paz-Bailey G, Ramaswamy M, Hawkes SJ, Geretti AM. Herpes simplex virus type 2: epidemiology and management options in developing countries. Sex Transm Infect. 2007;83(1):16–22.

28. Corey L, Adams HG, Brown ZA, Holmes KK. Genital herpes simplex virus infections: clinical manifestations, course, and complications. Ann Intern Med. 1983;98(6):958–72.

29. Kimberlin DW, Rouse DJ. Clinical practice. Genital herpes. N Engl J Med. 2004;350(19):1970–7.

30. Wald A, Zeh J, Selke S, Ashley RL, Corey L. Virologic characteristics of subclinical and symptomatic genital herpes infections. N Engl J Med. 1995;333(12):770–5.

31. Sauerbrei A. Herpes Genitalis: diagnosis, treatment and prevention. Geburtshilfe Frauenheilkd. 2016;76(12):1310–7.

32. Cernik C, Gallina K, Brodell RT. The treatment of herpes simplex infections: an evidence-based review. Arch Intern Med. 2008;168(11):1137–44.

33. Kimberlin DW. Herpes simplex virus infections of the newborn. Semin Perinatol. 2007;31(1):19–25.

34. Whitley R, Arvin A, Prober C, Corey L, Burchett S, Plotkin S, et al. Predictors of morbidity and mortality in neonates with herpes simplex virus infections. The National Institute of Allergy and Infectious Diseases Collaborative Antiviral Study Group. N Engl J Med. 1991;324(7):450–4.

35. Rudnick CM, Hoekzema GS. Neonatal herpes simplex virus infections. Am Fam Physician. 2002;65(6):1138–42.

36. Bernstein DI, Bellamy AR, Hook EW 3rd, Levin MJ, Wald A, Ewell MG, et al. Epidemiology, clinical presentation, and antibody response to primary infection with herpes simplex virus type 1 and type 2 in young women. Clin Infect Dis. 2013;56(3):344–51.

37. Jin F, Prestage GP, Mao L, Kippax SC, Pell CM, Donovan B, et al. Transmission of herpes simplex virus types 1 and 2 in a prospective cohort of HIV-negative gay men: the health in men study. J Infect Dis. 2006;194(5):561–70.

38. O'Brien JJ, Campoli-Richards DM. Acyclovir. An updated review of its antiviral activity, pharmacokinetic properties and therapeutic efficacy. Drugs. 1989;37(3):233–309.

39. Beauman JG. Genital herpes: a review. Am Fam Physician. 2005;72(8):1527–34.

40. Jiang YC, Feng H, Lin YC, Guo XR. New strategies against drug resistance to herpes simplex virus. Int J Oral Sci. 2016;8(1):1–6.

41. Piret J, Boivin G. Antiviral resistance in herpes simplex virus and varicella-zoster virus infections: diagnosis and management. Curr Opin Infect Dis. 2016;29(6):654–62.

42. Bacon TH, Levin MJ, Leary JJ, Sarisky RT, Sutton D. Herpes simplex virus resistance to acyclovir and penciclovir after two decades of antiviral therapy. Clin Microbiol Rev. 2003;16(1):114–28.

43. Straus SE, Ostrove JM, Inchauspe G, Felser JM, Freifeld A, Croen KD, et al. NIH conference. Varicella-zoster virus infections. Biology, natural history, treatment, and prevention. Ann Intern Med. 1988;108(2):221–37.

44. Ku CC, Zerboni L, Ito H, Graham BS, Wallace M, Arvin AM. Varicella-zoster virus transfer to skin by T cells and modulation of viral replication by epidermal cell interferon-alpha. J Exp Med. 2004;200(7):917–25.

45. Levin MJ. Varicella-zoster virus and virus DNA in the blood and oropharynx of people with latent or active varicella-zoster virus infections. J Clin Virol. 2014;61(4):487–95.

46. Heininger U, Seward JF. Varicella. Lancet. 2006;368(9544):1365–76.

47. Reynolds MA, Watson BM, Plott-Adams KK, Jumaan AO, Galil K, Maupin TJ, et al. Epidemiology of varicella hospitalizations in the United States, 1995–2005. J Infect Dis. 2008;197(Suppl 2):S120–6.

48. Arvin AM, Moffat JF, Redman R. Varicella-zoster virus: aspects of pathogenesis and host response to natural infection and varicella vaccine. Adv Virus Res. 1996;46:263–309.

49. Dworkin RH, Johnson RW, Breuer J, Gnann JW, Levin MJ, Backonja M, et al. Recommendations for the management of herpes zoster. Clin Infect Dis. 2007;44(Suppl 1):S1–26.

50. Tyring SK. Vaccination of older adults against herpes zoster is safe and effective. Evid Based Med. 2013;18(5):e43.

51. Lal H, Cunningham AL, Godeaux O, Chlibek R, Diez-Domingo J, Hwang SJ, et al. Efficacy of an adjuvanted herpes zoster subunit vaccine in older adults. N Engl J Med. 2015;372(22):2087–96.

52. Tricco AC, Zarin W, Cardoso R, Veroniki AA, Khan PA, Nincic V, et al. Efficacy, effectiveness, and safety of herpes zoster vaccines in adults aged 50 and older: systematic review and network meta-analysis. BMJ. 2018;363:k4029.

53. McGirr A, Widenmaier R, Curran D, Espie E, Mrkvan T, Oostvogels L, et al. The comparative efficacy and safety of herpes zoster vaccines: a network meta-analysis. Vaccine. 2019;37(22):2896–909.

54. Liesegang TJ. Herpes zoster ophthalmicus natural history, risk factors, clinical presentation, and morbidity. Ophthalmology. 2008;115(2 Suppl):S3–12.

55. Sweeney CJ, Gilden DH. Ramsay Hunt syndrome. J Neurol Neurosurg Psychiatry. 2001;71(2):149–54.

56. Kim SR, Khan F, Ramirez-Fort MK, Downing C, Tyring SK. Varicella zoster: an update on current treatment options and future perspectives. Expert Opin Pharmacother. 2014;15(1):61–71.

57. Gabutti G, Valente N, Sulcaj N, Stefanati A. Evaluation of efficacy and effectiveness of live attenuated zoster vaccine. J Prev Med Hyg. 2014;55(4):130–6.

58. Saint-Leger E, Caumes E, Breton G, Douard D, Saiag P, Huraux JM, et al. Clinical and virologic characterization of acyclovir-resistant varicella-zoster viruses isolated from 11 patients with acquired immunodeficiency syndrome. Clin Infect Dis. 2001;33(12):2061–7.

59. Balfour HH, Jr., Benson C, Braun J, Cassens B, Erice A, Friedman-Kien A, et al. Management of acyclovir-resistant herpes simplex and varicella-zoster virus infections. J Acquir Immune Defic Syndr (1988) 1994;7(3):254–260.

60. Miller GD, Tindall JP. Hand-foot-and-mouth disease. JAMA. 1968;203(10):827–30.

61. Berlin LE, Rorabaugh ML, Heldrich F, Roberts K, Doran T, Modlin JF. Aseptic meningitis in infants < 2 years of age: diagnosis and etiology. J Infect Dis. 1993;168(4):888–92.

62. Weller TH, Enders JF, Buckingham M, Finn JJ Jr. The etiology of epidemic pleurodynia: a study of two viruses isolated from a typical outbreak. J Immunol. 1950;65(3):337–46.

63. Lott JP, Liu K, Landry M-L, Nix WA, Oberste MS, Bolognia J, et al. Atypical hand-foot-and-mouth disease associated with coxsackievirus A6 infection. J Am Acad Dermatol. 2013;69(5):736–41.

64. Anh NT, Nhu LNT, Van HMT, Hong NTT, Thanh TT, Hang VTT, et al. Emerging Coxsackievirus A6 causing hand, foot and mouth disease, Vietnam. Emerg Infect Dis. 2018;24(4):654–62.

65. Osterback R, Vuorinen T, Linna M, Susi P, Hyypiä T, Waris M. Coxsackievirus A6 and hand, foot, and mouth disease, Finland. Emerg Infect Dis. 2009;15(9):1485–8.

66. Guimbao J, Rodrigo P, Alberto MJ, Omenaca M. Onychomadesis outbreak linked to hand, foot, and mouth disease, Spain, July 2008. Euro Surveill. 2010;15(37):19663.

67. Kimmis BD, Downing C, Tyring S. Hand-foot-and-mouth disease caused by coxsackievirus A6 on the rise. Cutis. 2018;102(5):353–6.

68. Hao C, Hao C, Luo J, Li J. Genomic features of coxsackievirus A6 correlate with herpangina and hand, foot and mouth disease. Futur Virol. 2016;11(4):259.

69. Vogels CBF, Ruckert C, Cavany SM, Perkins TA, Ebel GD, Grubaugh ND. Arbovirus coinfection and co-transmission: a neglected public health concern? (unsolved mystery). PLoS Biol. 2019;17(1):e3000130.

70. Martinez JD, Garza JAC-dL, Cuellar-Barboza A. Going Viral 2019. Dermatol Clin. 2019;37(1):95–105.

71. Burt FJ, Chen W, Miner JJ, Lenschow DJ, Merits A, Schnettler E, et al. Chikungunya virus: an update on the biology and pathogenesis of this emerging pathogen. Lancet Infect Dis. 2017;17(4):e107–e17.

72. Dutta SK, Tripathi A. Association of toll-like receptor polymorphisms with susceptibility to chikungunya virus infection. Virology. 2017;511:207–13.

73. WHO Guidelines Approved by the Guidelines Review Committee. Dengue: guidelines for diagnosis, treatment, prevention and control: new edition. Geneva: World Health Organization World Health Organization; 2009.

74. Prompetchara E, Ketloy C, Thomas SJ, Ruxrungtham K. Dengue vaccine: global development update. Asian Pac J Allergy Immunol. 2019;38(3):178–85.

75. Mizumoto K, Ejima K, Yamamoto T, Nishiura H. On the risk of severe dengue during secondary infection: a systematic review coupled with mathematical modeling. J Vector Borne Dis. 2014;51(3):153–64.

76. Sakuntabhai A, Turbpaiboon C, Casademont I, Chuansumrit A, Lowhnoo T, Kajaste-Rudnitski A, et al. A variant in the CD209 promoter is associated with severity of dengue disease. Nat Genet. 2005;37(5):507–13.

77. Wang L, Chen R-F, Liu J-W, Lee I-K, Lee C-P, Kuo H-C, et al. DC-SIGN (CD209) promoter −336 A/G polymorphism is associated with dengue hemorrhagic fever and correlated to DC-SIGN expression and immune augmentation. PLoS Negl Trop Dis. 2011;5(1):e934.

78. Lan NTP, Kikuchi M, Huong VTQ, Ha DQ, Thuy TT, Tham VD, et al. Protective and enhancing HLA alleles, HLA-DRB1*0901 and HLA-A*24, for severe forms of dengue virus infection, dengue hemorrhagic fever and dengue shock syndrome (HLA-DRB1*0901 and A*24 affect DHF/DSS). PLoS Negl Trop Dis. 2008;2(10):e304.

79. Loke H, Bethell DB, Phuong CXT, Dung M, Schneider J, White NJ, et al. Strong HLA class I–restricted T cell responses in dengue hemorrhagic fever: a double-edged sword? J Infect Dis. 2001;184(11):1369–73.

80. Chapter 1 – Origin of Zika Virus Disease. In: Qureshi AI, editor. Zika Virus Disease. Cambridge, Massachusetts: Academic Press; 2018. p. 1–25.

81. Zika. Aftab R. InnovAiT. 2017;10(4):224–7.

82. Faye O, Freire CC, Iamarino A, Faye O, de Oliveira JV, Diallo M, et al. Molecular evolution of Zika virus during its emergence in the 20(th) century. PLoS Negl Trop Dis. 2014;8(1):e2636.

83. Schuler-Faccini LRE, Feitosa IM, et al. Possible Association Between Zika Virus Infection and Microcephaly. MMWR Morb Mortal Wkly Rep 2016. 2015;65:59–62.

84. Yuan L, Huang X-Y, Liu Z-Y, Zhang F, Zhu X-L, Yu J-Y, et al. A single mutation in the prM protein of Zika virus contributes to fetal microcephaly. Science. 2017;358(6365):933–6.

85. Chapter 8 – Clinical manifestations and laboratory diagnosis of Zika virus disease. In: Qureshi AI, editor. Zika virus disease. Cambridge, Massachusetts: Academic Press; 2018. p. 103–115.

86. Parra B, Lizarazo J, Jimenez-Arango JA, Zea-Vera AF, Gonzalez-Manrique G, Vargas J, et al. Guillain-Barre syndrome associated with Zika virus infection in Colombia. N Engl J Med. 2016;375(16):1513–23.

87. da Silva IRF, Frontera JA, Bispo de Filippis AM, Nascimento O. Neurologic complications associated with the Zika virus in Brazilian adults. JAMA Neurol. 2017;74(10):1190–8.

88. Abad CL, Safdar N. The reemergence of measles. Curr Infect Dis Rep. 2015;17(12):51.

89. Huiming Y, Chaomin W, Meng M. Vitamin A for treating measles in children. Cochrane Database Syst Rev. 2005;4:CD001479.

90. McLean HQ, Fiebelkorn AP, Temte JL, Wallace GS. Prevention of measles, rubella, congenital rubella syndrome, and mumps, 2013: summary recommendations of the Advisory Committee on Immunization Practices (ACIP). MMWR Recomm Rep. 2013;62(Rr-04):1–34.

91. Understanding emerging and re-emerging infectious diseases. Bethesda: National Institutes of Health (US); 2007.

92. Eggertson L. Lancet retracts 12-year-old article linking autism to MMR vaccines. CMAJ. 2010;182(4):E199–200.

93. CDC Measles Cases in the United States [20 March 2020]. Available from: https://www.cdc.gov/measles/cases-outbreaks.html.

94. Chen T, Hedman L, Mattila PS, Jartti T, Ruuskanen O, Soderlund-Venermo M, et al. Serological evidence of Merkel cell polyomavirus primary infections in childhood. J Clin Virol. 2011;50(2):125–9.

95. Pastrana DV, Tolstov YL, Becker JC, Moore PS, Chang Y, Buck CB. Quantitation of human seroresponsiveness to Merkel cell polyomavirus. PLoS Pathog. 2009;5(9):e1000578.

96. van der Meijden E, Bialasiewicz S, Rockett RJ, Tozer SJ, Sloots TP, Feltkamp MC. Different serologic behavior of MCPyV, TSPyV, HPyV6, HPyV7 and HPyV9 polyomaviruses found on the skin. PLoS One. 2013;8(11):e81078.

97. Schowalter RM, Pastrana DV, Pumphrey KA, Moyer AL, Buck CB. Merkel cell polyomavirus and two previously unknown polyomaviruses are chronically shed from human skin. Cell Host Microbe. 2010;7(6):509–15.

98. Engels EA, Frisch M, Goedert JJ, Biggar RJ, Miller RW. Merkel cell carcinoma and HIV infection. Lancet. 2002;359(9305):497–8.

99. Gooptu C, Woollons A, Ross J, Price M, Wojnarowska F, Morris PJ, et al. Merkel cell carcinoma arising after therapeutic immunosuppression. Br J Dermatol. 1997;137(4):637–41.

100. Hampras SS, Giuliano AR, Lin HY, Fisher KJ, Abrahamsen ME, McKay-Chopin S, et al. Natural history of polyomaviruses in men: the HPV infection in men (HIM) study. J Infect Dis. 2015;211(9):1437–46.

101. Feng H, Shuda M, Chang Y, Moore PS. Clonal integration of a polyomavirus in human Merkel cell carcinoma. Science. 2008;319(5866):1096–100.

102. Shuda M, Feng H, Kwun HJ, Rosen ST, Gjoerup O, Moore PS, et al. T antigen mutations are a human tumor-specific signature for Merkel cell polyomavirus. Proc Natl Acad Sci U S A. 2008;105(42):16272–7.

103. Schmitt M, Wieland U, Kreuter A, Pawlita M. C-terminal deletions of Merkel cell polyomavirus large T-antigen, a highly specific surrogate marker for virally induced malignancy. Int J Cancer. 2012;131(12):2863–8.

104. Shuda M, Kwun HJ, Feng H, Chang Y, Moore PS. Human Merkel cell polyomavirus small T antigen is an oncoprotein targeting the 4E-BP1 translation regulator. J Clin Invest. 2011;121(9):3623–34.

105. Paulson KG, Lewis CW, Redman MW, Simonson WT, Lisberg A, Ritter D, et al. Viral oncoprotein antibodies as a marker for recurrence of Merkel cell carcinoma: a prospective validation study. Cancer. 2017;123(8):1464–74.

106. Fitzgerald TL, Dennis S, Kachare SD, Vohra NA, Wong JH, Zervos EE. Dramatic increase in the incidence and mortality from Merkel cell carcinoma in the United States. Am Surg. 2015;81(8):802–6.

107. Lemos BD, Storer BE, Iyer JG, Phillips JL, Bichakjian CK, Fang LC, et al. Pathologic nodal evaluation improves prognostic accuracy in Merkel cell carcinoma: analysis of 5823 cases as the basis of the first consensus staging system. J Am Acad Dermatol. 2010;63(5):751–61.

108. Heath M, Jaimes N, Lemos B, Mostaghimi A, Wang LC, Penas PF, et al. Clinical characteristics of Merkel cell carcinoma at diagnosis in 195 patients: the AEIOU features. J Am Acad Dermatol. 2008;58(3):375–81.

109. Harms KL, Healy MA, Nghiem P, Sober AJ, Johnson TM, Bichakjian CK, et al. Analysis of prognostic factors from 9387 Merkel cell carcinoma cases

forms the basis for the new 8th edition AJCC staging system. Ann Surg Oncol. 2016;23(11):3564–71.

110. Muirhead R, Ritchie DM. Partial regression of Merkel cell carcinoma in response to withdrawal of azathioprine in an immunosuppression-induced case of metastatic Merkel cell carcinoma. Clin Oncol (R Coll Radiol). 2007;19(1):96.

111. Wong HH, Wang J. Merkel cell carcinoma. Arch Pathol Lab Med. 2010;134(11):1711–6.

112. Jaeger T, Ring J, Andres C. Histological, immuno-histological, and clinical features of merkel cell carcinoma in correlation to merkel cell polyomavirus status. J Skin Cancer. 2012;2012:983421.

113. Leroux-Kozal V, Leveque N, Brodard V, Lesage C, Dudez O, Makeieff M, et al. Merkel cell carcinoma: histopathologic and prognostic features according to the immunohistochemical expression of Merkel cell polyomavirus large T antigen correlated with viral load. Hum Pathol. 2015;46(3):443–53.

114. Gardair C, Samimi M, Touze A, Coursaget P, Lorette G, Caille A, et al. Somatostatin receptors 2A and 5 are expressed in Merkel cell carcinoma with no association with disease severity. Neuroendocrinology. 2015;101(3):223–35.

115. Moshiri AS, Doumani R, Yelistratova L, Blom A, Lachance K, Shinohara MM, et al. Polyomavirus-negative Merkel cell carcinoma: a more aggressive subtype based on analysis of 282 cases using multimodal tumor virus detection. J Invest Dermatol. 2017;137(4):819–27.

116. Harrington C, Kwan W. Outcomes of Merkel cell carcinoma treated with radiotherapy without radical surgical excision. Ann Surg Oncol. 2014;21(11):3401–5.

117. Strom T, Carr M, Zager JS, Naghavi A, Smith FO, Cruse CW, et al. Radiation therapy is associated with improved outcomes in Merkel cell carcinoma. Ann Surg Oncol. 2016;23(11):3572–8.

118. Chen MM, Roman SA, Sosa JA, Judson BL. The role of adjuvant therapy in the management of head and neck merkel cell carcinoma: an analysis of 4815 patients. JAMA Otolaryngol Head Neck Surg. 2015;141(2):137–41.

119. D'Angelo SP, Bhatia S, Brohl AS, Hamid O, Mehnert JM, Terheyden P, et al. Avelumab in patients with previously treated metastatic Merkel cell carcinoma: long-term data and biomarker analyses from the single-arm phase 2 JAVELIN Merkel 200 trial. J Immunother Cancer. 2020;8(1)

120. Kaufman HL, Russell J, Hamid O, Bhatia S, Terheyden P, D'Angelo SP, et al. Avelumab in patients with chemotherapy-refractory metastatic Merkel cell carcinoma: a multicentre, single-group, open-label, phase 2 trial. Lancet Oncol. 2016;17(10):1374–85.

121. Kaufman HL, Russell JS, Hamid O, Bhatia S, Terheyden P, D'Angelo SP, et al. Updated efficacy of avelumab in patients with previously treated metastatic Merkel cell carcinoma after >/=1 year of follow-up: JAVELIN Merkel 200, a phase 2 clinical trial. J Immunother Cancer. 2018;6(1):7.

122. D'Angelo SP, Russell J, Lebbe C, Chmielowski B, Gambichler T, Grob JJ, et al. Efficacy and safety of first-line Avelumab treatment in patients with stage IV metastatic Merkel cell carcinoma: a preplanned interim analysis of a clinical trial. JAMA Oncol. 2018;4(9):e180077.

123. Nghiem PT, Bhatia S, Lipson EJ, Kudchadkar RR, Miller NJ, Annamalai L, et al. PD-1 blockade with Pembrolizumab in advanced Merkel-cell carcinoma. N Engl J Med. 2016;374(26):2542–52.

124. van der Meijden E, Janssens RW, Lauber C, Bouwes Bavinck JN, Gorbalenya AE, Feltkamp MC. Discovery of a new human polyomavirus associated with trichodysplasia spinulosa in an immunocompromised patient. PLoS Pathog. 2010;6(7):e1001024.

125. Chen T, Mattila PS, Jartti T, Ruuskanen O, Soderlund-Venermo M, Hedman K. Seroepidemiology of the newly found trichodysplasia spinulosa-associated polyomavirus. J Infect Dis. 2011;204(10):1523–6.

126. Wu JH, Simonette RA, Nguyen HP, Rady PL, Tyring SK. Small T-antigen of the TS-associated polyomavirus activates factors implicated in the MAPK pathway. J Eur Acad Dermatol Venereol. 2016;30(6):1061–2.

127. Nguyen HP, Patel A, Simonette RA, Rady P, Tyring SK. Binding of the trichodysplasia spinulosa-associated polyomavirus small T antigen to protein phosphatase 2A: elucidation of a potential pathogenic mechanism in a rare skin disease. JAMA Dermatol. 2014;150(11):1234–6.

128. Wu JH, Narayanan D, Simonette RA, Rady PL, Tyring SK. Dysregulation of the MEK/ERK/MNK1 signalling cascade by middle T antigen of the trichodysplasia spinulosa polyomavirus. J Eur Acad Dermatol Venereol. 2017;31(8):1338–41.

129. Haycox CL, Kim S, Fleckman P, Smith LT, Piepkorn M, Sundberg JP, et al. Trichodysplasia spinulosa–a newly described folliculocentric viral infection in an immunocompromised host. J Investig Dermatol Symp Proc. 1999;4(3):268–71.

130. Kazem S, van der Meijden E, Feltkamp MC. The trichodysplasia spinulosa-associated polyomavirus: virological background and clinical implications. APMIS. 2013;121(8):770–82.

131. Fischer MK, Kao GF, Nguyen HP, Drachenberg CB, Rady PL, Tyring SK, et al. Specific detection of trichodysplasia spinulosa-associated polyomavirus DNA in skin and renal allograft tissues in a patient with trichodysplasia spinulosa. Arch Dermatol. 2012;148(6):726–33.

132. Holzer AM, Hughey LC. Trichodysplasia of immunosuppression treated with oral valganciclovir. J Am Acad Dermatol. 2009;60(1):169–72.

133. Benoit T, Bacelieri R, Morrell DS, Metcalf J. Viral-associated trichodysplasia of immunosuppression: report of a pediatric patient with response to oral valganciclovir. Arch Dermatol. 2010;146(8):871–4.

134. Schwieger-Briel A, Balma-Mena A, Ngan B, Dipchand A, Pope E. Trichodysplasia spinulosa–a rare complication in immunosuppressed patients. Pediatr Dermatol. 2010;27(5):509–13.

135. Wanat KA, Holler PD, Dentchev T, Simbiri K, Robertson E, Seykora JT, et al. Viral-associated trichodysplasia: characterization of a novel polyomavirus infection with therapeutic insights. Arch Dermatol. 2012;148(2):219–23.

136. Laroche A, Allard C, Chababi-Atallah M, Masse M, Bertrand J. Trichodysplasia spinulosa in a renal transplant patient. J Cutan Med Surg. 2015;19(1):66–8.

137. Wieland U, Silling S, Hellmich M, Potthoff A, Pfister H, Kreuter A. Human polyomaviruses 6, 7, 9, 10 and Trichodysplasia spinulosa-associated polyomavirus in HIV-infected men. J Gen Virol. 2014;95(Pt 4):928–32.

138. Johne R, Buck CB, Allander T, Atwood WJ, Garcea RL, Imperiale MJ, et al. Taxonomical developments in the family Polyomaviridae. Arch Virol. 2011;156(9):1627–34.

139. Nguyen KD, Lee EE, Yue Y, Stork J, Pock L, North JP, et al. Human polyomavirus 6 and 7 are associated with pruritic and dyskeratotic dermatoses. J Am Acad Dermatol. 2017;76(5):932–40.e3.

140. Ho J, Jedrych JJ, Feng H, Natalie AA, Grandinetti L, Mirvish E, et al. Human polyomavirus 7-associated pruritic rash and viremia in transplant recipients. J Infect Dis. 2015;211(10):1560–5.

141. Wu JH, Simonette RA, Nguyen HP, Rady PL, Tyring SK. Molecular mechanisms supporting a pathogenic role for human polyomavirus 6 small T antigen: protein phosphatase 2A targeting and MAPK cascade activation. J Med Virol. 2017;89(4):742–7.

142. Schrama D, Groesser L, Ugurel S, Hafner C, Pastrana DV, Buck CB, et al. Presence of human polyomavirus 6 in mutation-specific BRAF inhibitor-induced epithelial proliferations. JAMA Dermatol. 2014;150(11):1180–6.

143. Benvenuto D, Giovanetti M, Ciccozzi A, Spoto S, Angeletti S, Ciccozzi M. The 2019-new coronavirus epidemic: evidence for virus evolution. J Med Virol. 2020;92(4):455–9.

144. Stadnytskyi V, Bax CE, Bax A, Anfinrud P. The airborne lifetime of small speech droplets and their potential importance in SARS-CoV-2 transmission. Proc Natl Acad Sci U S A. 2020;117(22):11875–7.

145. Zhou P, Yang XL, Wang XG, Hu B, Zhang L, Zhang W, et al. A pneumonia outbreak associated with a new coronavirus of probable bat origin. Nature. 2020;579(7798):270–3.

146. Bahl P, Doolan C, de Silva C, Chughtai AA, Bourouiba L, MacIntyre CR. Airborne or droplet precautions for health workers treating COVID-19? J Infect Dis. 2020, [online ahead of print].

147. Zhang Y, Cao W, Xiao M, Li YJ, Yang Y, Zhao J, et al. Clinical and coagulation characteristics of 7 patients with critical COVID-2019 pneumonia and acro-ischemia. Zhonghua Xue Ye Xue Za Zhi. 2020;41(0):E006.

148. Recalcati S. Cutaneous manifestations in COVID-19: a first perspective. J Eur Acad Dermatol Venereol. 2020;34(5):e212–e3.

149. Najarian DJ. Morbilliform Exanthem associated with COVID-19. JAAD Case Rep. 2020;6(6):493–4.

150. Sachdeva M, Gianotti R, Shah M, Lucia B, Tosi D, Veraldi S, et al. Cutaneous manifestations of COVID-19: report of three cases and a review of literature. J Dermatol Sci. 2020;98(2):75–81.

151. Marzano AV, Genovese G, Fabbrocini G, Pigatto P, Monfrecola G, Piraccini BM, et al. Varicella-like exanthem as a specific COVID-19-associated skin manifestation: multicenter case series of 22 patients. J Am Acad Dermatol. 2020;83(1):280–5.

152. Fernandez-Nieto D, Ortega-Quijano D, Jimenez-Cauhe J, Burgos-Blasco P, de Perosanz-Lobo D, Suarez-Valle A, et al. Clinical and histological characterization of vesicular COVID-19 rashes: a prospective study in a tertiary care hospital. Clin Exp Dermatol. 2020;45(7):872–5.

153. Freeman EE, McMahon DE, Lipoff JB, Rosenbach M, Kovarik C, Takeshita J, et al. Pernio-like skin lesions associated with COVID-19: a case series of 318 patients from 8 countries. J Am Acad Dermatol. 2020;83(2):486–92.

154. Andina D, Noguera-Morel L, Bascuas-Arribas M, Gaitero-Tristan J, Alonso-Cadenas JA, Escalada-Pellitero S, et al. Chilblains in children in the setting of COVID-19 pandemic. Pediatr Dermatol. 2020;37(3):406–11.

155. Docampo-Simon A, Sanchez-Pujol MJ, Juan-Carpena G, Palazon-Cabanes JC, Vergara-De Caso E, Berbegal L, et al. Are chilblain-like acral skin lesions really indicative of COVID-19? A prospective study and literature review. J Eur Acad Dermatol Venereol. 2020;34(9):e445–7.

156. Magro C, Mulvey JJ, Berlin D, Nuovo G, Salvatore S, Harp J, et al. Complement associated microvascular injury and thrombosis in the pathogenesis of severe COVID-19 infection: a report of five cases. Transl Res. 2020;220:1–13.

157. Zhang Y, Cao W, Xiao M, Li YJ, Yang Y, Zhao J, et al. Clinical and coagulation characteristics in 7 patients with critical COVID-2019 pneumonia and acro-ischemia. Zhonghua Xue Ye Xue Za Zhi. 2020;41(4):302–7.

158. Llamas-Velasco M, Munoz-Hernandez P, Lazaro-Gonzalez J, Reolid-Perez A, Abad-Santamaria B, Fraga J, et al. Thrombotic occlusive vasculopathy in skin biopsy from a livedoid lesion of a COVID-19 patient. Br J Dermatol. 2020;183(3):564–95.

159. Tang N, Li D, Wang X, Sun Z. Abnormal coagulation parameters are associated with poor prognosis in patients with novel coronavirus pneumonia. J Thromb Haemost. 2020;18(4):844–7.

160. Tang N, Bai H, Chen X, Gong J, Li D, Sun Z. Anticoagulant treatment is associated with decreased mortality in severe coronavirus disease 2019 patients with coagulopathy. J Thromb Haemost. 2020;18(5):1094–9.

Reemerging Viral Infections: Implications of Lack of Vaccination

Ritu Swali, Claire Wiggins, Sahira Farooq, Radhika A. Shah, and Emily Limmer

Abbreviations

AIDS	Acquired immunodeficiency syndrome
CCHF	Crimean-Congo hemorrhagic fever
CDC	Centers for Disease Control and Prevention
CRS	Congenital rubella syndrome
CSF	Cerebrospinal fluid
DFA	Direct fluorescent antibody
DNA	Deoxyribonucleic acid
ELISA	Enzyme-linked immunosorbent assay
HBV	Hepatitis B virus
HCV	Hepatitis C virus
HI	Hemagglutinin inhibition
HIV	Human immunodeficiency virus
HLA	Human leukocyte antigen
HPV	Human papillomavirus
HZ	Herpes zoster
IFN	Interferon
Ig	Immunoglobulin
MMR	Measles-mumps-rubella
MMRV	Measles-mumps-rubella-varicella
NSAID	Nonsteroidal anti-inflammatory drug
PCR	Polymerase chain reaction
PHN	Postherpetic neuralgia
PRN	Plaque reduction neutralization
RNA	Ribonucleic acid
RV	Rubella virus
SARS	Severe acute respiratory syndrome
SPS	Shingles Prevention Study
STI	Sexually transmitted infection
UV	Ultraviolet
VZV	Varicella-zoster virus
WHO	World Health Organization

R. Swali (✉)
Department of Dermatology, University of Nebraska Medical Center, Omaha, NE, USA

C. Wiggins
Baylor College of Medicine, Houston, TX, USA

S. Farooq
McGovern Medical School and UT Health, Houston, TX, USA

R. A. Shah
Texas A&M University, Dallas, TX, USA

E. Limmer
University of Texas Southwestern Medical Center, Dallas, TX, USA

Introduction

Mucocutaneous manifestations of viruses result from the replication of viral organisms either primarily in the epidermis or as a secondary effect of viral replication elsewhere [1]. Along with being the largest physical barrier against pathologic microorganisms, the skin has an innate antiviral immune system composed of endogenous antiviral proteins, e.g., interferons as well as interferon-independent pathways, and environmental factors [2]. However, in certain populations, a loss, lack of, or suppression of antiviral proteins will make way for viral diseases to manifest. Patients with inflammatory skin conditions, at extremes of age, and with an immunocompro-

© Springer Nature Switzerland AG 2021
S. K. Tyring et al. (eds.), *Overcoming Antimicrobial Resistance of the Skin*, Updates in Clinical Dermatology, https://doi.org/10.1007/978-3-030-68321-4_7

mised status could benefit from enhanced antiviral immunity [2].

The advent of vaccinations changed the face of modern medicine in 1796 when Edward Jenner noted that milkmaids who had bouts of cowpox did not contract smallpox. At the time, smallpox had a 30% mortality rate and left survivors with debilitating scars, including corneal scars, resulting in blindness [3]. After several years, he published his research in "On the Origin of the Vaccine Inoculation," documenting that variolation could, and would, eventually lead to the eradication of the "speckled monster" [3]. The smallpox vaccine with public health measures led to eradication of the number one infectious disease killer in the history of the world (until the last smallpox patient was treated in 1977). Since

then, the development of vaccines for other infections has markedly reduced morbidity and mortality from multiple fatal infectious diseases in many parts of the world (Fig. 7.1) [4].

Vaccines provide active immunity by introducing a modified component of a pathogen to the host, thus stimulating the host's immune system to memorize how to identify and attack the virus upon re-exposure. Passive immunity is developed by transferring antibodies from one host to another, giving the host tools to attack the virus without the ability to recognize it. Many primary and secondary viral skin diseases predominantly have been prevented with active immunization strategies [1].

The recent anti-vaccination movement is rooted in the miseducation of social media influ-

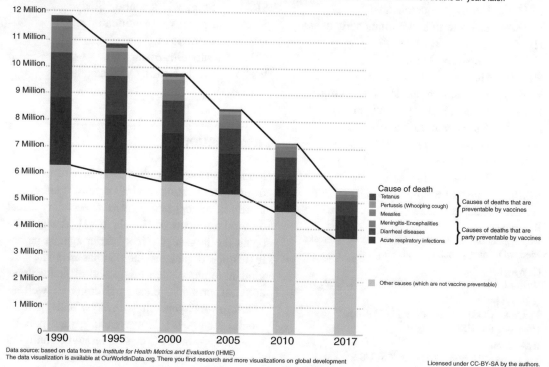

Global number of child deaths per year – by cause of death

Shown is the number of children younger than 5 year who died in a year. The height of the bar shows the total number of deaths with colored sections showing the number of children who died of diseases that are wholly or partially preventable by vaccines.
The number od child deaths for which there are vaccines available declined from 5.5 million deaths in 1990 to 1.8 million deaths 27 years later.

Data source: based on data from the *Institute for Health Metrics and Evaluation* (IHME)
The data visualization is available at OurWorldinData.org. There you find research and more visualizations on global development

Licensed under CC-BY-SA by the authors.

Fig. 7.1 Based on data from the Institute for Health Metrics and Evaluation, vaccine-preventable deaths have dramatically decreased over the past few decades. (Reprinted from Our World in Data: Vaccination, by Vanderslott S, Dadonaite B, and Roser M., 2015. https://ourworldindata.org/vaccination. Link to license: https://creativecommons.org/licenses/by/4.0. No changes were made to the original content)

encers combined with vulnerable parenting. A large role played by the healthcare industry was the publication of a paper in *The Lancet* in 1998 by British physician Andrew Wakefield, who suggested plausibility in the link between autism and the measles-mumps-rubella (MMR) vaccine [5]. The paper was retracted in 2010, accompanied by a detailed commentary in *The British Medical Journal* by Deer et al. the following year, documenting that Wakefield had been paid by anti-vaccine lobbyists to make false proclamations of the dangers of the MMR vaccine [6]. Wakefield subsequently lost his license to practice medicine in the United Kingdom; however, widespread fear of vaccinations had already spread throughout the world, resulting in vaccination refusal [7–10]. Common tactics used by "anti-vaxxers," including skewing science, censoring opposition, attacking critics, and claiming that vaccines are toxic, have been very effective in continuing this trend [11].

Consequentially, unfounded fears of vaccination are often attributed to Wakefield's discredited publication and to general distrust of the medical and pharmaceutical establishments. Fears of adverse effects and vaccine safety far outweigh other societal beliefs to avoid vaccinations (Fig. 7.2) [12]. Other facts, however, may play a role such as the fact most persons currently having children did not suffer these illnesses because their parents had them vaccinated [12]. Therefore, they have no firsthand knowledge of the morbidity and mortality that can result from measles or rubella infections. Furthermore, distrust of western medicine due to political reasons has prevented children from receiving MMR, polio, and other vaccines in conflict zones. For example, Doctors Without Borders were forced to leave certain areas of the Democratic Republic of Congo in 2019, because rebel groups burned their clinics and murdered healthcare workers [13]. Therefore, neither MMR nor the recently approved Ebola vaccine reached the susceptible individuals. Surprisingly, recent surveys on vaccine safety demonstrated higher percentages of distrust in vaccines in regions associated with higher education levels, such as Western Europe and North America, versus regions perceived to have lower education rates, including Africa and Central America (Fig. 7.3) [14].

Another reason that some persons avoid life-saving vaccines may be apathy or the belief that they are not susceptible to a particular infection [12]. The 2019–2020 influenza season is an example: thus far, >12,000 Americans, including 27 children, have died of influenza [15]. Many persons still will not receive the vaccine, citing such pseudo-reasons from previous influenza seasons that the vaccine was not 100% effective; therefore, "it is not worth the pain of the injection." Others may state that the "flu-like syndrome resulting from vaccination is worse than the flu." This statement is extremely misleading, because the cytokine storm that may result from vaccination is not fatal, but influenza kills [12].

Today, previously eliminated viral infections have reemerged, and implications of decreased herd immunity are becoming increasingly apparent.

Reemerging Primary Viral Infections of the Skin

Varicella-Zoster Virus: Primary Varicella (Chickenpox)

Primary varicella-zoster virus (VZV), or varicella, is a highly contagious member of the *Herpesvirus* family. Although only one serotype is known, five viral clades have been identified, spanning Europe (1, 3, and 5), Asia (2), and Africa (4) [16]. The virus evolved alongside early human ancestors, likely originating in Africa and spreading worldwide [17]. VZV is highly host-specific, naturally infecting only humans, primarily affecting pre-adolescent children. Varicella does not have a predilection for any race or gender [18]. The number of chickenpox cases is on the decline after the utilization of effective vaccines; however, as vaccination rates fall, the number of cases will subsequently increase [19, 20].

Historically, varicella was regarded as one of childhood's rites-of-passage, a mere nuisance compared to the threat of the similar appearing, but more sinister, smallpox. However, with small-

O. Yaqub et al. / Social Science & Medicine 112 (2014) 1–11

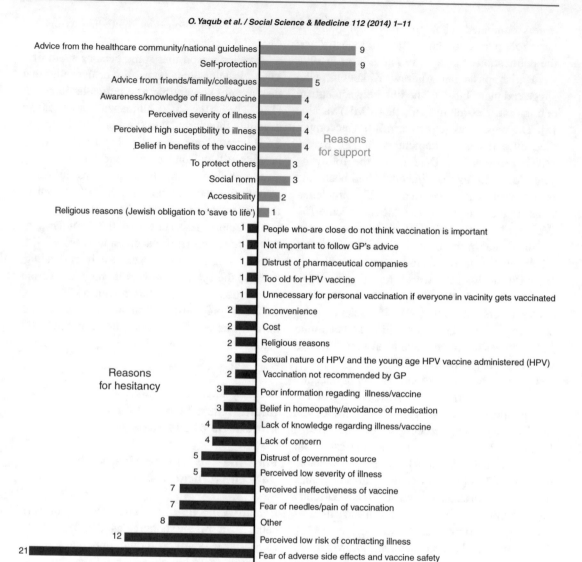

Fig. 7.2 Various reasons for vaccine hesitancy versus vaccine support reported in the literature. (Reprinted from Attitudes to vaccination: A critical review., by Yaqub O, Castle-Clarke S, Sevdalis N, and Chataway J. https://well-come.ac.uk/reports/wellcome-global-monitor/2018/chapter-5-attitudes-vaccines. No changes were made to the original content)

pox long eradicated, the notion of varicella as innocuous was challenged. In the setting of medical advances in pediatric cancer treatments in the 1960s, immunocompromised children, newly cured of cancer, were now at risk for severe morbidity and mortality from VZV [23]. Dr. Thomas Weller was the first to isolate and cell-culture VZV in 1954 and confirm that herpes zoster (HZ) and varicella are caused by the same vector

(VZV) [24]. Dr. Michiaki Takahashi from Japan created the first live attenuated VZV vaccine, approved in 1986. Japan and South Korea were among the first countries to vaccinate for chickenpox in 1988, with the United States following suit in 1995 [25]. The varicella vaccine is licensed and available worldwide but is only used routinely in a subset of countries. In the United States in 1995, there were over 120,000 cases of

Percentage of people who answered 'strongly agree', 'somewhat agree', 'neither agree nor disagree', 'somewhat disagree', 'strongly disagree' or 'no opinion'
Do you agree, disagree, or neither agree nor disagree with the following statement? Vaccines are safe

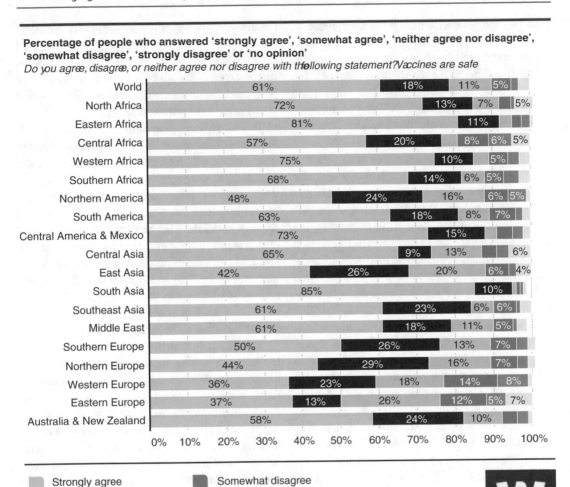

Source: **Wellcome Global Monitor, part of the Gallup World Poll 2018**

Fig. 7.3 Perceived safety of vaccines by region. (Reprinted from Wellcome Global Monitor 2018: Chap. 5: Attitudes to vaccines, by Wellcome Global Monitor. https://www.sciencedirect.com/science/article/pii/ S0277953614002421. Link to license: https://creative-commons.org/licenses/by/3.0/. No changes were made to the original content)

chickenpox and 115 deaths attributed to the virus. Less than 50,000 cases have been reported after 1998 and less than 40 deaths annually since 2000, due to the advent of the chickenpox vaccine [26].

Varicella initially manifests after a prodrome of fever, malaise, and loss of appetite. Over the next week, generalized pruritic papules develop and evolve into vesicles with surrounding erythema, pustules, and lastly crusted papules until

resolution occurs with residual hypopigmentation. Lesions appear in a series of crops so that the different stages of lesion development may be observed at one point in time. Distribution of the lesions is concentrated centrally rather than on distal extremities. In previously healthy patients, the symptoms usually last about 3–7 days. The scabs may take several weeks to heal, however, often leaving behind scars. The severity of disease can range from a barely noticeable rash to hundreds of vesicles. Complications include bacterial superinfection of skin lesions, pneumonia, sepsis, cerebellar ataxia, and encephalitis. Diagnosis is made clinically, but polymerase chain reaction (PCR) for VZV DNA is the laboratory test of choice to confirm the diagnosis when the presentation is atypical [23].

Although it is debated whether or not VZV is transmitted via respiratory droplets, the vesicular fluid is highly contagious. The transmission rate is directly proportional to the number of cutaneous lesions, with no spread of disease in the absence of lesions [27]. Once the virus reaches a susceptible host, the respiratory tract and adjacent lymphatics become infected. VZV then infects T lymphocytes, which migrate to the keratinocytes, among other cells in the body [28]. Although the innate immune system fights back against the virus with the production of alpha-interferon, viral proliferation surmounts this effort, resulting in the production of cutaneous lesions [29]. The incubation period for VZV can be several weeks, mediated by cell-to-cell spread rather than extracellular viral dissemination. It is for this reason that patients who lack a sufficient cell-mediated host response are particularly vulnerable to VZV, as T lymphocyte response is more important than the production of specific antibodies. During primary infection, the virus establishes dormancy in sensory ganglia, where it can be reactivated years later [30, 31].

Primary VZV infection is most common in unvaccinated children, although when it affects unvaccinated adolescents or adults, the clinical course is more severe. Vaccine effectiveness for preventing disease with one dose ranges from 55% to 87%, while two doses prevent 84% to 98% of disease. The United States and Canada are among the few countries that schedule two routine doses of the vaccine [19–22]. Prior to this vaccination policy in the United States, there were 100–150 annual deaths from VZV [32]. The vaccine has proven to be very safe and can even be used safely in select immunocompromised patients [19]. The most common reaction is a mild rash several weeks after vaccination, which

occurs in about 5% of patients [32]. More critical side effects, such as severe rash, pneumonia, and neurological symptoms, have been documented rarely around the globe in children who were immunocompromised without knowledge of this status prior to vaccination [23].

Because vaccination rates remain moderate to high, major decreases in varicella disease burden have been seen. However, as expansion of the vaccination programs continues, concern has been raised that vaccination produces weaker immunity than would be naturally derived through infection. This may translate to increased cost and morbidity associated with herpes zoster (HZ). The effects of preventing primary infection have yet to be fully realized, particularly in the setting of additionally vaccinating for HZ. There have been studies showing up to 72% reduced risk of HZ after VZV vaccine in pediatrics [33].

Therapy for varicella previously was supportive care to reduce inflammation and pruritus; however, well-tolerated oral antiviral medications, such as acyclovir, are commonly used today. Acyclovir-resistant VZV is rare, but in such cases foscarnet may be alternatively used. In healthy patients less than 12 years of age, antiviral treatment is not typically recommended, but is cost-effective, because it allows the child and parent to return to school and work sooner. Potential complications of varicella include bacterial superinfection of lesions, neurological symptoms, and maternal pneumonia and congenital transmission in pregnant women. Prognosis with treatment is favorable but is worse in immunocompromised and elderly patients [34].

Varicella-Zoster Virus: Herpes Zoster (Shingles)

Recognition of the dermatomal rash of herpes zoster (HZ)—also known as shingles—dates back to ancient times. HZ has been aptly named across cultures: in Spanish, Culebrilla literally means "small snake"; in Norwegian, Helvetesild translates to "hell's fire"; in German, Gürtelrose is "belt of rose(thorns)"; and in Arabic, Hezam innar describes a "belt of fire" [35]. In 1888, von Bokay suggested a relationship between chickenpox and HZ after he observed that children without varicella immunity developed chickenpox following exposure to HZ [36, 37].

HZ is highly prevalent and, per some studies, increasing in age-adjusted incidence worldwide, although precise epidemiologic data is difficult to obtain [38, 39]. Data from different populations within several countries estimate a median zoster incidence of 4 to 4.5 per 1000 person-years. In immunocompetent individuals, this rate is estimated at 1.2 to 3.4 cases per 1000 person-years, with an increased risk in those older than 65 years of age at 3.9 to 11.8 cases per 1000 person-years [35, 40]. Approximately 1 million cases of HZ occur annually in the United States, with 8% of those cases in immunocompromised patients. HZ risk increases with age. The average age of onset in adults is 50 years. Postherpetic neuralgia (PHN), the most common HZ complication, also increases with age, with 80% of cases occurring in patients older than 50 years [35]. As the percentage of elderly people in the global population increases, it is likely that more cases of HZ will be seen each year. Other than age and immune status, a family history of HZ is the best predictor of shingles [41, 42]. Through strategic adult vaccination for HZ, boosting the aging immune system to protect against viral reactivation, HZ complications can be prevented.

In contrast to varicella, which is caused by an acute varicella-zoster virus (VZV) infection, HZ is caused by a reactivation of the same virus, which commonly lies dormant in the dorsal root ganglia, autonomic ganglia, and cranial nerve ganglia [35]. VZV reactivation events are typically suppressed by T-cell-mediated immunity and remain subclinical [43]. However, in immunosuppressed or immunosenescent individuals with weakened cell-mediated immunity, VZV reactivation yields clinical HZ. Viral replication results in ganglionitis and local destruction of tissue, producing an inflammatory response that is the likely cause of the classic prodromal pain of HZ [35].

HZ patients typically experience a prodromal pain, often described as "burning," "stabbing," or "shooting," the cause of which becomes apparent once dermatomal skin lesions become visible days later [44]. The time from the onset of pain to the outbreak of skin lesions represents the transit time for the virus to spread from the ganglia, down the nerve endings, to the epidermal-dermal junction to finally replicate at the skin's surface. First, an erythematous, macular phase develops which progresses into papules and vesicles. HZ lesions can be seen at all stages of development once the vesicular phase is reached. Vesicular pustulation occurs within a week of rash onset, and after several more days, lesions ulcerate and crust over. These crusts take longer to resolve, usually after several weeks, potentially leaving behind areas of hypo-/hyper-pigmentation or scarring. If vesicular lesions continue to erupt for longer than a week, or if there is extensive involvement of multiple dermatomes, investigation for an underlying immunodeficiency should be conducted [35].

HZ is generally diagnosed clinically based on the characteristic rash and other accompanying signs and symptoms. However, in some cases, the diagnosis may be less obvious. The rash may be absent (as in zoster *sine* herpete), limited, or, in the case of immunocompromised patients, atypical [45]. These situations warrant further diagnostic testing. Polymerase chain reaction (PCR) is the preferred method as it provides results in about a day and is the most sensitive and specific laboratory test for detecting VZV [36]. PCR can test lesions of all stages and can aid in the diagnosis of vaccine-modified infection [46]. It can also test non-cutaneous specimens such as CSF and blood [45, 46]. If PCR is not available, direct fluorescent antibody (DFA) is an alternative, though it is significantly less sensitive than PCR and less useful if scrapings are from late-stage lesions [36, 45]. Viral culture is also less sensitive than PCR and requires a longer turnaround time [36]. Additionally, viral proteins remain after viral replication has ceased, so PCR and DFA can be positive when viral culture is negative [36].

Serologic tests such as the latex agglutination assay and enzyme-linked immunosorbent assays (ELISA) can be used to screen for immunity to varicella [36].

Latent VZV is kept from reactivation by a competent immune system. Increasing age correlates with a reduction in VZV-specific cell-mediated immunity and is the most important risk factor for herpes zoster and its complications, followed by a family history of shingles. The estimated lifetime risk in the general population is about 30% with risk increasing dramatically past the age of 50 [48]. On the opposite end of the age spectrum, varicella infection that occurs at a time when cellular immunity is not fully matured (i.e., in utero or early infancy) is associated with risk for pediatric herpes zoster [45]. Disease-related immunosuppression in HIV/AIDS, diabetes mellitus, or malignancies such as leukemia and lymphoma also increase risk [45, 48]. Organ or hematopoietic stem cell transplant patients as well as patients with autoimmune diseases (e.g., inflammatory bowel disease, rheumatoid arthritis, systemic lupus erythematosus, etc.) are also at increased risk due to use of immunosuppressant therapy. Additionally, risk of herpes zoster is reported to be higher in Caucasians more than those of African ancestry and in pregnant women. It is markedly higher in unvaccinated individuals and in those with a family history of herpes zoster [45, 47].

HZ can result in significant complications. PHN, defined as unresolved pain months after rash onset, occurs in about 20% of patients with HZ [49]. Both peripheral and central nervous system components can contribute to PHN, explaining the variety of pain types described by patients, such as burning, electric-shock-like, throbbing, and allodynia [50]. Thought to be due to a different mechanism, postherpetic itch is also a common complication. Significant physical and emotional disability associated with PHN and postherpetic itch is common, leading to impaired patient quality of life and increased healthcare costs. In the United States, gabapentin, lidocaine patches, pregabalin, tricyclic antidepressants,

and opioid analgesics are often used as first-line treatments, but many patients report inadequate symptom control with one or more of these treatments [50]. Acute and chronic VZV encephalitis is a rare but serious complication of HZ which can occur before or after rash onset, characterized by delirium and other neurological symptoms. Particularly in HZ ophthalmicus, VZV can invade the large cerebral arteries and cause necrosis, producing transient ischemic attacks or strokes several weeks after the initial disease. VZV can also directly invade the spinal cord, leading to myelitis, or invade the retina and cause retinitis [50].

In light of these complications and widespread incidence, defense against HZ is critical to public health. A live attenuated varicella vaccine was developed in Japan in 1974 and became the first licensed shingles vaccine in the United States in 2006 [36]. The Food and Drug Administration licensed Zostavax® (zoster live vaccine) which is now indicated for adults ages 50 and over [37]. The CDC has recommended that unless a contraindication exists, all adults age 60 and older should receive one dose of the shingles vaccine regardless of past varicella infection or immunity status. Contraindications to the vaccine include pregnancy, significant allergy to a vaccine component, and an immunocompromised state. The vaccine was derived from the original primary VZV vaccine after it was noted that, with increased potency, the Oka-derived varicella vaccine could improve T-cell-mediated immunity in older adults and thus protect against HZ outbreaks [51]. The Shingles Prevention Study (SPS) studied 38,546 immunocompetent subjects over 60 years old who were randomized to receive either a dose of the Oka/Merck VZV vaccine or a placebo injection. This multi-center trial revealed that the vaccine led to a 51.3% decrease in HZ, 39% decrease in PHN in those who did develop HZ, and overall decrease in disease burden by 61.1%. The vaccine was overall very well tolerated with mild side effects including injection site rash, headache, and zoster-like rash occurring several weeks after vaccination [51]. Additionally, a new recombinant zoster vaccine approved in 2017, Shingrix, is the current recommended vaccine for shingles in the United States due to the lack of live vaccine-related adverse effects and improved efficacy [52]. It is recommended for persons aged 50 years and older. A heat-treated vaccine, created from the same Oka/Merck viral strain as in Zostavax, is under development for use in immunocompromised patients.

Clinicians face common vaccination barriers in the prevention of shingles, especially since many patients do not recall episodes of primary VZV during childhood. However, nearly all adults have serologic evidence of prior VZV exposure and thus should be vaccinated regardless of prior chickenpox history. Even more so, now that there is increased refusal for the primary varicella vaccine, the incidence of shingles is expected to increase as this population ages. As the burden of disease is significant, cost coverage of the HZ vaccine is also advisable in order to provide coverage for all patients [49].

Treatment for HZ in immunocompetent patients should include systemic antiviral therapy and as-needed pain medication for patients over 50 years of age, with moderate to severe pain or moderate to severe rash. Gabapentin has shown to decrease chronic pain if initiated at acute onset of the rash [53]. Treatment with antiviral medications has been shown to decrease pain duration in multiple randomized and controlled clinical trials. Brivudine (not available in the United States), famciclovir, and valacyclovir have demonstrated greater efficacy than acyclovir in clinical trials, although other issues such as cost, dose frequency, and patient frailty should be considered. There is currently no evidence for the use of antiviral treatment after 72 hours of rash onset, unless vesicles are continuing to form. In immunocompromised patients, intravenous rather than oral acyclovir is the standard treatment, as there is limited data for outpatient oral medication use in these populations. HIV-positive patients need treatment until all lesions have healed due to increased risk for relapse. HZ ophthalmicus treatment should be overseen by an ophthalmologist with cool ocular compresses, antibiotic ophthalmic ointments, and topical steroids. Pregnant women can be treated when the benefit of antivirals outweighs the risk of harm to the fetus, while breast-feeding mothers are also treated cautiously, as acyclovir can be transmitted via breast milk [50].

Human Papillomavirus

Human papillomavirus (HPV) is the most common sexually transmitted infection; however, vaccines against the virus have shown to be very safe and effective in preventing disease. The bivalent, quadrivalent, and nonavalent vaccines prevent cervical and other anogenital cancers as well as some oral and other HPV-associated cancers, with the quadrivalent and nonavalent vaccines additionally protecting against condyloma accuminatum or anogenital warts. The World Health Organization (WHO) has recommended that HPV vaccines be included in all national immunization schedules since April 2009 [54]. Public and private organizations, such as Gavi, the Vaccine Alliance, have worked to provide subsidized and free vaccines to low- and low-middle-income countries given the extensive impact of preventing HPV-associated disease [55].

Although great policy strides have been made to promote HPV vaccines, about 35,000 cases of HPV-associated cancer and millions of other cases of non-cancerous disease are diagnosed in the United States annually [56]. Even when vaccines are made available to adolescent males and females, the ideal candidates for vaccination, they remain underutilized [57]. This is unfortunately due to gaps in guardian vaccine education, provider hesitancy to make strong recommendations for vaccination, and guardian refusal due to perceived stigma associated with the HPV vaccine [58–62]. The vaccine was initially approved for cervical cancer, so it is often mistaken to be only for females [61, 62]. Furthermore, guardian hesitancy related to the vaccine is in part due to the stigma of sexually transmitted infections (STIs) and reluctance to consider the minor in their care to be at risk for STIs [58–60].

Healthcare providers may not educate patients and their families appropriately on the vaccine [58–60]. Due to reasons such as these, only about half of recommended adolescents receive the vaccine [60]. More than 70% of adults are not aware the HPV causes cervical, oral, penile, and anal cancers [60]. Although screening via pap smears has greatly decreased cervical cancer rates, other forms of HPV-induced cancers are on the rise [60]. Men received healthcare provider recommendation for the HPV vaccine 19% of the time, where women received a recommendation 31.5% of the time [57]. Productive education about the relevance of HPV vaccination for cancer prevention is critical given the current lack of understanding [60].

If adolescent vaccination rates fail to improve in the United States, more than 4000 girls annually will develop cervical cancer later in life [63]. In addition to the devastating public health consequences, the financial burden of failing to vaccinate against HPV would be astounding. Additional provider visits; procedures such as pap smears, bronchoscopies, and colposcopies; and treatments for cancers and warts could be prevented through successful vaccination programs [64]. Improving provider training to encourage adolescent HPV vaccination rates is essential in protecting public health [65].

Although adverse effects (AE) following HPV vaccination are rare and generally no different than those following vaccination with a placebo, the perception of AEs has been distorted by social media. While serious AEs are exceedingly rare, a single report on social media, even if unsubstantiated, can instill fears on large segments of society, thus preventing vaccination or even official recommendations for vaccination [66].

Reemerging Systemic Diseases with Cutaneous Manifestations

Measles

Rubeola, more commonly known as measles, has been documented historically since the ninth century and likely dates back 5000–10,000 years.

Strides in measles pathophysiology began in 1957 with Dr. Francis Home's discovery of measles as a hematologic infectious process [67, 68]. A vaccine for measles was established by John Enders in 1963, after he and Dr. Thomas C. Peebles isolated blood-borne measles. The current US measles vaccine is a live, attenuated adaptation of this vaccine established in 1968 [67]. The CDC initiated serious efforts to eliminate measles in the late 1970s [67].

At the end of the twentieth century, over 1000,000 persons died from measles each year. The majority of these deaths were in unvaccinated, often malnourished, children. Deaths were usually secondary to measles pneumonia and/or secondary bacterial infections. From 2000 to 2015, the worldwide number of both measles cases and deaths fell by 70% and 79%, respectively [68]. However, while efforts in vaccination were able to logistically eliminate measles in the United States in 2000, the incidence of measles in the United States is on the rise, from 63 reported cases in 2010 to 372 reported cases in 2018, with most cases in unvaccinated patients [67]. Due to the "Anti-Vaxx" movement, there has been more resistance to vaccine use, especially in the United States since 2014 [69]. While trepidation with regard to vaccines is certainly not a new phenomenon, current momentum is largely rooted in the since-retracted and discredited 1998 article by Andrew Wakefield that linked autism to the MMR vaccine [69]. In the United States, it is thought that the most salient factor in measles outbreaks is travel to other countries (particularly Ukraine, Mexico, Cuba, Israel, Japan, Thailand, and the Philippines) and lack of vaccination [70]. From January 1 to December 31, 2019, there were 1282 cases of measles reported in the United States (including cases in 31 states), with approximately three quarters of cases diagnosed in Orthodox Jewish communities near New York City; this is the highest incidence rate of measles seen in the United States since the 1990s [67]. Yet, these numbers are miniscule compared to the epidemic that crippled the Democratic Republic of Congo in the same year, counting over 230,000 incidences and more than 6000 deaths [67]. According to 2019 preliminary

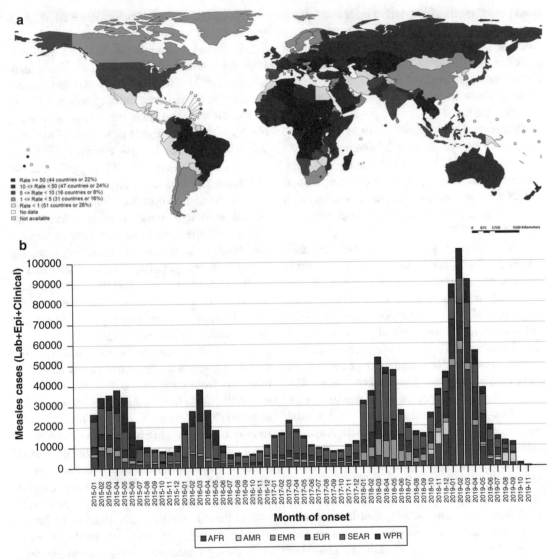

Fig. 7.4 (a, b) Incidence rate of measles across the world, per 2019 WHO measles surveillance data. Global Measles and Rubella Monthly Update. World Health Organization; [2020]. License: CC BY-NC-SA 3.0 IGO

WHO surveillance data, measles cases have hit a record high across the world (Fig. 7.4) [71].

Measles is a highly contagious viral illness of the *Paramyxoviridae* family. This negative-sense RNA virus is single-stranded and enveloped [68]. Transmission is through airborne inhalation of respiratory droplets containing the virus [67]. While the incubation period has been documented to be highly variable, it is roughly 10 days [68]. One to two weeks after exposure to the virus, pulmonary symptoms as well as viral manifestations like fever and coryza appear.

Conjunctivitis can also be present, completing the "three Cs": cough, coryza, and conjunctivitis [67, 68]. In the immediate 2 to 3 days following the onset of the previously described symptoms, small, white macules known as Koplik spots can be found on mucosal membranes of the oral cavity on an erythematous base [67]. The measles exanthem appears 3–5 days after the onset of symptoms. The rash consists of red macules and papules that spread in a craniocaudal manner; macules may coalesce [67]. Fever often breaks during the cutaneous exanthem [68]. The infectious period is defined as 4 days prior and following this exanthem [67]. Measles is transmitted from people with active infections to others; it does not remain latent [68]. Once a person has had measles, production of IgG antibodies to hemagglutinin is protective against subsequent infection [68].

Diagnosis is typically made clinically. Laboratory tests to confirm the diagnosis include detection of IgM or IgG antibodies in serum. Reverse transcriptase polymerase chain reaction (RT-PCR) can confirm diagnosis earlier with samples from the oropharynx, nasopharynx, or urine [68].

While measles generally resolves approximately 1 week after the cutaneous eruption appears, complications are often seen in patients less than 5 or greater than 20 years old or who are pregnant [67, 68]. Immunocompromised state and vitamin A deficiency are also risk factors for complications [68]. Less severe complications include pneumonia, laryngotracheobronchitis, otitis media, diarrhea, and keratoconjunctivitis. Pneumonia and diarrhea are often due to secondary viral or bacterial infections. In pregnant women, additional complications include spontaneous abortion, low birth weight, and intrauterine fetal death; the mother is also at increased risk of death [68]. Severe complications are less likely but more devastating. These include acute disseminated encephalomyelitis, measles inclusion body encephalitis, and subacute sclerosing panencephalitis [68]. Two recent studies on blood of unvaccinated Dutch children who contracted measles detail the concept of "immune amnesia," which explains that measles virus impairs on average 20% of previously acquired immunity by killing memory B cells. Additionally, measles virus was found to decrease the diversity of non-specific naive B cells, leading to impaired ability to form new immune memory [72]. This discovery helps explain the previously epidemiological observation that unvaccinated children who suffer from measles are subsequently more susceptible to unrelated infections compared to children vaccinated against measles [73].

Prevention of measles is achieved through vaccination. Vaccination options include the MMR (measles-mumps-rubella) and MMR-V (measles-mumps-rubella-varicella) immunization series [67]. The CDC guidelines recommend vaccination for children initially between 12 and 15 months and then again between 4 and 6 years old. Vaccination is highly protective of measles. The initial vaccine is 93% effective, while the second dose achieves 97% efficacy [67]. For the remaining 3%, herd immunity is essential to provide maximum protection. Unlike vaccines for viruses with low transmissibility, vaccines for highly infectious diseases like measles have a low threshold to becoming ineffective, requiring 96–99% of the population to be vaccinated to confer immunity. Once this is achieved, herd immunity extends to those who are not adequately vaccinated, including young infants and the immunocompromised [74].

There is currently no targeted antiviral drug despite numerous attempts due to a combination of factors from pragmatic cost of manufacturing and shelf-life to trouble in biochemical antiviral design [75]. Without a specific drug therapy, measles treatment is often supportive and directed at complication management. Treatments include vitamin A and appropriate antibiotics for secondary bacterial infections. With severe cases, antivirals such as ribavirin and interferon alpha can be helpful [68]. In studies, IFN-alpha and ribavirin have been shown to improve outcomes, especially through decreasing complication risk; likewise, vitamin A has been shown to be effective, particularly in patients less than 2 years old [75]. While complications from measles are quite common, cited in approximately 30%–40% of cases, death from measles or measles complications is rare, at 0.2% in the United States, but common in resource-limited parts of the world [76]. During outbreaks, methods such as isolation of infectious persons and persons who are not immune have been proved efficacious in decreasing the number of people who get the disease. Additionally, vaccinating outbreak populations even after exposure to the virus has been proven to be effective in limiting the number of diseased individuals. Use of immunoglobulin has also been shown to decrease risk of measles and should especially be considered in the immuno-compromised [77].

Rubella

Rubella virus is the causative agent in rubella disease, also known as "German measles," which was first described in the 1750s by German physicians De Bergen and Orlow. In 1866, Scottish physician Henry Veale coined the term "rubella," which he derived from the Latin word "rubellus," meaning "reddish" [78]. The virus was first isolated in culture in 1962, and in 1967, its structure was observed under electron microscopy using antigen-antibody complexes. Infection with the virus typically results in a self-limiting, measles-like disease; however, if the virus infects the fetus, especially during the first trimester, miscarriage or congenital rubella syndrome (CRS) may result. Maternal rubella infection and CRS were first linked by Dr. Norman Gregg, an Australian ophthalmologist [79].

Before the measles-mumps-rubella (MMR) live, attenuated vaccine was introduced, rubella manifested as an acute disease in children and young adults. Due to vaccine implementation strategies since 1969, the number of rubella cases worldwide has been greatly reduced. Widespread epidemics have since become extinct, and since 2009, endemic transmission in the World Health Organization's (WHO) Region of the Americas has come to a halt. The peak age of incidence during the pre-vaccination era was 5 to 14 years but has now shifted to 15 to 19 years [80]. In the period immediately before conception or during the first 8–10 weeks of gestation, infection with rubella can lead to multiple fetal defects, such as fetal wastage or stillbirth, in up to 90% of cases [79].

Rubella virus is a single-stranded positive-sense RNA virus and belongs to the *Togaviridae* family and *Rubivirus* genus. Person-to-person spread occurs via the respiratory route [79].

Detergents, temperatures greater than 56 °C (132.8 ° F), UV light, and pH extremes less than 6.8 but greater than 8.1 can easily destroy the virus. Rubella clinically manifests as an erythematous, pruritic, papular rash, appearing approximately 1 week after viremia and lasting 1 to 3 days [80, 81]. Onset of rash occurs concomitantly with the appearance of antibodies and resolution of viremia. The rash initially develops on the face and then spreads to the extremities, covering the entire body within a day, and typically resolves by the third day [80]. Diagnosing rubella clinically is a challenging feat, as the exanthema can take on an atypical, scarlatiniform, or morbilliform presentation, resembling that of other viral infections such as parvovirus B19 or roseola due to human herpesviruses 6 and 7 [81].

Since the manifestation of rubella disease can resemble several other infectious processes, it is important to use clinical features and specific viral testing, such as throat swabs, oral fluids, or nasopharyngeal secretions, to diagnose rubella through virus detection [80]. Other specimens, including cataract tissue and urine, may also be used. In postnatal rubella, the timing of specimen collection is vital. On the first day of the rash, RV-IgM is present in sera in only 50% of cases; however, RV-IgM is detectable approximately 5 days after the rash in most cases and disappears in 4 to 12 weeks [81]. Several tests that exist to detect viral RNA from clinical specimens, including RT-PCR, ELISA, hemagglutinin inhibition (HI), and plaque reduction neutralization (PRN), are available to detect RV-IgG. Since incidence has greatly decreased, most rubella testing is for immunity to the virus through antibody titers [79].

The biggest risk factor for rubella infection is the absence of vaccination. These individuals, especially expectant mothers and children, are not only at greater risk for infection but also at greater risk for CRS and other complications. Conditions associated with rubella infection include postnatal rubella, CRS, and maternal rubella [78]. CRS usually results from primary infection, and it may persist for months to years. Signs and symptoms of CRS can be grouped into three categories—transient (thrombocytopenic purpura), permanent (heart defects, cataracts, hearing loss), and developmental (behavioral disorders). The most common finding in CRS is deafness, which presents in up to 67% of cases. The classic cutaneous manifestation of CRS is a "blueberry muffin" purpuric rash, which represents extramedullary hematopoiesis [80]. Other complications that can result from infection include arthralgia or arthritis, carpal tunnel syndrome, tenosynovitis, miscarriage and intrauterine fetal death in pregnant women, hemolytic anemia, thrombocytopenia, purpura, orchitis, uveitis, Guillain-Barré syndrome, and post-infectious encephalopathy [78].

The key to rubella infection prevention continues to be immunization against the virus through vaccination. Rubella vaccines may be given subcutaneously as a single component, but they are most often given as combination vaccines, such as measles-mumps-rubella-varicella (MMRV) or MMR [78]. All children should receive their first dose of the MMR vaccine at 12 to 15 months and the second dose at 4 to 6 years [80]. The vaccine is 95% effective in prevention after just one dose and almost 100% effective after both [78]. Since the MMR vaccine is a live attenuated vaccine containing the RA 27/3 strain of rubella virus, it should not be administered to pregnant women or immuno-compromised persons. The vaccination should be administered to women of childbearing age before conception. These women are also advised to avoid pregnancy for 1 month following vaccination. Rubella-susceptible women who have not yet been vaccinated and become pregnant should be vaccinated in the immediate postpartum period [78]. Moreover, in children with CRS, disease can be transmitted for as long as the child sheds virus, up to the age of 1 in 20% of children. Exclusion from daycare or school is necessary for confirmed cases of rubella. Until these individuals have two negative throat swab or urine cultures, they should be kept in isolation [78].

Treating rubella becomes a consideration in individuals who have acquired the infection but have not been vaccinated. Postnatally acquired rubella is typically self-limiting, and treatment is symptomatic through use of NSAIDs for associated arthralgia and arthritis. In gravid individuals, treatment depends on the age of gestation at the time of infection. When termination of pregnancy is not an option, immune globulin may be administered in women with known rubella exposure. Treatment of CRS is managed similarly to post-natally acquired rubella, with focus on symptom management and organ-specific treatment. Children should be monitored with audiologic, ophthalmic, and neurodevelopmental follow-up on a long-term basis, since manifestations of the disorder may be delayed. Prognosis of rubella disease is variable, depending on the severity and number of organs affected. In children with CRS, those with thrombocytopenia, hepatosplenomegaly, pulmonary hypertension, and interstitial pneumonia have a high risk of mortality [78]. No effective antiviral treatment currently exists to treat rubella infection [82].

Looking Forward: The Future of Viral Infections

Common Cutaneous Viruses

As we move forward with our vaccination efforts, it is important to remember that areas of progress, if not maintained, can easily regress. Viruses for which we have vaccines, such as human papillomavirus and hepatitis B, would likely flourish without the use of vaccines or medical therapies.

Hepatitis B virus (HBV) is a major cause of disease worldwide, with an estimated 200–300 million people chronically infected [83]. In addition to the classic symptoms of acute hepatitis such as fever, fatigue, and anorexia, a serum sickness-related rash is not uncommonly observed [84]. Long-term sequelae of untreated infection include cirrhosis and hepatocellular carcinoma, demonstrating the need for coordinated vaccine and treatment efforts. Reduction in new cases of HBV over the past several decades has been achieved through safer sexual and drug practices as well as widespread vaccination efforts. The Centers for Disease Control and Prevention recommends a three-shot series for children: the first soon after birth, the second at 1–2 months, and the third at 6–18 months. Vaccination has proven to be a safe, effective, and inexpensive method of preventing disease; however, if vaccination efforts are discontinued, rates of maternal-fetal transmission of HBV would certainly rise [85].

The success and acceptance of the HBV vaccine can provide guidance for promotion of the HPV vaccine. For example, both viruses can be sexually transmitted, but neither vaccine is promoted as preventative for a sexually transmitted disease. In the case of HBV, the vaccine is viewed as preventative for liver failure and liver cancer. Likewise, if the HPV vaccine is viewed as prevention for cancer, acceptance may improve.

Vaccines in Development

As we struggle to keep reemerging viruses at bay, our ability to prevent other life-threatening viruses also remains tenuous. Since the start of the anti-vaccination movement, fighting to reeducate the public has also posed new obstacles. Antiviral vaccine development has been a challenge on the scientific forefront due to pathogen variability, escape from vaccine-induced immune responses, short effector memories, reactogenicity, and various environmental factors, among other reasons [86]. Availability of vaccines globally has been limited due to not only costs but also the logistics of delivery. Funding for vaccine development is often based on economic viability rather than need. For example, even though scientists have been aware of the Ebola virus since 1976, only in recent years has sufficient funding become available to accelerate vaccine development. Even once a vaccine has been discovered, product development and licensing to bring it to market costs between 500 million and 1 billion dollars over an average of 11.9 years [86]. The World Health Organization (WHO) has listed pathogens that are of top priority for research and

development, several of which are viral illnesses such as Crimean-Congo hemorrhagic fever (CCHF), Ebola virus, Marburg virus, SARS, and Rift Valley fever virus [87]. With increasing international networking and collaboration, efforts to bring about needed vaccines and strategic planning in the event of viral epidemics are underway.

Development of new viral vaccines requires dedicated research and creative thinking. Many RNA viruses, such as hepatitis C virus (HCV) and human immunodeficiency virus (HIV), undergo extremely rapid rates of mutation, making effective vaccine development difficult [88, 89]. Human genetic variability also impacts vaccine efficacy. For example, certain human leukocyte antigen (HLA) allele variants have been associated with decreased antibody generation to several vaccines [90]. This is relevant in the case of patients with certain HLA class II alleles who are completely unresponsive to the hepatitis B vaccine [91]. Further understanding of both viral and human biology is required to create effective new vaccines.

Improving current vaccines and expanding the number of serotypes covered is another area of development. In the elderly, defending against immunosenescence requires effective vaccines. For example, combining different immunostimulatory factors has shown improvement in the zoster glycoprotein vaccine by including the $AS01_B$ adjuvant system in a Phase III clinical trial, which led to herpes zoster risk reduction in adults greater than 70 years old [92]. In the field of tropical disease, a vaccine for dengue virus called Dengvaxia, a tetravalent dengue chimeric live attenuated vaccine, has been approved in several countries and recommended by WHO in ages 9 and older [93]. However, due to dengue virus's four different serotypes, each able to stimulate a cross-reactive and disease-enhancing antibody response against the other three serotypes, creating a very efficacious vaccine has been challenging [94, 95]. Therefore, the currently available quadrivalent dengue vaccine is recommended only for persons already infected with one strain of dengue [96].

Conclusion

The good news is that even with this resurgence of previously eradicated viruses, we are still at a mortality rate of less than 5%, compared to a century ago when infectious diseases were attributable to 50% of the nation's deaths. Advances in technology have foreseen bypasses for many of the hurdles our society faces with vaccinations today. For instance, genome editing tools that reprogram the immune system's B cells to produce antibodies against viruses may be the answer to random failure of vaccine-induced DNA rearrangement [97, 98]. To minimize the need for human resources and to maximize safety, needle-free delivery of vaccines, such as aerosolized routes, jet injectors, and microneedles, is being implemented [99]. Hopefully, with ease of accessibility and increased engagement of health benefits resulting in increased demand, the affordability of vaccinations can decrease the health burdens propagated by infectious diseases.

References

1. Vander straten M, Tyring SK. Mucocutaneous manifestations of viral diseases in children. Clin Dermatol. 2002;20(1):67–73.
2. Handfield C, Kwock J, Macleod AS. Innate antiviral immunity in the skin. Trends Immunol. 2018;39(4):328–40.
3. CDC. History of Smallpox. Centers for Disease Control and Prevention. https://www.cdc.gov/smallpox/history/history.html. Published 30 Aug 2016.
4. Vanderslott S, Dadonaite B, Roser M. Vaccination. Our World in Data. https://ourworldindata.org/vaccination. Published May 10, 2013. Accessed 19 Jan 2020.
5. Wakefield AJ, Murch SH, Anthony A, Linnell, Casson DM, Malik M, et al. Ileal lymphoid nodular hyperplasia, non-specific colitis, and pervasive developmental disorder in children. Lancet. 1998;351:637–41 [retracted].
6. Editors of the Lancet. Retraction: ileal lymphoid nodular hyperplasia, non-specific colitis, and pervasive developmental disorder in children. Lancet. 2010;375:445.
7. Deer B. How the case against the MMR vaccine was fixed. BMJ. 2011;342:c5347.
8. Deer B. Secrets of the MMR scare. The Lancet's two days to bury bad news. BMJ. 2011;342:c7001.
9. Maisonneuve H, Floret D. Wakefield's affair: 12 years of uncertainty whereas no link between autism and MMR vaccine has been proved. Presse Med. 2012;41(9 Pt 1):827–34.
10. Battistella M, Carlino C, Dugo V, Ponzo P, Franco E. Vaccines and autism: a myth to debunk? Ig Sanita Pubbl. 2013;69(5):585–96.
11. Hussain A, Ali S, Ahmed M, Hussain S. The antivaccination movement: a regression in modern medicine. Cureus. 2018;10(7):e2919.
12. Chapter 5: Attitudes to vaccines. Wellcome. https://wellcome.ac.uk/reports/wellcome-global-monitor/2018/chapter-5-attitudes-vaccines. Accessed 6 Feb 2020.
13. DRC: MSF shuts down Ebola treatment center following violent attack. Doctors without borders - USA. https://www.doctorswithoutborders.org/what-we-do/news-stories/story/drc-msf-shuts-down-ebola-treatment-center-following-violent-attack. Published February 26, 2019. Accessed 19 Jan 2020.
14. Yaqub O, Castle-Clarke S, Sevdalis N, Chataway J. Attitudes to vaccination: a critical review. Soc Sci Med. https://www.sciencedirect.com/science/article/pii/S0277953614002421. Published April 16, 2014. Accessed 6 Feb 2020.
15. CDC. 2019–2020 U.S. Flu season: preliminary burden estimates. Centers for Disease Control and Prevention. https://www.cdc.gov/flu/about/burden/preliminary-in-season-estimates.htm. Published January 10, 2020. Accessed 19 Jan 2020.
16. Breuer J, Grose C, Norberg P, Tipples G, Schmid DS. A proposal for a common nomenclature for viral clades that form the species varicella-zoster virus: summary of VZV nomenclature meeting 2008, Barts and the London School of Medicine and Dentistry, 24–25 July 2008. J Gen Virol. 2010;91:821–8.
17. Wagenaar TR, Chow VT, Buranathai C, Thawatsupha P, Grose C. The out of Africa model of varicella-zoster virus evolution: single nucleotide polymorphisms and private alleles distinguish Asian clades from European/North American clades. Vaccine. 2003;21(11–12):1072–81.
18. Sadzot-Delvaux C, Merville-Louis M-P, Delree P, Marc P, Moonen G, Rentier B. An in vivo model of varicella-zoster virus latent infection of dorsal root ganglia. J Neurosci Res. 1990;26:83–9.
19. Spackova M, Wiese-posselt M, Dehnert M, Matysiak-klose D, Heininger U, Siedler A. Comparative varicella vaccine effectiveness during outbreaks in day-care centres. Vaccine. 2010;28(3):686–91.
20. Vázquez M, Larussa PS, Gershon AA, et al. Effectiveness over time of varicella vaccine. JAMA. 2004;291(7):851–5.
21. Mahamud A, Wiseman R, Grytdal S, et al. Challenges in confirming a varicella outbreak in the two-dose vaccine era. Vaccine. 2012;30(48):6935–9.
22. Shapiro ED, Vazquez M, Esposito D, et al. Effectiveness of 2 doses of varicella vaccine in children. J Infect Dis. 2011;203(3):312–5.

23. Gershon AA, Gershon MD. Pathogenesis and current approaches to control of varicella-zoster virus infections. Clin Microbiol Rev. 2013;26(4):728–43. Weller T, Stoddard MB. 1952. Intranuclear inclusion bodies in cultures of human tissue inoculated with varicella vesicle fluid. J. Immunol. 68:311–319

24. Takahashi M, Asano Y, Kamiya H, et al. Development of varicella vaccine. J Infect Dis. 2008;197(Suppl 2):S41–4.

25. CDC. Reported Cases and Deaths from Vaccine Preventable Diseases, United States, 1950-2013. Centers for Disease Control and Prevention. https://www.cdc.gov/vaccines/pubs/pinkbook/downloads/appendices/E/reported-cases.pdf. Published May 2019. Accessed 1 Sept 2014.

26. Tsolia M, Gershon AA, Steinberg SP, Gelb L. Live attenuated varicella vaccine: evidence that the virus is attenuated and the importance of skin lesions in transmission of varicella-zoster virus. National Institute of Allergy and Infectious Diseases Varicella Vaccine Collaborative Study Group. J Pediatr. 1990;116(2):184–9.

27. Arvin AM, Moffat JF, Sommer M, et al. Varicella-zoster virus T cell tropism and the pathogenesis of skin infection. Curr Top Microbiol Immunol. 2010;342:189–209.

28. Ku CC, Zerboni L, Ito H, Graham BS, Wallace M, Arvin AM. Varicella-zoster virus transfer to skin by T cells and modulation of viral replication by epidermal cell interferon-alpha. J Exp Med. 2004;200(7):917–25.

29. Malavige GN, Jones L, Kamaladasa SD, et al. Viral load, clinical disease severity and cellular immune responses in primary varicella zoster virus infection in Sri Lanka. PLoS One. 2008;3(11):e3789.

30. Jean-philippe P, Freedman A, Chang MW, et al. Severe varicella caused by varicella-vaccine strain in a child with significant T-cell dysfunction. Pediatrics. 2007;120(5):e1345–9.

31. Plotkin SA, Orenstein WA, Offit PA. Vaccines E-book. 6th Ed. Philadelphia: Elsevier Health Sciences-Saunders; 2012.

32. Galea SA, Sweet A, Beninger P, et al. The safety profile of varicella vaccine: a 10-year review. J Infect Dis. 2008;197(Suppl 2):S165–9.

33. Weinmann S, Naleway AL, Koppolu P, et al. Incidence of Herpes Zoster among children: 2003-2014. Pediatrics. 2019;144:1.

34. Kim SR, Khan F, Ramirez-fort MK, Downing C, Tyring SK. Varicella zoster: an update on current treatment options and future perspectives. Expert Opin Pharmacother. 2014;15(1):61–71.

35. Yawn BP, Gilden D. The global epidemiology of herpes zoster. Neurology. 2013;81(10):928–30.

36. CDC. Epidemiology and Prevention of Vaccine-Preventable Diseases. Centers for Disease Control and Prevention. https://www.cdc.gov/vaccines/pubs/pinkbook/index.html. Published 2017. Accessed 1 Sept 2019.

37. Voelker R. Increasing cases of Shingles in the eye raise key questions. JAMA. 2019;322:712.

38. Mullooly JP, Riedlinger K, Chun C, Weinmann S, Houston H. Incidence of herpes zoster, 1997-2002. Epidemiol Infect. 2005;133(2):245–53.

39. Yawn BP, Saddier P, Wollan PC, St sauver JL, Kurland MJ, Sy LS. A population-based study of the incidence and complication rates of herpes zoster before zoster vaccine introduction. Mayo Clin Proc. 2007;82(11):1341–9.

40. Brisson M, Edmunds WJ, Gay NJ, Law B, De serres G. Modelling the impact of immunization on the epidemiology of varicella zoster virus. Epidemiol Infect. 2000;125(3):651–69.

41. Hicks LD, Cook-norris RH, Mendoza N, Madkan V, Arora A, Tyring SK. Family history as a risk factor for herpes zoster: a case-control study. Arch Dermatol. 2008;144(5):603–8.

42. Hernandez PO, Javed S, Mendoza N, Lapolla W, Hicks LD, Tyring SK. Family history and herpes zoster risk in the era of shingles vaccination. J Clin Virol. 2011;52(4):344–8.

43. Klein NP, Holmes TH, Sharp MA, et al. Variability and gender differences in memory T cell immunity to varicella-zoster virus in healthy adults. Vaccine. 2006;24(33–34):5913–8.

44. Gnann JW, Whitley RJ. Clinical practice. Herpes zoster. N Engl J Med. 2002;347(5):340–6.

45. Cohen JI. Clinical practice: Herpes zoster. N Engl J Med. 2013;369(3):255–63.

46. Leung J, Harpaz R, Baughman AL, et al. Evaluation of laboratory methods for diagnosis of varicella. Clin Infect Dis. 2010;51(1):23–32.

47. Harpaz R. Do varicella vaccination programs change the epidemiology of herpes zoster? A comprehensive review, with focus on the United States. Expert Rev Vaccines. 2019;18(8):793–811.

48. Schmader K. Herpes Zoster. Ann Intern Med. 2018;169(3):ITC19–31.

49. Willison CB, Morrison LK, Mendoza N, Tyring SK. Shingles vaccine. Expert Opin Biol Ther. 2010;10(4):631–8.

50. Dworkin RH, Portenoy RK. Pain and its persistence in herpes zoster. Pain. 1996;67:241–51.

51. Oxman MN, Levin MJ, Johnson GR, et al. A vaccine to prevent herpes zoster and postherpetic neuralgia in older adults. N Engl J Med. 2005;352(22):2271–84.

52. CDC. Shingrix Shingles Vaccination. What You Should Know. Centers for Disease Control and Prevention. https://www.cdc.gov/vaccines/vpd/shingles/public/shingrix/index.html. Published January 25, 2018. Accessed 15 Aug 2019.

53. Lapolla W, Digiorgio C, Haitz K, et al. Incidence of postherpetic neuralgia after combination treatment with gabapentin and valacyclovir in patients with acute herpes zoster: open-label study. Arch Dermatol. 2011;147(8):901–7.

54. Human papillomavirus vaccines. WHO position paper. Wkly Epidemiol Rec. 2009;84(15):118–31.

55. Gavi, the Vaccine Alliance. More than 30 million girls to be immunised with HPV vaccines by 2020 with GAVI support. 2012. http://www.gavi.org/library/news/press-releases/2012/more-than-30-million-girls-immunised-with-hpv-by-2020/.

56. Dunne EF, Park IU. HPV and HPV-associated diseases. Infect Dis Clin N Am. 2013;27(4):765–78.

57. Suk R, Montealegre JR, Nemutlu GS, et al. Public knowledge of human papillomavirus and receipt of vaccination recommendations. JAMA Pediatr. 2019;173(11):1099–101.

58. Attia AC, Wolf J, Núñez AE. On surmounting the barriers to HPV vaccination: we can do better. Ann Med. 2018;50(3):209–25.

59. Bonanni P, Zanella B, Santomauro F, Lorini C, Bechini A, Boccalini S. Safety and perception: what are the greatest enemies of HPV vaccination programmes? Vaccine. 2018;36(36):5424–9.

60. Patty NJS, Van dijk HM, Wallenburg I, et al. To vaccinate or not to vaccinate? Perspectives on HPV vaccination among girls, boys, and parents in the Netherlands: a Q-methodological study. BMC Public Health. 2017;17(1):872.

61. Apaydin KZ, Fontenot HB, Shtasel D, et al. Facilitators of and barriers to HPV vaccination among sexual and gender minority patients at a Boston community health center. Vaccine. 2018;36(26):3868–75.

62. Radisic G, Chapman J, Flight I, Wilson C. Factors associated with parents' attitudes to the HPV vaccination of their adolescent sons: a systematic review. Prev Med. 2017;95:26–37.

63. Chesson HW, Ekwueme DU, Saraiya M, Dunne EF, Markowitz LE. The estimated impact of human papillomavirus vaccine coverage on the lifetime cervical cancer burden among girls currently aged 12 years and younger in the United States. Sex Transm Dis. 2014;41(11):656–9.

64. Chesson HW, Ekwueme DU, Saraiya M, Watson M, Lowy DR, Markowitz LE. Estimates of the annual direct medical costs of the prevention and treatment of disease associated with human papillomavirus in the United States. Vaccine. 2012;30(42):6016–9.

65. Rahman M, Laz TH, Mcgrath CJ, Berenson AB. Provider recommendation mediates the relationship between parental human papillomavirus (HPV) vaccine awareness and HPV vaccine initiation and completion among 13- to 17-year-old U.S. adolescent children. Clin Pediatr (Phila). 2015;54(4):371–5.

66. Morimoto A, Ueda Y, Egawa-takata T, et al. Effect on HPV vaccination in Japan resulting from news report of adverse events and suspension of governmental recommendation for HPV vaccination. Int J Clin Oncol. 2015;20(3):549–55.

67. CDC. Measles (Rubeola). Centers for Disease Control and Prevention. https://www.cdc.gov/measles/index.html. Published May 13, 2019. Accessed 17 Aug 2019.

68. Moss WJ. Measles. Lancet. 2017;390(10111):2490–502.

69. Benecke O, Deyoung SE. Anti-vaccine decision-making and Measles resurgence in the United States. Glob Pediatr Health. 2019;6:2333794X19862949.

70. Sarkar S, Zlojutro A, Khan K, Gardner L. Measles resurgence in the USA: how international travel compounds vaccine resistance. Lancet Infect Dis. 2019;19(7):684–6.

71. Measles and Rubella Surveillance Data. World Health Organization. https://www.who.int/immunization/monitoring_surveillance/burden/vpd/surveillance_type/active/measles_monthlydata/en/. Published January 10, 2020. Accessed 6 Feb 2020.

72. Petrova VN, Sawatsky B, Han AX, et al. Incomplete genetic reconstitution of B cell pools contributes to prolonged immunosuppression after measles. Sci Immunol. 2019;4(41):eaay6125.

73. Jensen A, Andersen PK, Stensballe LG. Early childhood vaccination and subsequent mortality or morbidity: are observational studies hampered by residual confounding? A Danish register-based cohort study. BMJ Open. 2019;9(9):e029794.

74. Hendrix KS, Sturm LA, Zimet GD, Meslin EM. Ethics and childhood vaccination policy in the United States. Am J Public Health. 2016;106(2):273–8.

75. Plemper RK, Snyder JP. Measles control – can measles virus inhibitors make a difference? Curr Opin Investig Drugs. 2009;10(8):811–20.

76. Bester JC. Measles and measles vaccination: a review. JAMA Pediatr. 2016;170(12):1209.

77. Gastañaduy PA, Banerjee E, Debolt C, et al. Public health responses during measles outbreaks in elimination settings: strategies and challenges. Hum Vaccin Immunother. 2018;14(9):2222–38.

78. Leung AKC, Hon KL, Leong KF. Rubella (German measles) revisited. Hong Kong Med J. 2019;25(2):134–41.

79. Lambert N, Strebel P, Orenstein W, Icenogle J, Poland GA. Rubella. Lancet. 2015;385(9984):2297–307.

80. Vander straten MR, Tyring SK. Rubella. Dermatol Clin. 2002;20(2):225–31.

81. Bouthry E, Picone O, Hamdi G, Grangeot-keros L, Ayoubi JM, Vauloup-fellous C. Rubella and pregnancy: diagnosis, management and outcomes. Prenat Diagn. 2014;34(13):1246–53.

82. CDC. Rubella (German Measles, Three-Day Measles). Centers for Disease Control and Prevention. https://www.cdc.gov/rubella/index.html. Reviewed September 15, 2017. Accessed 1 Sept 2019.

83. Matthews PC, Barnes E. Hepatitis B vaccine shortage: another symptom of chronic neglect? BMJ. 2017;359:j4686.

84. Dienstag JL. Immunopathogenesis of the extrahepatic manifestations of hepatitis B virus infection. Springer Semin Immunopathol. 1981;3(4):461–72.

85. Nemerofsky SL, Akingboye B, Ferguson C, Africa D. Sustained improvement in administration of the Hepatitis B vaccine birth dose: a quality improvement initiative. Am J Med Qual. 2018;33(3):313–20.

86. Pronker ES, Weenen TC, Commandeur HR, Osterhaus AD, Claassen HJ. The gold industry standard for risk and cost of drug and vaccine development revisited. Vaccine. 2011;29(35):5846–9.

87. Lambe T, Bowyer G, Ewer KJ. A review of phase I trials of Ebola virus vaccines: what can we learn from the race to develop novel vaccines? Philos Trans R Soc Lond Ser B Biol Sci. 2017;372(1721):20160295.

88. Cuevas JM, Geller R, Garijo R, López-aldeguer J, Sanjuán R. Extremely high mutation rate of HIV-1 in vivo. PLoS Biol. 2015;13(9):e1002251.

89. Ribeiro RM, Li H, Wang S, et al. Quantifying the diversification of hepatitis C virus (HCV) during primary infection: estimates of the in vivo mutation rate. PLoS Pathog. 2012;8(8):e1002881.

90. Posteraro B, Pastorino R, Di giannantonio P, et al. The link between genetic variation and variability in vaccine responses: systematic review and meta-analyses. Vaccine. 2014;32(15):1661–9.

91. Li ZK, Nie JJ, Li J, Zhuang H. The effect of HLA on immunological response to hepatitis B vaccine in healthy people: a meta-analysis. Vaccine. 2013;31(40):4355–61.

92. Cunningham AL, Lal H, Kovac M, et al. Efficacy of the Herpes Zoster subunit vaccine in adults 70 years of age or older. N Engl J Med. 2016;375(11):1019–32.

93. Torres JR, Falleiros-arlant LH, Gessner BD, et al. Updated recommendations of the International Dengue Initiative expert group for CYD-TDV vaccine implementation in Latin America. Vaccine. 2019;37(43):6291–8.

94. Khetarpal N, Khanna I. Dengue fever: causes, complications, and vaccine strategies. J Immunol Res. 2016;2016:6803098.

95. Anderson KB, Endy TP, Thomas SJ. The dynamic role of dengue cross-reactive immunity: changing the approach to defining vaccine safety and efficacy. Lancet Infect Dis. 2018;18(10):e333–8.

96. Wilder-smith A. Dengue vaccine development: status and future. Bundesgesundheitsblatt Gesundheitsforschung Gesundheitsschutz. 2020;63(1):40–4.

97. Plotkin SA. Increasing complexity of vaccine development. J Infect Dis. 2015;212(Suppl 1):S12–6.

98. Lau CH. Applications of CRISPR-Cas in bioengineering, biotechnology, and translational research. CRISPR J. 2018;1:379–404.

99. National Vaccine Advisory Committee, Enhancing the work of the HHS National Vaccine Program in global immunizations. 2013. www.hhs.gov/nvpo/nvac/reports/index.html.

Part III

Emerging Resistance to Antifungals

Mechanisms of Antifungal Drug Resistance

8

Fabio Francesconi, Alex Panizza Jalkh, Omar Lupi, and Yasmin Khalfe

Abbreviations

ABC	Adenosine triphosphate-binding cassette
AmB	Amphotericin B
BMD	Broth microdilution
CLSI	Clinical and Laboratory Standards Institute
CYP	Cytochrome P450
EUCAST	European Committee on Antimicrobial Susceptibility Testing
MDR	Multidrug resistance
MFS	Major facilitator superfamily
MIC	Minimum inhibitory concentrations
NBD	Nucleotide-binding domains
PDR	Pleiotropic drug resistance
PMNs	Polymorphonuclear leukocytes
TMS	Transmembrane span domains

F. Francesconi
Dermatology Section - Federal University of the State of Amazonas (UFAM), Manaus, Brazil

Dermatologist - Hospital de Medicina Tropical, Manaus, Brazil

A. P. Jalkh
Dermatologist - FMTHVD/State University of Amazonas, Manaus, Brazil

O. Lupi
Associate Professor of Dermatology - Federal University of the State of Rio de Janeiro (UNIRIO), Rio de Janeiro, Brazil

Immunology Section - Federal University of Rio de Janeiro (UFRJ), Rio de Janeiro, Brazil

Titular Professor & Chairman - Policlinica Geral do Rio de Janeiro (PGRJ), Rio de Janeiro, Brazil

Ibero Latin American College of Dermatology (CILAD), Buenos Aires, Argentina

International League of Dermatological Societies (ILDS), London, UK

Y. Khalfe (✉)
School of Medicine, Baylor College of Medicine, Houston, TX, USA
e-mail: yasmin.khalfe@bcm.edu

Introduction

Fungi are strict aerobic eukaryotes that require an exogenous source of organic carbon for growth. They have a defined nucleus enclosed by a nuclear membrane and possess a fungal cell membrane. This cell membrane is composed of the central lipid, ergosterol, in contrast to the mammalian membrane primarily composed of cholesterol. Another essential structure in fungi is the cell wall predominantly made of chitin, mannan, and glucan, which is structurally different from the cell walls of bacteria and plants [1]. The "basement layer" of the cell wall is made of chitin, which creates a robust, shell-like scaffold that counterattacks the cytoplasm's internal osmotic pressure. The outer layer of the cell wall is glucan-based and helps establish chemical diversity among different fungal species [1]. The

© Springer Nature Switzerland AG 2021
S. K. Tyring et al. (eds.), *Overcoming Antimicrobial Resistance of the Skin*, Updates in Clinical Dermatology, https://doi.org/10.1007/978-3-030-68321-4_8

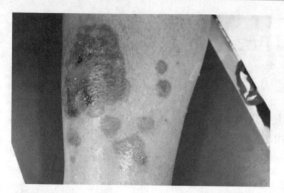

Fig. 8.1 Erythematous, well-circumscribed lesions on a patient's right arm due to cutaneous fungal infection. (Source: CDC PHIL)

four main categories of fungi that cause human disease (distinguished by their cellular structures) are yeasts, filamentous fungi, dimorphic fungi, and dermatophytes.

Most human fungal infections are superficial mycosis, predominantly infecting the skin and appendages of healthy individuals (Fig. 8.1). On the other end of the spectrum, there are systemic (invasive) fungal infections, including opportunistic infections in the immunocompromised. Invasive fungal infections have a lower incidence than superficial infections; however, these systemic infections are known to cause considerable human morbidity, mortality, and economic burden [2]. Invasive fungal infections are a substantial global health issue, resulting in 1.7 million deaths every year [3]. Almost all fungal-related deaths (over 90%) are related to *Cryptococcus*, *Candida*, *Aspergillus*, *Histoplasma*, and *Pneumocystis* [2]. These infections occur mostly commonly in immunocompromised patients undergoing chemotherapy, in HIV-positive persons, or in organ transplant recipients. As such, the world saw an upsurge of fungal disease associated with AIDS, increasing use of immunosuppressive therapies, and greater number of organ transplantations. A growing number of opportunistic fungal pathogens have emerged as well, including molds such as *Fusarium* spp., *Scedosporium* spp., *Penicillium* spp., *Lomentospora* spp., and the *Mucorales* [2].

As the diversity and spread in fungal infections continue to grow, the need for newer therapeutic drugs continues as well. However, fungi offer fewer pathogen-specific targets as they have a eukaryotic metabolism that is closer in resemblance to humans than to bacteria. This lack of pathogen-specific targets has limited the development of novel antifungal drugs when compared to the development of antibacterial treatment [2]. Currently, the three most common classes of antifungals used for the treatment of invasive infections are the polyenes, azoles, and echinocandins [2]. Other antifungal therapies include allylamines, flucytosine, griseofulvin, and potassium iodide.

Because of the serious fatalities associated with fungal infection and the limited number of therapeutic drug options, antifungal drug resistance is a major clinical concern that has been on the rise in recent years. With the number of effective treatment options being so restricted, resistance development to even one class of antifungal drugs drastically limits opportunities for successful therapy. In the last decade, resistance has been a growing problem that has been associated with indiscriminate antifungal use in agriculture, extensive prophylactic treatment, and abuse of empirical therapy [2].

Fungi resistance mechanisms show both inherent reduced drug susceptibility and acquired resistance. Mechanisms of acquired resistance include mutations in target proteins, overexpression of target proteins, upregulation of efflux pumps, and decreased access to targets. Other mechanisms such as biofilms, cellular stress response, and genetic abnormalities have also been identified as contributors to resistance. Given the seriousness of fungal infections and limited therapeutic options, an understanding of the mechanisms of antifungal resistance is imperative to effectively treat infection and develop novel therapeutics in the future.

Antifungal Agents

The antifungal drug classes include polyenes, azoles, echinocandins, allylamines, flucytosine, griseofulvin, and potassium iodide. Each class has a distinct mechanism of action. The antifungal drugs either target specific structural components of the cell membrane or cell wall, or they disrupt cellular processes such as DNA and RNA synthesis and mitosis.

Polyenes

Polyenes are naturally occurring macrolides produced by *Streptomyces* spp., gram-positive bacteria, and include amphotericin B and nystatin. Amphotericin B (AmB) is the first and most potent drug in the polyene group [1]. AmB's mechanism of action is twofold and dependent on the presence of sterols within the fungal cell membrane. Firstly, it binds ergosterol, a fungal-specific sterol, therefore targeting fungal membranes. Polyenes insert a pore-like structure into the cell membrane, leading to disruption. With this, the proton gradient of the cell membrane is destroyed, and ions leak across the cell creating osmotic instability and cell death. Secondly, reactive oxygen species accumulate due to AmB, which results in DNA, protein, mitochondrial, and membrane damage [4].

While the drug preferentially targets ergosterol, cholesterol is structurally and functionally similar; polyenes can interact with cholesterol and frequently show higher levels of toxicity in humans [4]. Still, AmB has historically been the "gold standard" for systemic fungal infections, particularly those that are severe and life-threatening [1]. Prevalent side effects of amphotericin use include infusion reactions and significant dose-limiting nephrotoxicity [5].

Azoles

Azoles act primarily by blocking the synthesis of ergosterol, causing accumulation of a toxic methylated sterol that stops cell growth. Specifically, azoles block lanosterol 14α-demethylase, the enzyme that converts lanosterol to ergosterol. This leads to the accumulation of methylated sterols in fungal cells, ultimately interfering with the integrity and functionality of the cell membrane. Other reported effects of azoles on fungal structures are related to metabolite pools, oxidative damage, and mitochondrial dysfunction [4].

Structurally, the azoles are either an imidazole or a triazole attached to a quaternary carbon. The imidazole-based azoles were introduced first and included miconazole, clotrimazole, econazole, ketoconazole, tioconazole, and sulconazole and, more recently, serconazole and luliconazole [1]. The triazoles have a nitrogen-containing ring and, with this, possess greater specificity against the fungal cytochrome P450 (CYP) enzyme. These include terconazole, fluconazole, itraconazole, voriconazole, posaconazole, efinaconazole, and isavuconazonium [1].

Azoles have a broad spectrum of coverage and are often first-line therapy for many invasive fungal infections. Drug-level monitoring is necessary as azoles are associated with cytochrome P450 inhibition which can cause unsafe interactions with other medications. This drug class can also cause toxicities such as hallucinations, hepatotoxicity, and QTc prolongation [5].

Echinocandins

Echinocandins are semi-synthetic lipopeptides that inhibit β-1,3-glucan synthase. This enzyme is necessary for the biosynthesis of β-1,3-glucan, a major structural component of the fungal cell wall that helps maintain cell wall integrity [1]. The cell wall protects fungal cells from environmental stress, and without this structure, cells are subject to damage [4]. Because the cell wall is specific to fungi, echinocandins can reduce the thickness of the cell wall, targeting the fungal cells without being toxic to mammalian cells. Drugs in this class include caspofungin, micafungin, and anidulafungin [4]. The next-generation echinocandin, rezafungin, is currently in phase III clinical trials [1].

Echinocandins have very low activity against endemic mycoses and are mainly used for yeasts and mold infections, particularly for invasive candidiasis [5]. It is overall a well-tolerated drug class, with limited adverse effects as less than 1% experience flushing, fever, or chills. The lack of oral formulations limits its usage [5].

Allylamines

The allylamines are a man-made antifungal drug class that inhibit the enzyme, squalene epoxidase. This enzyme is critical for the biosynthesis of ergosterol as it catalyzes the reaction of squalene to lanosterol and ultimately ergosterol [1]. Drugs in this class include terbinafine, naftifine, and butenafine. Allylamines are commonly used as a topical agent, and terbinafine is the only oral, approved drug used for treating onychomycosis [1].

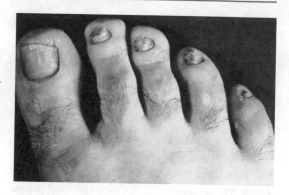

Fig. 8.3 Onychomycosis caused by the dermatophytic fungal organism, *Epidermophyton floccosum*

Flucytosine (5-Fluorocytosine)

Flucytosine (5-fluorocytosine) inhibits pyrimidine metabolism and DNA synthesis. As a pyrimidine analog, it is converted to 5-fluorouracil and selectively interferes with fungal RNA and protein synthesis. Flucytosine is available as an oral medication, but it has a high level of toxicity, and adverse effects are mainly related to bone marrow suppression [5]. Resistance development limits its use as monotherapy, and it is used sparingly and in combination with AmB [1]. The major indications for this drug are for the management of cryptococcal meningitis, urinary candidiasis, or chromoblastomycosis (Fig. 8.2) [5].

Other Drugs

Griseofulvin is a mycotoxin produced by *Penicillium* spp. that is effective against *Microsporum*, *Trichophyton*, and *Epidermophyton* (Fig. 8.3) [6]. The drug interferes with microtubule aggregation and function [7]. By interacting with the fungal cell microtubules, griseofulvin inhibits mitosis [6].

Potassium iodide is another agent shown to work against fungi but has an unclear mechanism of action. It is not certain whether it acts as a fungicidal agent or by enhancing the body's immunologic and nonimmunologic defense mechanisms.

Antifungal Drug Therapy Rational

In order to choose the appropriate antifungal therapy, clinicians must consider the correct indications for drug classes and specific drugs. For example, the classes that target ergosterol (polyenes, azoles, allylamines) are consequently ineffective against *P. jirovecii*, as the fungus contains cholesterol instead of ergosterol.

Another essential consideration is related to the host's immune response. In some infections, the drug alone is not enough to eliminate the microorganism, and the immunological influence of the drug must be evaluated. Multiple drugs affect the activity of polymorphonuclear leukocytes (PMNs). For example, AmB increases the

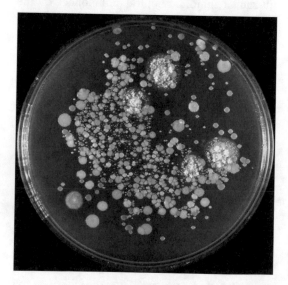

Fig. 8.2 Culture producing numerous colonies of *Cryptococcus neoformans*, the organism that causes cryptococcal meningitis

aggregation, adherence, and fungicidal activity of PMNs. Additionally, allylamines also can increase the fungicidal activity of PMNs, and azoles can inhibit chemotaxis and superoxide production of PMNs [7].

Other clinical features also influence the treatment outcome. In cases with indwelling catheters, artificial heart valves, and other implanted devices, biofilm formation may block the drug from reaching the necessary site and can cause continued or new infection [8]. Lastly, pharmacokinetics affect drug penetration at different infection locations in the body. This can lead to delivery of suboptimal concentration of the drug and ultimately induce fungal resistance. Inappropriate dosage, poor compliance, drug exposure in the form of prophylaxis, and repeated or long-term therapy are all associated with the emergence of resistance [8].

Antifungal Drug Resistance

Inevitably, some fungal strains develop resistance to antifungal drugs during treatment. This resistance can be caused by either inherently less susceptible strains, or it can be caused by an acquired drug resistance [9]. Drug resistance is a major concern with antifungals as this has led to limited treatment options and, subsequently, altered patient management [8]. Losing the effectiveness of one antifungal drug class can reduce treatment options by 33% or 50%, and an even greater concern is the emergence of fungi resistant to multiple drug classes [10]. Antifungal resistance can be categorized as microbiological resistance or clinical resistance (or both). Understanding the mechanisms behind antifungal resistance is key to better diagnosing and treating fungal infections and to developing effective, novel therapies.

Microbiologic drug resistance is defined as a strain of pathogen requiring an antimicrobial concentration that exceeds the normal concentration range needed to inhibit the growth of pathogen for the wild-type strain [11]. Microbiological resistance can be either primary (intrinsic among fungi without previous exposure) or secondary (acquired).

Clinical resistance is defined as a resistance in which the pathogen is unable to be inhibited by an antimicrobial concentration that can be safely achieved through regular dosing. Resistance is measured clinically as an increase in the MIC of an antifungal drug when tested according to approved methods [10].

Susceptibility Testing

With this, there is a need for antifungal susceptibility tests that are reproducible and clinically relevant. The current tests include two independent standards, the Clinical and Laboratory Standards Institute (CLSI) method and the European Committee on Antimicrobial Susceptibility Testing (EUCAST) method. Both are methods that use broth microdilution (BMD) susceptibility testing of *Candida* and filamentous fungi, and minimum inhibitory concentration is measured and referenced to a clinical breakpoint [12]. While there are some differences in inoculum size and minimum inhibitory concentrations (MIC), these methods show close agreement and provide a way to differentiate strains with no resistance (wild-type) from strains with intrinsic or acquired resistance [11].

Microbiology laboratory testing predicts susceptibility to an antifungal agent only to a limited degree. Some drugs, for example, caspofungin, and fungal species are not reliable in testing; additionally, most common pathogens have drug- and species-specific breakpoints, but these do not exist for rare yeasts and molds [12]. It is important to note that the in vitro minimum inhibitory concentration is not conclusively linked with clinical response. The result indicates one of the following: a high probability of treatment success, the uncertain effect of treatment, or a high probability of treatment failure [12]. This testing can aid with identifying trends in susceptibility changes or new drug resistance mechanisms. While yeast susceptibility testing is routine, the Infectious Diseases Society of America does not formally recommend testing of *Aspergillus*.

Inherent Resistance

Fungal resistance to drug treatment occurs with all antifungal drug classes. However, resistance is relatively infrequent, as most fungi are susceptible to the commonly used antifungals. Intrinsic resistance to one class of antifungals can be seen; however, it is rare for fungi to be pan-resistant to all drug classes; *C. auris* is one exception that is found to be resistant to the main three classes of antifungals [1]. Inherent resistance occurs from selection of less susceptible species. In *Candida*, a shift has been documented in global epidemiological studies toward less susceptible strains due to the impact of widespread triazole use [9]. The shift has been toward non-*C. albicans* species including *Candida krusei* and *Candida glabrata*, the latter of which is well-known to have inherent reduced susceptibility to fluconazole [9]. Often, *Candida* strains that are inherently resistant to fluconazole show resistance to higher activity azoles as well (Fig. 8.4). For *Aspergillus*, this

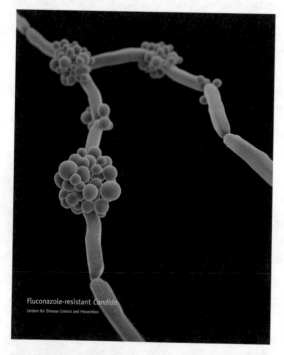

Fluconazole-resistant *Candida*
Centers for Disease Control and Prevention

Fig. 8.4 Illustration depicting a three-dimensional (3D) computer-generated image of a fluconazole-resistant *Candida*. (Source: https://phil.cdc.gov/Details.aspx?pid=16871)

resistance does not always hold true, as species may be fluconazole-resistant but susceptible to higher activity azoles like voriconazole [9]. One exception in the Netherlands was the development of a multidrug-resistant *A. fumigatus* variant caused by the prevalent use of agricultural fungicides [13].

Acquired Resistance

In contrast to inherent resistance, acquired (secondary) resistance is gained during therapy. Acquired resistance to the azoles and echinocandin drug classes is a growing issue globally, and the possibility of multidrug resistance is a major concern given the limited number of available antifungal drugs. Antifungal resistance mechanisms have been studied to better understand drug susceptibility [9].

Fungi employ four main strategies to resist drug therapy:

1. Mutations induced in targeted proteins (observed in azoles and echinocandins)
2. Overexpression of targeted proteins (observed in azoles)
3. Upregulation of biosynthesis of efflux pumps or augmented insertion of efflux pumps in cell membranes (observed in azoles)
4. Decreased access to targets as in the sequestration of ergosterol (observed in polyenes)

1. Mutations in Targeted Proteins

One mechanism of antifungal resistance seen with echinocandins and azole is genetic modification of the drug target protein. This type of mutation leads to reduced affinity of the drug for the target site.

Echinocandin resistance is based in amino acid substitutions in the FKS1 and FKS2 subunits of glucan synthase. Amino acid substitutions at *Fks*1 positions Phe641 and Ser645 are the most common modifications in *C. albicans*, and these mutations in target proteins decrease enzyme affinity for echinocandins by several thousand-fold. Other *Candida* species have similar mutations. *C. glabrata* is found to have both FKS1 (Phe625, Ser629) and FKS2 (Phe659, Ser663) mutations [9]. Reversal of FKS2-dependent resistance in *C. glabrata* is possible by treatment with the calcineurin inhibitor, tacrolimus. Additionally, *C. parapsilosis* shows a proline-to-alanine mutation in FKS1 due to naturally occurring polymorphisms [14]. In the *Scedosporium* species, echinocandin resistance is found to be due to a Trp-to-Phe substitution at position 695 [14].

Triazoles have varied affinities for drug targets, and this causes differences in their activity. Fluconazole has the broadest resistance as it has weak drug target interaction and a narrow spectrum, with activity only against yeasts and not molds. Conversely, triazoles such as voriconazole and posaconazole are highly active, interact with the drug target strongly, and have activity against both yeasts and molds – displaying a narrower spectrum of resistance mutations [9].

Azole resistance is commonly due to mutations in *ERG11*, as this gene encodes lanosterol 14α-demethylase, the enzyme targeted by azoles. Over 140 amino acid substitutions have been reported in *Candida* which have an additive effect [15]. In *C. albicans*, two common alterations are R467K and G464S, near the heme-binding site [8].

In *Aspergillus*, resistance can be caused by mutations in *Cyp51A*, but in *C. glabrata*, mutations in *CgERG11* do not cause resistance [9]. In *C. auris*, azole resistance has been thought to stem from *ERG11* polymorphisms [10]. The *Fusarium* species (especially *F. solani* complex, *F. oxysporum*, and *F. fujikuroi* complex) are resistant to multiple drugs, and the CYP51A amino acid substitution and/or gene overexpression may be involved in azole resistance [14]. *Mucormycetes* are resistant to azoles through the Phe129 substitution for Tyr in the *CYP51 F5* gene and the possible contribution of Val-to-Ala substitutions at positions 291 and 293 [14].

2. Overexpression of Targeted Proteins

In azole-resistant *C. albicans*, overexpression of ERG11 is frequent and contributes directly to resistance as an increase in target protein requires more drug for inhibition [16]. There are many mechanisms responsible for the overexpression of *ERG11* in azole-resistant fungi. The *EFGR* gene is located on chromosome 5. It can be amplified if two copies of the left arm of chromosome 5 are formed (i(5L)) or if the whole chromosome 5 is duplicated. Another mechanism causing overexpression of *ERG11* is through activating mutations of Upc2, a transcription factor involved with ergosterol biosynthesis [8].

Other species including *C. glabrata*, *C. parapsilosis*, *C. tropicalis*, and *C. krusei* have also been reported to show overexpression of *ERG11*. Azole resistance has also been seen in *A. fumigatus* with mutations in the promoter region of *Cyp51A*, thus causing overexpression of the target protein [11].

3. Upregulation of Biosynthesis of Efflux Pumps or Augmented Insertion of Efflux Pumps in Cell Membranes

The most common mechanism of azole resistance is increased activity of drug efflux pumps in fungi; most often this type of resistance is caused by gain-of-function mutations in transcription factors that regulate transporters [10]. There are two drug efflux systems that cause azole resistance in fungi: the adenosine triphosphate-binding cassette (ABC) superfamily and the major facilitator superfamily (MFS). These systems are both membrane-associated efflux pumps that can cause multidrug resistance (MDR) [8].

The ABC proteins are made up of two cytoplasmic nucleotide-binding domains (NBD) that catalyze ATP hydrolysis, as well as two transmembrane span domains (TMS). Different fungi have been found to have varying numbers of ABC transporters. One category of ABC transporter, the pleiotropic drug resistance (PDR) class, includes transporters involved with azole resistance in *C. albicans*. CDR1 and CDR2 are two such transporters that, when upregulated, enhance drug efflux and reduce azole accumulation [8].

In contrast, MFS transporters have multiple TMS domains, but no cytoplasmic domains. They have been found to use electrochemical potential and proton-motive force to regulate drug efflux [17]. While there are multiple MFS transporters, only one MFS, *MDR1*, has shown to be correlated with azole resistance in *C. albicans*. However, unlike CDR gene-encoded efflux pumps which affect all azole drugs, pumps encoded by MDR genes are usually selective for fluconazole [11]. In *A. fumigatus*, the MFS transporter that is encoded by *Afu*MDR3 is upregulated in some itraconazole-resistant mutants [18].

4. Decreased Access to Target as in the Sequestration of Ergosterol

The polyenes, which work by targeting plasma membrane sterols, are used for systemic infection, particularly in severe cases. The mechanisms of resistance are not well understood; however, resistance has been associated with a lower amount of ergosterol content in the cell membrane, as well as increased filamentation [1].

Fungi that can survive without ergosterol would have decreased susceptibility to polyenes. Studies suggest that fungi can develop resistance by utilizing zymosterol instead of ergosterol in the cell membrane [1]. This would lead to increased membrane integrity. Decreased access to ergosterol can also occur in polyenes resistance due to increased filamentation through hyphae. As such, these structures play a crucial role in virulence and nutrient acquisition [1]. Decreased access to ergosterol can ultimately lead to resistance.

Other Mechanisms of Resistance

Biofilms

One mechanism by which fungi avoid detection by the immune system is through the production of biofilms. Biofilms serve as a physical barrier and are often seen on mucus membranes and medical devices (such as catheters) [1]. The biofilm produced by fungi is characterized by an extracellular matrix that contains substances such as glucan and mannan. Glucan synthase produces ß-1,3-glucan which serves as a key component and is regulated by components of the yeast PKC pathway, such as Smi1, Rlm1, Rho1, and Fsk1. Other proteins and glucoamylases that affect matrix production and resistance phenotypes are Zap1, alcohol dehydrogenases Adh5, Csh1, Ifd6, CaGca1, and CaGca2 [8].

Functionally, the biofilm extracellular matrix serves an adhesive role and causes resistance to antifungal drugs by directly trapping them within the biofilm area. Due to this, the fungal cells are consequently less exposed to the drug by the physical barrier [10]. Biofilms not only sequester drugs within the matrix but can also induce drug efflux pumps by upregulation of *CDR* and *MDR* genes. This can cause as much as a 10,000-fold decrease in antifungal susceptibility for fungi with biofilms in comparison to susceptibility of planktonic (free-floating) fungal cells [1].

Stress Responses and Drug Adaptation

Fungi are known to have a robust response against cellular stressors, and adaptations will often result in increased in vitro MICs [9]. This cellular response can allow for survival from stress caused by drug exposure, and over time, resistance is developed [8]. Hsp90 and calcineurin are two regulators that play a major role in the drug-induced stress response of fungi which was first described with azoles [9]. Hsp90 stabilizes calcineurin, a protein phosphatase involved with calcineurin-Crz1 signaling which works on multiple cellular responses including ion homeostasis and cell wall integrity pathway, Mkc1 [8]. Therefore, by inhibiting Hsp90 or calcineurin, azoles can gain efficacy against fungi that are resistant [9].

Adaptive cellular responses also impact echinocandin resistance, and genetic or chemical modulation of Hsp90 reduces echinocandin tolerance [19]. PKC, HOG, and calcineurin signaling coordinate chitin synthesis, which has also been found to increase as a compensatory response to echinocandin action. Chitin replaces β-1,3-glucan which helps maintain structural integrity of the cell wall and decreases sensitivity to echinocandins; a link has been observed between increased chitin levels and paradoxical growth with very high levels of echinocandins [19]. Additionally, sphingolipids in the membrane can interact with echinocandins, and this can control enzyme sensitivity through echinocandin-Fks interaction [19].

Chromosomal Abnormalities

Genetic alterations and chromosomal anomalies have been found to be associated with azole resistance in fungi [9]. One mechanism that can cause resistance is through loss of heterozygosity. In particular, this is seen with mutations in the genes, *ERG11*, *TAC1*, and *MRR1*. Analysis of *C. albicans* with clinical resistance has shown that mutations in these genes often begin in a heterozygous state and then are converted to homozygous by loss of heterozygosity [8].

Another mechanism of resistance is through chromosome copy number variations, including aneuploidies. Azole resistance in *C. albicans* has been seen through these larger-scale changes. For example, *ERG11* and *TAC1* are two genes that confer resistance to azoles in *C. albicans*. These genes are located on the left arm of chromosome 5, and the formation of isochromosome i(5L) creates resistance by increasing the chromosome copy number [9]. One variant of i(5L) incorporates *CDR1* and *MRR1* from the right arm region of chromosome 3 [8]. These genes encode for a major ABC transporter and a transcriptional activator of the major facilitator superfamily transporter, which ultimately facilitates increased efflux and resistance development [10].

Additionally, increased stress promotes chromosome changes and aneuploidy. It has been found that azole exposure causes aberrant cell cycle regulation in *C. albicans*, and a tetraploid intermediate precedes aneuploid formation when exposed to fluconazole [20].

Lastly, *C. glabrata* and *C. neoformans* have also shown resistance through chromosomal modifications. An increase in *ERG11* copy number has been found in *C. glabrata* azole resistance, as well as the formation of novel chromosome configurations and aneuploidies [8]. Disomies of chromosomes 1 and 4 have been associated with azole resistance in *C. neoformans*, in which *ERG11* and *AFR1* can be altered in copy number [8].

Mitochondrial Defects

C. glabrata has been shown to have high-frequency azole-resistant mutants that lack a mitochondrial genome; these mutants resemble multidrug-resistant *S. cerevisiae* that also lack a mitochondrial genome [8]. Mutants that lack mitochondrial DNA ("petite mutants") are resistant to azoles due to transcription activation upregulation, including *PDR3* in *S. cerevisiae* and *CgPDR1* in *C. glabrata* [8]. With *C. glabrata*, mutants that lack mitochondrial DNA upregulate ABC transporter genes causing increased azole resistance, and these petite mutants have shown increased virulence in studies [21]. Contrastingly, *C. albicans* is "petite negative," as it cannot lose its mitochondrial DNA. Overall, the difference in resistance versus susceptibility in different *Candida* species demonstrates the complexities of mitochondrial defects as a mechanism of resistance in various fungi.

Conclusion

As fatalities associated with fungal infections continue to grow as a major global health issue, the need for effective antifungal treatment is crucial. The current number of effective therapeutic drug options, however, is limited. With this, the documented rise in antifungal drug resistance in recent years is a critical concern, as resistance development severely limits the ability to successfully treat fatal infection. Resistance has been found to be inherent or acquired, and common mechanisms of acquired resistance include mutations in target proteins, overexpression of targets, upregulation of efflux pumps, and decreased access to target proteins. Furthermore, the potential for multidrug resistance in fungi is of major concern. With a lack of numerous antifungal treatments available and the known fatalities associated with fungal infection, continued research into effective drug therapy is necessary. With this, an understanding of the mechanisms of antifungal resistance is imperative in order to effectively diagnose infection, treat patients, and ultimately develop novel and successful therapeutics against fungal infection in the future.

References

1. Howard KC, Dennis EK, Watt DS, Garneau-Tsodikova S. A comprehensive overview of the medicinal chemistry of antifungal drugs: perspectives and promise. Chem Soc Rev. 2020;49(8):2426–80.

2. Rauseo AM, Coler-Reilly A, Larson L, Spec A. Hope on the Horizon: novel fungal treatments in development. Open Forum Infect Dis. 2020;7(2):ofaa016.

3. Bongomin F, Gago S, Oladele RO, Denning DW. Global and Multi-National Prevalence of fungal diseases-estimate precision. J Fungi (Basel). 2017;3(4):57.

4. Lee H, Lee DG. Novel approaches for efficient antifungal drug action. J Microbiol Biotechnol. 2018;28(11):1771–81.

5. Gintjee TJ, Donnelley MA, Thompson GR. Aspiring antifungals: review of current antifungal pipeline developments. J Fungi (Basel). 2020;6(1):28.

6. De carli L, Larizza L. Griseofulvin. Mutat Res. 1988;195(2):91–126.

7. Georgopapadakou NH. Antifungals: mechanism of action and resistance, established and novel drugs. Curr Opin Microbiol. 1998;1(5):547–57.

8. Cowen LE, Sanglard D, Howard SJ, Rogers PD, Perlin DS. Mechanisms of antifungal drug resistance. Cold Spring Harb Perspect Med. 2014;5(7):a019752.

9. Perlin DS, Shor E, Zhao Y. Update on antifungal drug resistance. Curr Clin Microbiol Rep. 2015;2(2):84–95.

10. Berman J, Krysan DJ. Drug resistance and tolerance in fungi. Nat Rev Microbiol. 2020;18(6):319–31.

11. Pfaller MA. Antifungal drug resistance: mechanisms, epidemiology, and consequences for treatment. Am J Med. 2012;125(1 Suppl):S3–13.

12. Perlin DS, Rautemaa-Richardson R, Alastruey-Izquierdo A. The global problem of antifungal resistance: prevalence, mechanisms, and management. Lancet Infect Dis. 2017;17(12):e383–e92.

13. Verweij PE, Snelders E, Kema GH, Mellado E, Melchers WJ. Azole resistance in Aspergillus fumigatus: a side-effect of environmental fungicide use? Lancet Infect Dis. 2009;9(12):789–95.

14. Houst J, Spizek J, Havlicek V. Antifungal Drugs. Meta. 2020;10(3):106.

15. Morio F, Loge C, Besse B, Hennequin C, Le pape P. Screening for amino acid substitutions in the Candida albicans Erg11 protein of azole-susceptible and azole-resistant clinical isolates: new substitutions and a review of the literature. Diagn Microbiol Infect Dis. 2010;66(4):373–84.

16. Lee Y, Puumala E, Robbins N, Cowen LE. Antifungal drug resistance: molecular mechanisms in and beyond. Chem Rev. 2020.

17. Sá-Correia I, dos Santos SC, Teixeira MC, Cabrito TR, Mira NP. Drug:H+ antiporters in chemical stress response in yeast. Trends Microbiol. 2009;17(1):22–31.

18. Nascimento AM, Goldman GH, Park S, et al. Multiple resistance mechanisms among Aspergillus fumigatus mutants with high-level resistance to itraconazole. Antimicrob Agents Chemother. 2003;47(5):1719–26.

19. Perlin DS. Mechanisms of echinocandin antifungal drug resistance. Ann N Y Acad Sci. 2015;1354:1–11.

20. Harrison BD, Hashemi J, Bibi M, et al. A tetraploid intermediate precedes aneuploid formation in yeasts exposed to fluconazole. PLoS Biol. 2014;12(3):e1001815.

21. Ferrari S, Sanguinetti M, De bernardis F, et al. Loss of mitochondrial functions associated with azole resistance in Candida glabrata results in enhanced virulence in mice. Antimicrob Agents Chemother. 2011;55(5):1852–60.

Emerging and Re-emerging Fungal Infections

Fabio Francesconi, Valeska Francesconi, Omar Lupi, and Yasmin Khalfe

Abbreviations

anti-IFN-γ	Anti-interferon-gamma
CAPA	COVID-19-associated pulmonary aspergillosis
HM	Hematologic malignancies
IA	Invasive pulmonary aspergillosis
IFI	Invasive fungal infection
TNFα	Tumor necrosis factor α

F. Francesconi
Dermatology Section - Federal University of the State of Amazonas (UFAM), Manaus, Brazil

Dermatologist - Hospital de Medicina Tropical, Manaus, Brazil

V. Francesconi
Dermatology Section - State University of Amazonas, Manaus, Brazil

Dermatologist - Hospital de Medicina Tropical, Manaus, Brazil

O. Lupi
Associate Professor of Dermatology - Federal University of the State of Rio de Janeiro (UNIRIO), Rio de Janeiro, Brazil

Immunology Section - Federal University of Rio de Janeiro (UFRJ), Rio de Janeiro, Brazil

Titular Professor & Chairman - Policlinica Geral do Rio de Janeiro (PGRJ), Rio de Janeiro, Brazil

Ibero Latin American College of Dermatology (CILAD), Buenos Aires, Argentina

International League of Dermatological Societies (ILDS), London, UK

Y. Khalfe (✉)
School of Medicine, Baylor College of Medicine, Houston, TX, USA
e-mail: yasmin.khalfe@bcm.edu

Introduction

Medical mycology is an ever-changing and fascinating branch of medicine. With recent advances in medical treatment, life expectancy has improved but simultaneously increased risk factors for fungal infections. With this, pathogens have new opportunities to cause human disease. New immunosuppressive therapies, widespread use of antimicrobials, and more sophisticated methods of identifying fungi (including new species) are the leading causes of changing trends and clinical manifestations observed in human fungal infections.

Dermatology is one of the specialties that studies and deals the most with clinical mycology. With that in mind, the modern dermatologist must be proficient in identifying the many presentations of skin manifestations related to fungal infection. This chapter aims to highlight the most striking changes regarding taxonomy, epidemiology, and clinical manifestations of emerging and re-emerging fungal skin infection.

© Springer Nature Switzerland AG 2021
S. K. Tyring et al. (eds.), *Overcoming Antimicrobial Resistance of the Skin*, Updates in Clinical Dermatology, https://doi.org/10.1007/978-3-030-68321-4_9

Invasive Fungal Infections and the Skin

Invasive fungal infection (IFI) occurs when the pathogen reaches the bloodstream and causes systemic infection. It is a life-threatening complication and requires swift diagnosis to prevent complications and fatal outcomes [1]. Diagnosis of IFI is based on clinical symptoms, imaging, and confirmation of the causative agent. It is a multisystemic disease that usually involves the lungs as a primary focus [2]. Patients most often report nonspecific symptoms such as fever, cough, chest pain, and hemoptysis; however, rash and oral lesions can also be seen. Thus, dermatologists can help identify and diagnose cases of IFI.

Certain clinical conditions are risk factors for developing IFI. In general, any type of immunosuppression can predispose a patient to systemic fungal infections, especially those related to cellular immunity. With the development of novel immunomodulators, certain drugs have been found to be more commonly associated with fungal infections:

- Ibrutinib is a Bruton's tyrosine kinase inhibitor that is used to treat B-cell malignancies. It is associated with severe fungal infection, particularly *Aspergillus* and *Cryptococcus* [3].
- Fingolimod is a syphingosine-1-phosphate receptor used for treating relapsing-remitting multiple sclerosis. Fingolimod has been suggested as a possible risk factor for the development of cryptococcosis and histoplasmosis [3].
- Cell cycle checkpoint inhibitors are used to treat cancers such as melanoma, non-small cell lung cancer, and hematologic malignancies. They are hypothesized to have antifungal effects because of upregulation of the immune system. In contrast, invasive aspergillosis and candidiasis have been shown to occur after use of the checkpoint inhibitor, nivolumab [3].

Dermatophytosis

Dermatophytes (tinea) are found globally and cause fungal infections that commonly affect the skin, hair, and nails [4]. The *Arthrodermatacea* family contains multiple genera of dermatophytes, and in 2017, a new taxonomic classification came into force. Now there are seven genera described: *Trichophyton*, *Epidermophyton*, *Nannizzia*, *Paraphyton*, *Lophophyton*, *Microsporum*, and *Arthroderma* [5]. Recently, *Epidermophyton* has been described as a sister genus of *Nannizzia*, and further extensive studies are needed to obtain conclusive results as to whether *Epidermophyton* falls within the *Nannizzia* clade [5].

Invasive Dermatophyte Infections

Invasive dermatophytosis is a rare infection; however, it is valuable to remember that it presents as a dermatophyte infection that reaches the dermis. Tricophytic invasion is the most common cause of invasive dermatophyte infection but is not necessarily an opportunistic infection [4]. In some cases, local trauma predisposes toward infection, while in others, topical or systemic immunosuppression is the predisposing factor. Clinically the infection presents as papules or nodules with a variable degree of suppuration. More severe cases can resemble kerion celsi.

The other type of infection includes deep dermatophytosis. In these cases, fungal structures reach the dermis in the context of an opportunistic infection. With few published cases, post-transplant patients are the leading risk group [6]. Other associations include HIV infection, diabetes mellitus, immunosuppressive therapeutics, and chronic liver disease [6]. CARD9 deficiency is due to a mutation that leads to an immunological deficit, and it is also associated with deep dermatophytosis (as well as other fungal infections including candidiasis and phaeohyphomycosis) [7]. Clinically, profound dermatophytosis manifests with nodular dermal or subcutaneous lesions and typical superficial infection including onychomycosis (Fig. 9.1). Lymphatic involvement is also reported. Rarely, invasion of other organs occurs, usually by local extension [7].

Pseudomycetoma

Dermatophytic pseudomycetomas are fungal infections characterized by deep dermal infiltra-

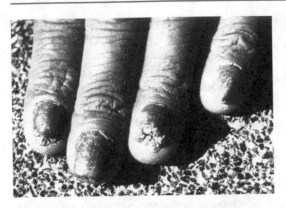

Fig. 9.1 The fingers on the left hand of a patient displaying symptoms of onychomycosis. (Source: CDC PHIL/ Dr. Libero Ajello (https://phil.cdc.gov/Details. aspx?pid=15714))

tion. Mycetomas show a triad of nodular swelling, draining sinuses, and "grain formation" of clustered organisms; these infections may be fungal or bacterial [8]. While its name suggests a fungal origin, botryomycosis is a bacterial mycetoma most commonly caused by *Staphylococcus aureus* followed by *Pseudomonas aeruginosa*. Unlike mycetomas, dermatophytic pseudomycetomas usually lack sinus tracts and commonly involve the scalp [8]. They are a rare cause of infection; however, an increase in recent reports in the literature suggests that these infections are an emerging cause of disease. Pseudomycetomas may not respond to antifungal treatment; therefore, having proper knowledge regarding the clinicopathological findings of this fungal infection is crucial [8].

Epidemiological Shift of Dermatophyte Infections

Over the last 20 or more years, *T. mentagrophytes* complex surpassed *T. rubrum* as the primary causative agent of dermatophytosis in India. *T. mentagrophytes* now represents about 90% of the dermatophyte cases in this region [9]. This epidemic in India showed more efficient human-to-human transmission and inflammatory and eruptive lesions were more common compared to previous infections [3]. It was found that in one

hospital, 78% of all skin lesions were due to dermatophytosis [10]. This increase in prevalence is likely due to environmental features such as tropical climate and poorer living standards in rural areas that can increase the risk of cutaneous dermatophyte infections [10].

Chronic Dermatophytosis

Chronic dermatophytosis is defined as infection that lasts for 6 or more months. Previously, chronic dermatophytosis was very rare, but with the epidemic of dermatophytosis in India, cases have been increasing over the last 40 years [11]. Chronic dermatophytosis is seen with relapse of the disease or when treatment is ineffective. In the first scenario, one of the main causes is familial dermatophytosis. In this case, the infection afflicts one or more members of the home due to everyday habits, and the entire family must be treated in order to control the infection. Patients afflicted with recurrent or chronic dermatophytosis do, in fact, usually have affected family members [11].

Drug-Resistant Dermatophytes

Resistance to antifungal treatment is the other cause of increasing dermatophyte infection, and although it is a rare phenomenon, the number of reports has been increasing with time. Most reported cases of drug-resistant dermatophyte infections are related to the *Trichophyton* genera, especially recalcitrant superficial dermatophytosis in India [10]. The multidrug resistance found in India may cause both treatment failure and relapses.

Candidiasis

Candida albicans is the most significant species within the *Candida* genus. However, in recent years, there has been a shift in infection patterns toward non-albicans *Candida* species, as well as the emergence of antifungal resistance.

Changes in *Candida* Species

C. albicans is well-established as the most prevalent species of *Candida* in cases of invasive candidiasis. However, in a 20-year surveillance study on invasive candidiasis, it was found that infections responsible by *C. albicans* decreased from 57.4% to 46.4% in recent years [12]. *C. glabrata* has also shown an increase in antifungal resistance and was found to be attributable for 30% of invasive candidemia in the United States [13]. Another worrisome species is *C. parapsilosis*, which has been found to be responsible for 15% of candidemia in the United States [14]. *C. parapsilosis* is related to inadequate infection control programs, and with its ability to develop resistance, it can be a concerning cause nosocomial infections [3].

Candida auris Emergence

First described in 2009, *Candida auris* is a multidrug-resistant organism that has been the subject of concern due to invasive candidiasis and potential for causing outbreaks in healthcare settings (nosocomial infection). It has many virulence factors, including a biofilm that allows itself to withstand environmental stress [15]. Other virulence factors include its production of phospholipases and proteinases, its proclivity to colonize patients and surfaces, and its resistance to antifungals [3]. *C. auris* is largely resistant to fluconazole, and additionally, 30% of isolates are resistant to amphotericin B and 5% are resistant to echinocandins [3]. The potential for multidrug resistance is an alarming aspect of this emerging fungi. Mortality rates for bloodstream infection have been found to be between 30 and 60% [16]. With the high possibility of mortality and potential for resistance, it is important that those who may have a *C. auris* infection be tested for susceptibility and closely monitored for clinical improvement [17].

Cryptococcosis

Although *Cryptococcus neoformans* has been studied since the nineteenth century, it was not until the HIV pandemic that it became universally recognized as an important cause of meningoencephalitis in AIDS patients. On the Pacific Northwest coast, another cryptococcus species, *C. gattii*, is an emerging fungus found to cause significant disease in both immunocompromised and immunocompetent hosts [3].

The new subdivision of the *Cryptococcus* genus was divided into seven groups based on molecular typing, and each has been found to have unique features [18]:

- *Cryptococcus neoformans* sensu stricto (formerly *C. neoformans* serotype A) causes most cases of cryptococcal meningoencephalitis.
- *Cryptococcus deneoformans* (previously *C. neoformans* serotype D or C) is more often involved with soft tissue and cutaneous infections. Infection is most common with HIV patients and those over 60 years old.
- *Cryptococcus gattii* sensu stricto infection is primarily found in Australia and has been seen mostly in healthy individuals.
- *Cryptococcus bacillisporus* has been found to affect those with HIV and other immunocompromised people.
- *Cryptococcus deuterogattii* affects immunocompetent people. It is an emerging fungus that is associated with previous outbreaks in Vancouver Island and the Pacific Northwest of the United States.
- *Cryptococcus tetragattii*, which previously belonged to the *C. gattii* classification, is a relatively rare species.
- *Cryptococcus decagattii* is another species that was previously categorized within the *C. gattii* classification and is a rare species, with few isolates found.

Aspergillosis

Aspergillus fumigatus and Non-fumigatus *Aspergillus*

Aspergillus fumigatus is the most common cause of invasive aspergillosis, an infection that normally affects the lungs and sinuses and has a high mortality rate in immunocompromised patients. Since the late 1990s, *A. fumigatus* has been associated with antimicrobial resistance, particularly with the azole class of drugs, and has caused global concern [19]. The majority of resistance is caused by mutations in the *cyp51A* gene which is usually associated with environmental exposure to azoles, but many other mechanisms have been implicated as well [20]. The species is, however, usually susceptible to newer-generation triazole antifungals which have greatly improved clinical outcomes. Nevertheless, continued development of resistance is a greatly emerging concern. Given the widespread use of azole fungicides globally, efforts have been discussed in recent years to curb growing resistance [21].

Aspergillus flavus is the second most common cause of invasive aspergillosis in immunocompromised patients. In immunocompetent patients, cutaneous, subcutaneous, and mucosal infections are seen. Infections with *A. flavus* have been increasing; this species is predominantly seen in Asia, the Middle East, and Africa [22]. Unlike *A. fumigatus*, triazole resistance is rare; however, data supports that *A. flavus* may be intrinsically resistant to amphotericin B [22]. A continued investigation into the diagnosis and pharmacologic treatment of *A. flavus* is important, and further understanding into its mechanisms of resistance is necessary as this fungal species continues to increase in incidence.

Influenza-Associated Invasive Pulmonary Aspergillosis

Invasive pulmonary aspergillosis (IA) is described as a complication of severe influenza infection, otherwise referred to as influenza-associated IA [23]. These cases often have no other risk factor for invasive aspergillosis. In the intensive care setting, the presence of influenza pneumonia has been shown to raise the risk of developing IA to 14% from 5% [24]. Additionally, it was found that mortality in immunocompetent patients with influenza-associated IA was 50%, while mortality in patients with severe influenza but without IA was 29% [24]. As an emerging cause of infection, further investigation is needed to understand the mechanism of damage of this disease and potential antifungal treatments.

COVID-19-Associated Invasive Pulmonary Aspergillosis

Just as critically-ill patients have been associated with influenza-associated IA, recently there have been reports describing fatal invasive aspergillosis associated with COVID-19 in patients [25]. This novel infection, known as COVID-19-associated pulmonary aspergillosis (CAPA), has emerged as a major concern. In a recent report from an ICU in the Netherlands, a high incidence (19.4%) of ICU patients with COVID-19 developed invasive pulmonary aspergillosis, suggesting that COVID-19 patients are at risk of developing IA [26]. In another report from Germany, 26.3% of ICU patients were reported to have developed CAPA, and mortality of these patients was 60% [27].

The risk of IA in COVID-19 patients is a newly emerging issue that is currently being further investigated. Because of the high mortality rates that have been reported, early diagnosis and systematic testing are important considerations in COVID-19 patients. A two-step process was proposed by Gangneux et al. that associates a molecular approach of qPCR for *Aspergillus*, *Pneumocystis jirovecii*, and *Mucorales* with culture for respiratory samples. If positive, a confirmatory test with blood biomarkers can be used [28]. Effective, rapid treatment with antifungals is necessary until the associated risks are better understood. As the COVID-19 pandemic continues globally, further assessment is needed to assess COVID-19-associated invasive pulmonary aspergillosis.

Blastomycosis

Blastomycosis is a dimorphic fungal infection that is caused by inhaling fungal spores and can lead to pulmonary infections. Until recently, this infection was thought to be caused by the sole agent *Blastomyces dermatitidis*, a fungus that is seen in areas of North America surrounding the Ohio and Mississippi River valleys and the Great Lakes [29]. In recent years, taxonomy has changed as researchers have divided *Blastomyces* into two species. In 2013, Brown et al. described

Blastomyces gilchristii, a novel species that along with *B. dermatitidis* makes up the species complex [30]. Since then, research describing *B. gilchristii* has been limited. It has been reported to have caused at least one case of fatal ARDS in humans [31]. Research on the ecological niches of these fungi have shown *B. dermatitidis* to be recovered from areas throughout North America, while *B. gilchristii* has been recovered only in Canada and some northern US states; both species are associated with major freshwater drainage basins [32].

Atypical blastomycosis can be caused by *Blastomyces helicus* in western North America and *Blastomyces percursus* in Africa [33]. *B. helices*, initially known as *Emmonsia helica*, most commonly affects immunocompromised patients, particularly those with HIV, malignancy, organ transplant, or autoimmune disease [33, 34]. *Blastomyces percursus* was initially described in 2015 and is characterized by secondary conidiospores that display an appearance of florets [33].

Histoplasmosis

Histoplasmosis is a dimorphic fungal infection caused by the *Histoplasma capsulatum* and often presents with respiratory symptoms, although it can disseminate to other organs including the skin, brain, gastrointestinal tract, adrenal glands, and bone marrow (Fig. 9.2)

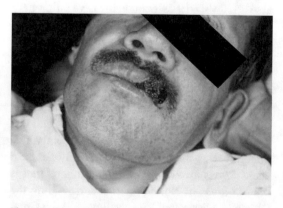

Fig. 9.2 Disseminated histoplasmosis manifesting as an ulcer on the upper lip. (Source: CDC PHIL/Susan Lindsley, VD (https://phil.cdc.gov/Details.aspx?pid=6840))

[35]. The fungus is predominantly found in North and South America, particularly the Ohio and Mississippi River valleys in the United States, and in recent years, there has been substantial increased burden on the healthcare system due to histoplasmosis-associated hospitalizations [36]. Disseminated histoplasmosis is more commonly seen in patients with HIV/AIDS and other immunosuppressive disorders or those taking immunosuppressive agents [37]. Studies suggest that handling bird or bat droppings is a risk factor for patients with AIDS and antiretroviral therapy and fluconazole are protective [38]. While *Histoplasma* has been recognized for many years, it has shown an increase in prevalence in recent years, and its re-emergence can be associated with the expansion in the susceptible population [39].

In terms of classification, Sepúlveda et al. suggested in 2017 that the *Histoplasma* genus is composed of at least four different cryptic species [40]. It was proposed that the originally described *Histoplasma* in Panama be named *H. capsulatum* sensu stricto and the other three *Histoplasma* found mainly around the Mississippi River, Ohio River, and South America be named *H. mississippiense*, *H. ohiense*, and *H. suramericanum*, respectively [40]. Further understanding of the differences between species is crucial to identifying the virulence factors of each and, in turn, the pathogenicity and resistance patterns of each species.

Sporotrichosis

The dimorphic fungi species, *Sporothrix*, causes a chronic granulomatous infection called sporotrichosis that was originally described in 1898 and has a global distribution [39]. Previously, *Sporothrix schenckii* was thought to be the only species causing human disease. However, recent advances in technology have allowed for further taxonomy research and shown that *Sporothrix* actually is a complex comprised of many taxons including *Sporothrix globosa* and *Sporothrix brasiliensis* [41].

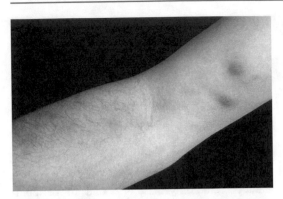

Fig. 9.3 Erythematous, papulosquamous lesions with lymphatic involvement, diagnosed as sporotrichosis due to *Sporothrix schenckii*. (Source: CDC PHIL/Dr. Libero Ajello (https://phil.cdc.gov/Details.aspx?pid=16820))

Classically, sporotrichosis had been associated with transmission through trauma with contaminated plants and was known as "rosebush mycosis" or the "gardener's mycosis" [42]. Cutaneous findings, most often nodules, usually appear 2 to 4 weeks after trauma and progress along lymphangitic channels (Fig. 9.3) [42]. Infection can also involve mucous membranes, with the ocular mucous being the most commonly affected. Ocular disease can lead to endophthalmitis, retinal granuloma, granulomatous uveitis, and choroiditis [43]. While many patients' *Sporothrix* infections resolve spontaneously, others may develop nonspecific cutaneous reactions such as erythema nodosum, erythema multiforme, and Sweet's syndrome [42, 44, 45]. Recent case reports of these reactions show the importance of identifying the infection in order to provide proper treatment.

Zoonotic Sporotrichosis in Brazil

In recent years, zoonotic transmission of *Sporothrix* has been reported. Particularly, in the last two decades in Brazil, there has been in an increase in incidence of infection found to be mainly transmitted through cats. Between 1992 and 2015, there was a documented emergence of this disease with 782 hospitalizations and 65 deaths in Brazil [46]. *S. brasiliensis* has been associated with feline transmission, showing a

higher virulence and a tendency to escalate to outbreaks or epidemics as seen in Brazil [47]. With this rise in zoonotic sporotrichosis, it is necessary to further study and understand both human and animal health as it relates to reducing the transmission of *Sporothrix*.

Re-emerging Mycoses due to Immunosuppressive Conditions

In recent years, emerging and re-emerging mycoses have evolved in epidemiology due to immunosuppressive conditions such as HIV, solid organ transplantation, diabetes mellitus, and iatrogenic immunosuppression. Here, emerging fungal infections that have shown changes in relation to immunosuppressive conditions and treatment are discussed.

Coccidioidomycosis

Coccidioides immitis in a dimorphic fungus found in desert regions of the southwest United States that causes coccidioidomycosis (also known as "valley fever") which usually present with infection of the lungs [48]. Occasionally, infection can disseminate and cause secondary cutaneous coccidioidomycosis (Fig. 9.4). In rare instances, primary cutaneous coccidioidomyco-

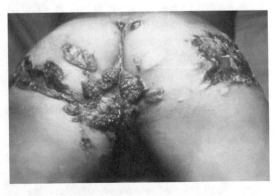

Fig. 9.4 A patient with cutaneous coccidioidomycosis caused by the fungal organism, *Coccidioides immitis*. (Source: CDC PHIL/ Dr. Brodsky (https://phil.cdc.gov/Details.aspx?pid=20552))

sis have been reported in literature and have resulted from trauma or laboratory inoculation [48]. Most commonly, those infected with *Coccidioides* do not show symptoms; however, patients who are immunocompromised are at a higher risk of developing severe illness. Patients at a higher risk include those with HIV/AIDS, organ transplant patients, persons taking immunosuppressive medications, pregnant women, and diabetic patients. Since the HIV epidemic, coccidioidomycosis has been recognized as an opportunistic infection that causes significant morbidity and mortality. With the introduction of antiretroviral therapy, rates of coccidioidomycosis among people with HIV/AIDS were shown to have decreased in Arizona [49]. Additionally, in the same study, those who did not receive antiretroviral therapy were three times more likely to develop symptomatic coccidioidomycosis than other HIV-infected persons [49]. In transplant patients, immunosuppression has long been known to be a risk factor for coccidioidomycosis. In the 1970s, increased mortality was documented in renal transplant patients on high-dose corticosteroid who had disseminated coccidioidomycosis [50]. There is an increased risk of coccidioidomycosis after organ transplantation when there is a past history of coccidioidomycosis or any positive serological findings just before transplantation; this risk may be reduced by initiating antifungal prophylactic therapy [50]. Additionally, as biologic agents increase in popularity, it has been found that the most commonly used agent, tumor necrosis factor α (TNFα) antagonists, causes a higher risk of developing symptomatic coccidioidomycosis [51]. Pregnancy is an established risk factor for coccidioidomycosis; however, the rate of infection appears to be decreasing for unknown reasons, and outcome has improved with amphotericin B treatment [52]. Lastly, it has been found that patients with diabetes mellitus are more likely to have severe coccidioidomycosis and commonly have lung disease [53]. Researchers have hypothesized that this could potentially be due to immune alteration [53]. As rates of diabetes mellitus increase worldwide, understanding the relationship between glycemic control and coccidioidomycosis is imperative.

Paracoccidioidomycosis

Paracoccidioides brasiliensis is a fungus endemic to South America that is usually associated with rural environments and agriculture [54]. Approximately 80% of the patients who are diagnosed each year with *P. brasiliensis* acquire the disease in Brazil, while others acquire it in different South American countries, mainly Colombia, Venezuela, Argentina, and Ecuador [54]. Paracoccidioidomycosis is found to be commonly associated with other compromising diseases, including tuberculosis in up to 20% of patients [55]. While *Paracoccidioides* is related to rural environments, the HIV epidemic was related to urban centers; therefore, there was overlap between HIV and *Paracoccidioides* infections during that time period, but mycoses such as histoplasmosis and coccidioidomycosis were more frequently associated with HIV [56]. Despite the advanced immunosuppression seen in HIV patients, the frequency of paracoccidioidomycosis is similar to that observed in non-HIV individuals in endemic areas [56]. In terms of immunosuppression due to hematologic malignancies (HM), lymphoma has been found to be the most commonly reported HM with paracoccidioidomycosis [56]. Overall, immunocompromised patients traveling to endemic areas should avoid high-risk exposures, and clinicians should keep paracoccidioidomycosis on the differential for patients with T-cell immunodeficiency who present with pulmonary infiltrates with nodules, cavitation or chronic alveolar consolidation, or skin or mucocutaneous lesions with a chronic evolution (Fig. 9.5) [56].

Mucormycosis

Mucormycosis (previously known as zygomycosis) is a fungus in the *Mucorales* order that has emerged in the past few decades as an infection associated with high mortality rates [57]. In developed countries, mucormycosis is relatively uncommon and mainly associated with diabetes mellitus, hematological malignancies undergoing chemotherapy, and allogeneic stem cell transplants [57]. Within hematologic malignancies,

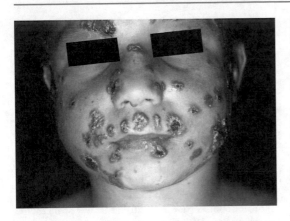

Fig. 9.5 Cutaneous manifestations of paracoccidioidomycosis caused by the fungus, *Paracoccidioides brasiliensis*. (Source: CDC PHIL/ Dr. Martins Castro, San Paulo, Brazil; Dr. Lucille K. Georg (https://phil.cdc.gov/Details.aspx?pid=12156))

acute myelogenous leukemia is the highest risk factor for mucormycosis [58]. As organ transplantation continues to increase, surveillance for mucormycosis is crucial as it is associated with a high mortality rate, and incidence ranges from 0.4% to 16.0% depending on organ type [57]. Classically, diabetes mellitus has been known as a risk factor for mucormycosis. However, in recent years, there has been a paradoxical increase in diabetes prevalence worldwide with a concomitant decrease in mucormycosis in diabetics [59]. It is hypothesized that the increased use of statins has led to this trend as statins have been found to work against some *Zygomycetes* [57, 59]. However, overall there is still a high annual incidence of mucormycosis in diabetics globally, and the strong association between diabetes control and socioeconomic status predisposes patients in these groups to life-threatening mucormycosis that could otherwise be prevented.

Talaromycosis

Talaromyces marneffei, previously known as *Penicillium marneffei*, is a fungus historically associated with causing infection in Southeast Asia, China, and India [60]. It was initially discovered in 1956 in bamboo rats and became increasingly frequent in humans in the 1980s

[61]. When the HIV epidemic reached Asia, the incidence of *Talaromyces marneffei* sharply increased in correlation with HIV/AIDS cases in Asia [62]. Fortunately, since the 1980s, antiretroviral therapy and improved control of the HIV/AIDS epidemic have reduced HIV transmission in certain areas of Asia, and infection with *Talaromyces marneffei* has subsequently decreased in prevalence [60]. However, there has been an increase in cases of *T. marneffei* in non-HIV-infected patients with other immunocompromising conditions [62]. In the 1990s, an increase in the use of immunosuppressive drugs occurred as organ transplantation increased and treatment of autoimmune diseases developed [62]. In children, non-HIV-associated *T. marneffei* infection became more frequently recognized as genetic testing for primary immunodeficiencies improved [62]. Additionally, *T. marneffei* was found to be associated with the acquired immunodeficiency syndrome caused by anti-interferon-gamma (anti-IFN-γ) autoantibodies [63]. Lastly, *T. marneffei* has recently been seen in patients who received monoclonal antibodies against CD20 and kinase inhibitors [64, 65]. For patients with weakened immune systems, *Talaromyces marneffei* can be fatal and requires swift and appropriate antifungal treatment [60]. Therefore, further studies to optimize surveillance of this disease are necessary.

Conclusion

In recent years, medical mycology has seen major changes in the taxonomy, epidemiology, clinical manifestations, and resistance development of many fungal species. Globally, emerging and re-emerging fungal infections have become a substantial concern. While technology has increased life expectancy, risk factors for fungal infection have subsequently increased. Certain fungal conditions such as invasive infections have grown in prevalence, and many of these infections show a concerning rate of mortality. As a specialty that deals with mycology on a regular basis, dermatology is a field that must be adept at diagnosing and treating fungal infections. It is imperative for dermatologists to be aware of the striking changes that have occurred within mycology in recent years, particularly those of emerging and re-emerging fungal infections.

References

1. Eades CP, Armstrong-James DPH. Invasive fungal infections in the immunocompromised host: mechanistic insights in an era of changing immunotherapeutics. Med Mycol. 2019;57(Supplement_3):S307–17. https://doi.org/10.1093/mmy/myy136.
2. Zhang H, Zhu A. Emerging invasive fungal infections: clinical features and controversies in diagnosis and treatment processes. Infect Drug Resist. 2020;13:607–15.
3. Friedman DZP, Schwartz IS. Emerging fungal infections: new patients, new patterns, and new pathogens. J Fungi (Basel). 2019;5(3):67.
4. Enoch DA, Yang H, Aliyu SH, Micallef C. The changing epidemiology of invasive fungal infections. Methods Mol Biol. 2017;1508:17–65.
5. Baert F, Stubbe D, D'hooge E, Packeu A, Hendrickx M. Updating the taxonomy of dermatophytes of the BCCM/IHEM collection according to the new standard: a phylogenetic approach. Mycopathologia. 2020;185(1):161–8.
6. Chastain MA, Reed RJ, Pankey GA. Deep dermatophytosis: report of 2 cases and review of the literature. Cutis. 2001;67(6):457–62.
7. Rouzaud C, Hay R, Chosidow O, et al. Severe dermatophytosis and acquired or innate immunodeficiency: a review. J Fungi (Basel). 2015;2(1):4.
8. Castro-echeverry E, Fiala K, Fernandez MP. Dermatophytic Pseudomycetoma of the Scalp. Am J Dermatopathol. 2017;39(2):e23–5.
9. Nenoff P, Verma SB, Vasani R, et al. The current Indian epidemic of superficial dermatophytosis due to Trichophyton mentagrophytes-A molecular study. Mycoses. 2019;62(4):336–56.
10. Upadhyay V, Kumar A, Singh AK, Pandey J. Epidemiological characterization of dermatophytes at a tertiary care hospital in Eastern Uttar Pradesh. India Curr Med Mycol. 2019;5(1):1–6.
11. Tuknayat A, Bhalla M, Kaur A, Garg S. Familial dermatophytosis in India: a study of the possible contributing risk factors. J Clin Aesthet Dermatol. 2020;13(2):58–60.
12. Pfaller MA, Diekema DJ, Turnidge JD, Castanheira M, Jones RN. Twenty years of the SENTRY antifungal surveillance program: results for species from 1997-2016. Open Forum Infect Dis. 2019;6(Suppl 1):S79–94.
13. Lamoth F, Lockhart SR, Berkow EL, Calandra T. Changes in the epidemiological landscape of invasive candidiasis. J Antimicrob Chemother. 2018;73(suppl_1):i4–i13.
14. Cleveland AA, Harrison LH, Farley MM, et al. Declining incidence of candidemia and the shifting epidemiology of Candida resistance in two US metropolitan areas, 2008-2013: results from population-based surveillance. PLoS One. 2015;10(3):e0120452.
15. Uppuluri P. Candida auris biofilm colonization on skin niche conditions. mSphere. 2020;5(1):e00972.
16. Spivak ES, Hanson KE. Candida auris: an emerging fungal pathogen. J Clin Microbiol. 2018;56(2):e01588.
17. Ostrowsky B, Greenko J, Adams E, et al. Candida auris isolates resistant to three classes of antifungal medications - New York, 2019. MMWR Morb Mortal Wkly Rep. 2020;69(1):6–9.
18. Hagen F, Khayhan K, Theelen B, et al. Recognition of seven species in the Cryptococcus gattii/Cryptococcus neoformans species complex. Fungal Genet Biol. 2015;78:16–48.
19. Denning DW, Venkateswarlu K, Oakley KL, et al. Itraconazole resistance in Aspergillus fumigatus. Antimicrob Agents Chemother. 1997;41(6):1364–8.
20. Wiederhold NP, Verweij PE. Aspergillus fumigatus and pan-azole resistance: who should be concerned? Curr Opin Infect Dis. 2020;33(4):290–7.
21. Meis JF, Chowdhary A, Rhodes JL, Fisher MC, Verweij PE. Clinical implications of globally emerging azole resistance in Aspergillus fumigatus. Philos Trans R Soc Lond Ser B Biol Sci. 2016;371(1709):20150460.
22. Rudramurthy SM, Paul RA, Chakrabarti A, Mouton JW, Meis JF. Invasive aspergillosis by : epidemiology, diagnosis, antifungal resistance, and management. J Fungi (Basel). 2019;5(3):55.
23. Garcia-vidal C, Barba P, Arnan M, et al. Invasive aspergillosis complicating pandemic influenza A (H1N1) infection in severely immunocompromised patients. Clin Infect Dis. 2011;53(6):e16–9.
24. Schauwvlieghe AFAD, Rijnders BJA, Philips N, et al. Invasive aspergillosis in patients admitted to the intensive care unit with severe influenza: a retrospective cohort study. Lancet Respir Med. 2018;6(10):782–92.
25. Blaize M, Mayaux J, Nabet C, et al. Fatal invasive aspergillosis and coronavirus disease in an immunocompetent patient. Emerg Infect Dis. 2020;26(7):1636–7.
26. van Arkel ALE, Rijpstra TA, Belderbos HNA. Van wijngaarden P, Verweij PE, Bentvelsen RG. COVID-19-associated Pulmonary Aspergillosis. Am J Respir Crit Care Med. 2020;202(1):132–5.
27. Koehler P, Cornely OA, Böttiger BW, et al. COVID-19 associated pulmonary aspergillosis. Mycoses. 2020;63(6):528–34.
28. Gangneux JP, Bougnoux ME, Dannaoui E, Cornet M, Zahar JR. Invasive fungal diseases during COVID-19: we should be prepared. J Mycol Med. 2020;30(2):100971.
29. Centers for Disease Control and Prevention. Sources of Blastomycosis. Available online: https://www.

cdc.gov/fungal/diseases/blastomycosis/causes.html. Accessed on 12 July 2020.

30. Brown EM, Mctaggart LR, Zhang SX, Low DE, Stevens DA, Richardson SE. Correction: phylogenetic analysis reveals a cryptic species Blastomyces gilchristii, sp. nov. within the human pathogenic fungus Blastomyces dermatitidis. PLoS One. 2016;11(12):e0168018.

31. Dalcin D, Rothstein A, Spinato J, Escott N, Kus JV. Blastomyces gilchristii as cause of fatal acute respiratory distress syndrome. Emerg Infect Dis. 2016;22(2):306–8.

32. Mctaggart LR, Brown EM, Richardson SE. Phylogeographic analysis of Blastomyces dermatitidis and Blastomyces gilchristii reveals an association with North American freshwater drainage basins. PLoS One. 2016;11(7):e0159396.

33. Schwartz IS, Kauffman CA. Blastomycosis. Semin Respir Crit Care Med. 2020;41(1):31–41.

34. Jiang YP, Dukik K, Munoz JF, et al. Phylogeny, ecology and taxonomy of systemic pathogens and their relatives in Ajellomycetaceae (Onygenales): Blastomyces, Emergomyces, Emmonsia, Emmonsiellopsis. Fungal Divers. 2018;90:245–91.

35. Assi MA, Sandid MS, Baddour LM, Roberts GD, Walker RC. Systemic histoplasmosis: a 15-year retrospective institutional review of 111 patients. Medicine (Baltimore). 2007;86(3):162–9.

36. Benedict K, Derado G, Mody RK. Histoplasmosis-associated hospitalizations in the United States, 2001-2012. Open Forum Infect Dis. 2016;3(1):ofv219.

37. Myint T, Leedy N, Villacorta cari E, Wheat LJ. HIV-associated histoplasmosis: current perspectives. HIV AIDS (Auckl). 2020;12:113–25.

38. Hajjeh RA, Pappas PG, Henderson H, et al. Multicenter case-control study of risk factors for histoplasmosis in human immunodeficiency virus-infected persons. Clin Infect Dis. 2001;32(8):1215–20.

39. Lockhart SR, Guarner J. Emerging and reemerging fungal infections. Semin Diagn Pathol. 2019;36(3):177–81.

40. Sepúlveda VE, Márquez R, Turissini DA, Goldman WE, Matute DR. Genome sequences reveal cryptic speciation in the human pathogen. MBio. 2017;8(6):e01339.

41. Galhardo MC, De Oliveira RM, Valle AC, et al. Molecular epidemiology and antifungal susceptibility patterns of Sporothrix schenckii isolates from a cat-transmitted epidemic of sporotrichosis in Rio de Janeiro, Brazil. Med Mycol. 2008;46(2):141–51.

42. Orofino-costa R, Macedo PM, Rodrigues AM, Bernardes-engemann AR. Sporotrichosis: an update on epidemiology, etiopathogenesis, laboratory and clinical therapeutics. An Bras Dermatol. 2017;92(5):606–20.

43. Ramírez soto MC. Differences in clinical ocular outcomes between exogenous and endogenous endophthalmitis caused by : a systematic review of published literature. Br J Ophthalmol. 2018;102(7):977–82.

44. Papaiordanou F, Da silveira BR, Abulafia LA. Hypersensitivity reaction to Sporothrix schenckii: erythema nodosum associated with sporotrichosis. Rev Soc Bras Med Trop. 2015;48(4):504.

45. Zhang Y, Pyla V. Sweet's syndrome-like sporotrichosis. Int J Dermatol. 2014;53(5):e324–5.

46. Falcão EMM, et al. Hospitalizations and deaths related to sporotrichosis in Brazil (1992-2015). Cad Saude Publica. 2019;35(4):e00109218.

47. Gremião ID, Miranda LH, Reis EG, Rodrigues AM, Pereira SA. Zoonotic epidemic of Sporotrichosis: cat to human transmission. PLoS Pathog. 2017;13(1):e1006077.

48. Chang A, Tung RC, Mcgillis TS, Bergfeld WF, Taylor JS. Primary cutaneous coccidioidomycosis. J Am Acad Dermatol. 2003;49(5):944–9.

49. Woods CW, Mcrill C, Plikaytis BD, et al. Coccidioidomycosis in human immunodeficiency virus-infected persons in Arizona, 1994-1997: incidence, risk factors, and prevention. J Infect Dis. 2000;181(4):1428–34.

50. Blair JE, Logan JL. Coccidioidomycosis in solid organ transplantation. Clin Infect Dis. 2001;33(9):1536–44.

51. Bergstrom L, Yocum DE, Ampel NM, et al. Increased risk of coccidioidomycosis in patients treated with tumor necrosis factor alpha antagonists. Arthritis Rheum. 2004;50(6):1959–66.

52. Bercovitch RS, Catanzaro A, Schwartz BS, Pappagianis D, Watts DH, Ampel NM. Coccidioidomycosis during pregnancy: a review and recommendations for management. Clin Infect Dis. 2011;53(4):363–8.

53. Santelli AC, Blair JE, Roust LR. Coccidioidomycosis in patients with diabetes mellitus. Am J Med. 2006;119(11):964–9.

54. Martinez R. New trends in Paracoccidioidomycosis epidemiology. J Fungi (Basel). 2017;3(1):1.

55. Quagliato júnior R, Grangeia Tde A, Massucio RA, De capitani EM, Rezende Sde M, Balthazar AB. Association between paracoccidioidomycosis and tuberculosis: reality and misdiagnosis. J Bras Pneumol. 2007;33(3):295–300.

56. Almeida FA, Neves FF, Mora DJ, et al. Paracoccidioidomycosis in Brazilian patients with and without human immunodeficiency virus infection. Am J Trop Med Hyg. 2017;96(2):368–72.

57. Petrikkos G, Skiada A, Lortholary O, Roilides E, Walsh TJ, Kontoyiannis DP. Epidemiology and clinical manifestations of mucormycosis. Clin Infect Dis. 2012;54(Suppl 1):S23–34.

58. Funada H, Matsuda T. Pulmonary mucormycosis in a hematology ward. Intern Med. 1996;35(7):540–4.

59. Reed C, Bryant R, Ibrahim AS, et al. Combination polyene-caspofungin treatment of rhino-orbital-cerebral mucormycosis. Clin Infect Dis. 2008;47(3):364–71.

60. Vanittanakom N, Cooper CR, Fisher MC, Sirisanthana T. Penicillium marneffei infection and recent advances in the epidemiology and molecular biology aspects. Clin Microbiol Rev. 2006;19(1):95–110.

61. Piehl MR, Kaplan RL, Haber MH. Disseminated penicilliosis in a patient with acquired immunodeficiency syndrome. Arch Pathol Lab Med. 1988;112(12):1262–4.

62. Chan JF, Lau SK, Yuen KY, Woo PC. Talaromyces (Penicillium) marneffei infection in non-HIV-infected patients. Emerg Microbes Infect. 2016;5:e19.

63. Tang BS, Chan JF, Chen M, et al. Disseminated penicilliosis, recurrent bacteremic nontyphoidal salmonellosis, and burkholderiosis associated with acquired immunodeficiency due to autoantibody against gamma interferon. Clin Vaccine Immunol. 2010;17:1132–8.

64. Chan JF, Chan TS, Gill H, et al. Disseminated infections with *Talaromyces marneffei* in non-AIDS patients given monoclonal antibodies against CD20 and kinase inhibitors. Emerg Infect Dis. 2015;21:1101–6.

65. Tse E, Leung RY, Kwong YL. Invasive fungal infections after obinutuzumab monotherapy for refractory chronic lymphocytic leukemia. Ann Hematol. 2015;94:165–7.

Mechanisms of Anti-protozoan/ Helminth Drug Resistance

10

Fabio Francesconi, Valeska Francesconi, Omar Lupi, and Yasmin Khalfe

Abbreviations

AADs	Amino acetonitrile derivatives
ABC	ATP-binding cassette
ACR2	Arsenate reductase
ACT	Artemisinin-based combination therapy

F. Francesconi
Dermatology Section - Federal University of the State of Amazonas (UFAM), Manaus, Brazil

Dermatologist - Hospital de Medicina Tropical, Manaus, Brazil

V. Francesconi
Dermatology Section - State University of Amazonas, Manaus, Brazil

Dermatologist - Hospital de Medicina Tropical, Manaus, Brazil

O. Lupi
Associate Professor of Dermatology - Federal University of the State of Rio de Janeiro (UNIRIO), Rio de Janeiro, Brazil

Immunology Section - Federal University of Rio de Janeiro (UFRJ), Rio de Janeiro, Brazil

Titular Professor & Chairman - Policlinica Geral do Rio de Janeiro (PGRJ), Rio de Janeiro, Brazil

Ibero Latin American College of Dermatology (CILAD), Buenos Aires, Argentina

International League of Dermatological Societies (ILDS), London, UK

Y. Khalfe (✉)
School of Medicine, Baylor College of Medicine, Houston, TX, USA
e-mail: yasmin.khalfe@bcm.edu

AmB	Amphotericin B
APOC	African Programme for Onchocerciasis Control
AQP1	Aquaporin 1
BZs	Benzimidazoles
CDTI	Community-directed treatment with ivermectin
CR	Cure rate
DEC	Diethylcarbamazine
DHFR-TS	Dihydrofolate reductase-thymidylate synthase
FR	Flavin reductase
GluCl	Glutamate-gated chloride
GST	Glutathione S-transferase
IL-10	Interleukin 10
IVM	Ivermectin
LEV	Levamisole
LF	Lymphatic filariasis
MDA	Mass drug administration
MDR	Multidrug resistance
MIL	Miltefosine
MLs	Macrocyclic lactones
MRPs	Multidrug resistance proteins
NTR	Nitroreductase
P-gp	P-glycoprotein
PRP1	Pentamidine resistance protein 1
PYR	Pyrimethamine
PZQ	Praziquantel
SDZ	Sulfadiazine
SNP	Single point mutations
SP	Sulfadoxine-pyrimethamine
SSG	Sodium stibogluconate

© Springer Nature Switzerland AG 2021
S. K. Tyring et al. (eds.), *Overcoming Antimicrobial Resistance of the Skin*, Updates in Clinical Dermatology, https://doi.org/10.1007/978-3-030-68321-4_10

STH)	Soil-transmitted helminths
TcCPR	Trypanosomal cytochrome P450 reductase
TDR1	Thiol-dependent reductase
WHO	World Health Organization

Introduction

Parasites are organisms that require a host and can infect multiple tissue and organ systems, commonly involving the gastrointestinal tract and the skin. They are divided into three main classes: helminths, protozoa, and ectoparasites. Helminths are large and multicellular, and they can be grouped into the flatworms (platyhelminthes), thorny-headed worms (acanthocephalins), and roundworms (nematodes) [1]. Protozoa are microscopic organisms that multiply in humans and typically infect through a fecal-oral route [1]. Ectoparasites are arthropods such as lice, mites, ticks, and fleas. Parasitic infections are a major health risk, currently infecting millions of people worldwide and causing thousands of deaths every year [2]. Drugs against parasites have been developed and have effectively treated many diseases. However, novel drugs have not been discovered in recent decades, and the reliance on the small number of current therapeutics is concerning. In recent years, the development of resistance against anti-parasitic drugs has emerged in human medicine. Here, mechanisms of resistance to drugs against helminths, protozoa, and ectoparasites are reviewed, and recommendations for slowing the spread of resistance are discussed.

Mechanisms of Anti-helminthic Drug Resistance

Anti-helminthic drug resistance is an emerging concern that came about in the last few decades. While it has been established as a major issue in livestock, there are fewer reports of helminth resistance in humans [3]. However, the incidence of anti-helminthic resistance is constantly changing and has evolved into an emerging issue. As veterinary research has already drawn attention to the issue of anti-helminthic resistance, the medical community has the opportunity to monitor resistance mechanisms and patterns and develop strategies to hamper the development and growth of resistant helminths [3].

Community- and population-based treatment has been implemented for multiple helminthic diseases on the recommendation of the World Health Organization (WHO). In endemic areas, drug selection is crucial because of the concern for failure and resistance. Refugium is an important, relatively new concept that has served as an approach to slowing anti-helminthic resistance. It is the practice of preserving some of the parasite population unexposed to treatment and serves as a recommended strategy for resistance control in livestock. The success of generating refugia is dependent on factors that vary such as fitness cost of resistance, degree of parasite mixing, parasite genetics, and the environment of the population treated [4]. The size of refugia is defined by the proportion of the population treated, treatment frequency, and percentage of parasite population in the community not subject to drug action [5].

The most commonly used anti-helminthic drugs belong to one of three classes: benzimidazoles, imidazothiazoles, and macrocyclic lactones. Because of the lack of many efficacious therapeutics, resistance to one drug class, as well as multidrug resistance, is a major concern. Additionally, specific helminthic diseases including filariasis, schistosomiasis, and onchocerciasis have recently shown emerging mechanisms of resistance.

Common Anti-helminthic Drugs

Benzimidazoles

Benzimidazoles (BZs) are a group of anti-helminthic drugs that are commonly used in both human and veterinary medicine because of their ease of administration, low cost, and wide range of effectiveness. The primary mechanism of action of these drugs is the inhibition of microtubule formation [6]. BZ selectively bind to the cytoskeletal protein beta-tubulin, while the microtubule is losing a heterodimer, which impedes polymerization and blocks matrix formation [6]. Microtubules are important for many cell functions including mitosis, cell motility, and transport; therefore, inhibiting microtubules is ovicidal, larvicidal, and adulticidal.

Benzimidazole resistance in veterinary parasites has been found to be caused by single point mutations (SNP) at codons 167 (phenylalanine to tyrosine), 198 (glutamic acid to alanine), and 200 (phenylalanine to tyrosine) of the beta-tubulin gene [6]. Those mutations cause conformational changes that impede the association of the drug with its binding site, and they may be present alone or in combination [6].

In human soil-transmitted helminths (STH), there is limited evidence of resistance to benzimidazoles. Mass drug administration (MDA) has become more prevalent due to public health recommendations. However, long-term use of BZ has raised concern about the emergence of genetic resistance. BZ has been found to have limited efficacy against *T. trichiura*, the now most prevalent STH in Latin America [7, 8]. This has caused alarm that there may be genetic resistance to BZ. In a recent study in Honduras, STH prevalence was documented, and genetic sequences containing codons 200, 198, and 167 were sequenced [9]. Researchers did not find SNPs in the sample. While this does not exclude the possibility of their existence, it suggested that STH control issues that Honduras currently faces are likely not due to drug resistance, but rather low drug efficacy, environmental conditions, and factors permitting reinfections [9].

This study was in accordance with previous studies done in Asia and Africa in which researchers could not identify SNPs, as well as a Brazilian study in which codons 198 and 167 from *A. lumbricoides* did not show SNPs [10–12]. In comparison, elevated frequency of SNPs has been found in Haiti, Kenya, and Panama, particularly in codon 200 in *T. trichiura* [13, 14]. With this and the knowledge available about the emergence of resistance in veterinary helminths, it is important to monitor for BZ resistance and potential emergence of SNPs particularly in areas where mass drug administration (MDA) is used.

Imidazothiazoles

The imidazothiazole anti-helminthic drug class targets nicotinic acetylcholine-gated channels. This drug class mediates synaptic signaling and increases the flow of cations, leading to rigid paralysis [15]. Levamisole (LEV) is an imidazothiazole that is commonly used, and pyrantel is a tetrahydropyrimidine. Other drugs in this class include the quaternary amines and the amino acetonitrile derivatives (AADs) [15].

Resistance to levamisole is thought to be due to loss of cholinergic receptors. In studying *Caenorhabditis elegans*, it was found that the levamisole receptor is made of a pentameric ring of three essential subunits, UNC-63, UNC-38, and UNC-29, as well as two nonessential subunits, LEV-1 and LEV-8 [16]. In resistant strains of *Oesophagostomum dentatum*, researchers found fewer active levamisole receptors [17]. They concluded that the strains were made up of different channels whose averaged properties caused resistance [17].

Pyrantel resistance in livestock helminths develops mainly as cross-resistance due to the widespread use of levamisole [3]. In pyrantel-resistant *O. dentatum*, it has been found that nicotinic acetylcholine receptor properties are altered and changes in channel opening probability contribute to resistance [18].

On a molecular level, studies have shown that multiple genes may cause resistance, including a sex-linked gene in *T. colubriformis* and *O. dentatum*; however, further studies are needed to better understand parasite nicotinic acetylcholine receptors and characterize resistance, particularly in humans [19].

Macrocyclic Lactones

Macrocyclic lactones (MLs) are broad-spectrum anti-helminthics that treat infections in livestock and humans. Ivermectin is a common ML that is largely used to treat onchocerciasis and lymphatic filariasis. MLs work by allosterically modulating glutamate-gated chloride (GluCl) channels [20]. Secondary targets include GABA-gated chloride channels and some cation channels. Overall, MLs cause hyperpolarization of the nematode neuromuscular system, which can lead to inhibition of pharyngeal pumping/feeding, motility, reproduction, and egg-laying [20].

In recent years, there has been evidence of development of ivermectin (IVM) or macrocyclic lactone (ML) resistance in *Onchocerca volvulus* and *Dirofilaria immitis* [21–23]. Resistance against ML is likely associated with the ATP-binding cassette (ABC) transporters, a system that functions to transport compounds, including drugs. The multidrug resistance ABC transport protein P-glycoprotein (P-gp) and multidrug resistance proteins (MRPs) are found to be involved with resistance [24]. P-gp is responsible for controlling tissue distribution of ivermectin within the body and prevents it from entering brain tissue [25]. Resistance to macrocyclic lactones could be caused by a gain-of-function mutation in P-gp or ABC transporter genes, which would cause rapid removal of the drug from the worm [19].

In Ghana specifically, treatment of *Onchocerca volvulus* with ivermectin has been used for many years. However, the recent reports of suboptimal response suggested resistance to ivermectin rather than an issue with pill or host factors [26]. Further research has suggested that polymorphism in MDR1 and CYP3A genes may explain the suboptimal response seen. There has been a relationship between MDR1/CYP3A4 variants and ivermectin treatment response established; however, larger studies are needed to confirm findings and optimize treatment [27].

Overall, the mechanisms of ML resistance are complex and require further investigation to develop an understanding of helminth biology and drug pharmacology. Understanding markers of ML resistance would allow for better treatment and prevention of future resistance.

Cross-Resistance and Multidrug Resistance

Cross-resistance and multidrug resistance are major concerns given the increasing reports of anti-helminthic treatment failure. In veterinary medicine, helminth resistance to broad-spectrum medications is so widespread that sheep farming in areas of South America and Africa has been majorly impacted [3]. The current spread of drug resistance in livestock has been a rapid development, and its implications for human medicine are alarming.

The possibility of a link between BZ and ML resistance is of significant concern. Selection for resistance with one drug has been found to predispose toward resistance against the other drug [15]. De Lourdes Mottier et al. found a correlation between repeated exposure or resistance to MLs and an increase in frequency of beta-tubulin alleles that are a determinant for BZ resistance [28]. This suggests the possibility of cross-resistance and that ML resistance may predispose to multidrug resistance.

Multidrug resistance (MDR) occurs primarily through active efflux of drugs by membrane transporters [29]. These transporters include the ATP-binding cassette (ABC) system, which transport drugs using energy derived from hydrolysis of the terminal phosphate of ATP [29]. P-glycoprotein (P-gp) is an integral membrane protein that is a member of the ABC transporter family that mediates export of drugs [30]. Cellularly, changes in gene expression can cause alterations to ABC transporters causing resistance. These mechanisms include overexpression of efflux transporters, downregulation of target genes, or changes in mRNA stability [29]. It is thought that inhibition of P-gp can induce additional resistance including activation of co-existing drug transporters MRP1, MR2, and MRP3, breast cancer resistance protein, and bile salt exporter protein [29]. Further evidence of the influence of the transporters in resistance strains is the use of MDR/P-gp reversal agents, such as verapamil, which can restore sensitivity to the drug [31]. Better understanding of helminth P-gp inhibition could allow for improved therapeutic treatments.

Resistance in Helminthic Diseases

Filariasis

Lymphatic filariasis is a neglected tropical disease that is most commonly caused by the filarial nematode *Wuchereria bancrofti* and spread by a wide range of mosquitoes [32]. Patients can present with lymphedema and elephantiasis, and often the disease can be severe and disfiguring (Fig. 10.1). Filarial hydrocele is also seen in men. Treatment is dependent on appropriate drug administration. As no vaccine is available, the World Health Organization began annual

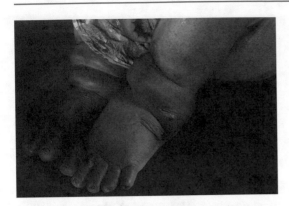

Fig. 10.1 Lymphatic filariasis (LF) is a neglected tropical disease. (Source: CDC; https://www.cdc.gov/dotw/lymphatic-filariasis/index.html)

treatment of communities with mass drug administration (MDA) in 2000 with the goal of eliminating lymphatic filariasis [33]. This included the use of three drugs: ivermectin, albendazole, and diethylcarbamazine. As global programs aimed at eliminating lymphatic filariasis have grown, so has the concern about resistance to anti-helminthics.

The primary agent used to treat filariasis is diethylcarbamazine (DEC), a piperazine derivative that has been used since 1947 [33]. DEC is thought to exert its microfilaricidal effect by disrupting the eicosanoid production of the parasite, which leads to immobilization and death. DNA breaks leading to apoptosis (likely attributed to altered function of microtubules) are also related to DEC's function [33]. However, the mechanism of action of the drug is still not fully understood, and while it has the best activity against microfilariae, it is not 100% effective against adult worms [34]. Eberhard et al. showed that treatment failure of DEC in *W. bancrofti* was not due to incomplete drug regimens, serum-level differences, or inadequate drug dosage, but rather due to nonsusceptibility and parasite tolerance for DEC [35]. Further research is needed to fully understand DEC's mechanism of action to better characterize mechanisms of resistance to the drug. Mechanisms of resistance to albendazole (benzimidazole) and ivermectin (macrocyclic lactone) have been studied and established as previously discussed in this chapter. Taken together, the use of MDA can lead to strong selective pressure on helminths and could cause resistance

leading to treatment failure [33]. Further studies should be undertaken to understand mechanisms of resistance, to develop new potential therapeutics, and to monitor for emergence of drug resistance in this parasite population.

Schistosomiasis

Schistosomiasis is a neglected tropical disease caused by trematode flukes in the *Schistosoma* genus and infects millions of people most commonly in sub-Saharan Africa, the Middle East, South America, and Southeast Asia [36, 37]. Infection can present nonspecifically as malaise, fever, and fatigue, or it can affect specific organ systems including the skin, intestinal, hepatosplenic, urogenital, pulmonary, or nervous systems [36]. Infection has been found to concentrate in focal areas geographically and is governed by the interactions of humans, intermediate host snails, and human-water contact patterns. Global community-based schistosomiasis control programs have focused on MDA, particularly with the drug, praziquantel [36].

Praziquantel (PZQ), the most common drug for the treatment of schistosomiasis, is active against all the *Schistosoma* species – *S. mansoni*, *S. haematobium*, *S. japonicum*, *S. intercalatum*, and *S. mekongi* [3]. In endemic areas, treatment with praziquantel is given indiscriminately to the entire population. In Egypt, for example, all school-age children and millions of adults are screened and treated every 6–12 months [3]. Because of concern for drug failure and resistance, Egypt has an elaborate national monitoring system that tests stool samples from treatment failures. As PZQ is the only current agent that works against all species causing schistosomiasis, drug resistance is an alarming concern.

The first report indicating resistance to PZQ came from a localized focus in Northern Senegal, a region with a cure rate (CR) of only 18% [38]. While drug resistance could not be ruled out, the low cure rate could alternatively be explained by heavy initial infection, intense transmission, prepatent parasites, and immunologic naivety. In Egypt, parasites were isolated that showed a three- to fivefold reduced susceptibility to PZQ [39]. However, more recent studies have failed to show any resistance to PZQ in the same area despite a decade of drug pressure [40]. Newer approaches are focusing on mechanisms underlying possible drug resistance such as ABC multidrug transporters [41].

It is difficult to discern between reduced susceptibility and resistance because measurements of infection burden are insensitive [42]. A major issue is that there is no reliable in vitro test to determine PZQ resistance [3]. However, the findings of reduced susceptibility to PZQ1 in schistosomes could foreshadow the development of resistance. It is important to develop better diagnostic tests as well as drugs and vaccines against schistosomiasis in order to prepare for the possible effects of PZQ resistance.

Onchocerciasis

Onchocerciasis is an infection also known as "river blindness" that is caused by the parasite, *Onchocerca volvulus*, and is transmitted to humans through blackflies [43]. Microfilariae migrate to the organs, most commonly the skin and the eyes. In the skin, nodules can form around adult worms, and in the eyes, lesions can form that lead to permanent blindness. Onchocerciasis is most commonly found in sub-Saharan Africa, and multiple programs have been launched in the area to quell the spread of infection [43]. In 1995, the African Programme for Onchocerciasis Control (APOC) was launched which aimed to control infection by establishing community-directed treatment with ivermectin (CDTI) [43]. Since then, multiple other programs have been started that use IVM to treat large populations with the goal of eliminating onchocerciasis. With the widespread use of IVM, the possibility of resistance in humans has become an emerging concern.

Possible human resistance was reported in 2004 in Ghana, in reports of patients failing to respond to IVM therapy [26]. In a 2007 report, Osei-Atweneboana et al. showed that IVM suppression of skin microfilariae was reported in communities that had gotten 6–18 years of MDA of IVM, suggesting recrudescence of disease

[21]. As previously discussed, polymorphisms in the MDR1 and CYP3A genes may explain suboptimal responses, and a relationship between MDR1/CYP3A4 variants and ivermectin treatment response has been established [27]. Additionally, genetic markers including beta-tubulin genes are under investigation. IVM treatment in resistant *H. contortus* has also been shown to cause a loss of polymorphism at genes encoding the gamma-aminobutyric acid receptor, glutamate-gated chloride channel, and ATP-binding cassette transporter; therefore, further understanding of these genes and other potential polymorphisms in *O. volvulus* are needed [44, 45]. With the development of IVM resistance, efforts are necessary to develop vaccines and drugs with novel mechanisms of action, which is now a goal of the WHO [45].

Mechanisms of Anti-protozoan Drug Resistance

Protozoan infection treatment with drugs likely began with Paul Ehrlich at the end of the nineteenth century when he successfully treated two malaria patients with methylene blue. Since then, understanding of anti-protozoan therapeutics has grown substantially. However, the burden of infectious disease remains, and protozoal diseases have emerged as major detriments to health, economy, and social well-being globally. With the lack of vaccines and other preventative measures, controlling protozoan infection has been challenging and dependent on effective available drugs. Because of this, the emergence of anti-protozoan drug resistance is now of major concern. Resistance mechanisms in many protozoan diseases have recently been discovered, and measures to reduce resistance as well as development of novel therapeutic drugs are necessary.

Resistance in Protozoan Diseases

Malaria

Malaria is one of the most important protozoan diseases, accounting for over 200 million cases

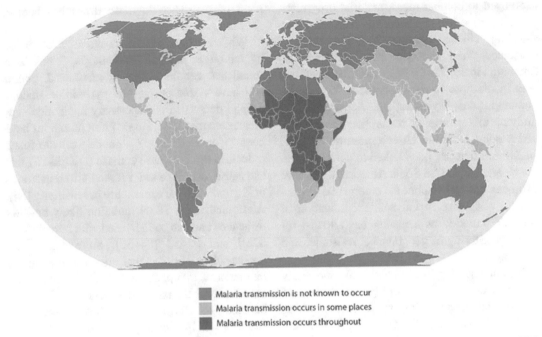

Fig. 10.2 Map showing an approximation of the parts of the world where malaria transmission occurs. (Source: CDC; https://www.cdc.gov/malaria/about/distribution.html)

annually in recent years [46]. Nearly half of the world's population is at risk (Fig. 10.2). Most cases and deaths occur in sub-Saharan Africa [46]. Malaria is a complex disease caused by a protozoan of the *Plasmodium* genera. Although malaria does not affect the skin, it is essential to understand the impact of antimalarial drug resistance, as it has emerged as one of the most significant challenges facing parasite control today.

In the last few years, nearly all antimalarial drugs have considerably decreased in efficacy. Resistance in malaria has spread as it confers a survival advantage, and resistant infections are more likely to recrudesce [47]. Drug resistance has been observed in *Plasmodium falciparum*, *P. vivax*, and *P. malariae*, three of the five malaria species that infect humans [47]. *Plasmodium falciparum* is the deadliest form of malaria and is responsible for a majority of malaria infection-associated mortality.

Chloroquine, an aminoquinolone, became the gold standard therapeutic against *P. falciparum* in the two decades after World War II [47]. Unfortunately, chloroquine is no longer efficacious in many parts of the world because of wide-spread resistance globally [48]. Chloroquine resistance was first reported in Southeast Asia and South America in the 1950s and is now seen in almost all endemic areas [49, 50]. A similar situation was seen with the antimalarial drug, sulfadoxine-pyrimethamine (SP), as its resistance also spread from Asia and South America to Africa and became widespread over the last few decades [47]. In order to combat resistance, chloroquine and SP were used in combination for a short period of time. Additionally, *P. falciparum* has shown resistance to the alkaloid, quinine, first in South America and since then more frequently reported in Southeast Asia and western Oceania [47]. Mefloquine, which was initially synthesized from quinine, has shown frequent resistance in Southeast Asia, as well as the Amazon region and parts of Africa [47].

The most recent and pressing concern is the development of resistance against the newer class of malarial drug, artemisinin. Its derivatives, artesunate, artemether, and dihydroartemisinin, are widely used as artemisinin-based combination therapy (ACT), the now recommended treatment for falciparum malaria [48] Because ACT has been used to combat recent malarial drug resistance, the prospect of artemisinin resistance is an alarming, emerging threat. The first cases of resistance were reported near Thailand and Cambodia in 2007 [51]. Resistance has now been seen in multiple countries including Cambodia, Thailand, Laos, Myanmar, and Vietnam [47]. In studying this resistance, researchers have identified a point mutation on chromosome 13 of *P. falciparum* that has been linked to delayed parasite clearance [52]. In South America, there have also been concerns about the emergence of artemisinin resistance in Guyana. Identification of the K13 mutation as a marker has allowed for better monitoring of geographical resistance and mapping.

Monitoring for drug resistance and early detection is crucial as keeping the efficacy of antimalarial drugs is imperative to controlling malaria globally. The WHO has partnered with many countries and research institutions globally to track and work to slow spread of resistance. In 2015, the WHO developed the *Strategy for malaria elimination in the Greater Mekong subregion (2015–2030)*, which advocates for elimination of all malaria species across the region by 2030, with priority for areas where multidrug-resistant malaria has developed. Understanding the impact of drug resistance in malaria and being able to extrapolate these lessons to other protozoan infections will help develop future clinical strategies that minimize the impact of resistance and better optimize parasitic cure.

Toxoplasmosis

Toxoplasma gondii is a protozoan parasite that infects humans through ingestion of cysts in undercooked meat, by consumption of food or water contaminated with oocysts, or from mother to fetus transmission. Severe disease may occur in immunocompromised patients. The odds ratios for *Toxoplasma* in HIV/AIDS are reported to be high [53]. *Toxoplasma* is treated with the two drugs, pyrimethamine (PYR) and sulfadiazine (SDZ), which inhibit the pyrimidine biosynthesis enzymes, dihydrofolate reductase, and dihydropteroate synthase. In recent years, the development of resistance to these drugs has been a growing concern.

While PYR and SDZ work against *Toxoplasma* by inhibiting nucleotide synthesis, it has been found that certain strains of resistant *T. gondii* still have viable purine and pyrimidine analogs despite defects in the necessary nucleotide synthesis enzymes [54]. Single point mutations have been identified in *T. gondii* dihydrofolate reductase-thymidylate synthase (DHFR-TS) that can cause resistance to PYR, and different strains of *T. gondii* can vary markedly in sensitivity [55]. Additionally, the T83N mutation likely bestows resistance and can be increased with mutations of S36R and F245S [54–56]. Sulfonamides are another class of drugs that are used in mainstay treatment of toxoplasmosis. Drug resistance has been seen for the past few decades and has been induced to form sulfamethoxazole-resistant strains [54]. In recent years, strains have been isolated from livestock and newborns showing resistance to sulfadiazine. Ck3 and Pg1 *T. gondii* isolates are two such strains collected from livestock [57]. The *T. gondii* isolate TgCTBr11 was found in newborns with congenital toxoplasmosis and was associated with polymorphisms in the DHPS gene, a gene known to bring about resistance to SDZ and sulfamethoxazole [54, 58]. While many studies have shown an increase in reporting SDZ resistance, the mechanism of action is not fully understood yet [54]. The emergence of *T. gondii* resistance is a developing concern, and ongoing studies suggest increases in treatment failure to established drugs. With the severity of toxoplasmosis in immunocompromised patients, resistance to current drugs is a major cause of alarm. Further studies are needed to fully understand mechanisms of resistance, and development of novel drugs to treat toxoplasmosis in patients is crucial.

Trichomoniasis

Trichomoniasis, caused by *Trichomonas vaginalis*, is the most prevalent sexually transmitted infection in the United States and commonly presents with no or minimal symptoms, allowing for unknowing transmission between sexual partners. Metronidazole has been the drug of choice for the treatment of *T. vaginalis* infection since its development, and the CDC recommends the use of either metronidazole or tinidazole (another 5-nitroimidazole) to treat trichomoniasis [59]. Resistance to metronidazole in *T. vaginalis* has been reported since the early 1960s [60], and currently metronidazole resistance occurs in 4–10% of cases, while tinidazole resistance is seen in 1% of cases [61, 62]. If a patient consistently fails treatment with a nitroimidazole and is unlikely to have non-adherence or reinfection, metronidazole/tinidazole susceptibility testing is recommended by the CDC.

Clinical drug resistance to metronidazole has been seen typically under aerobic conditions and occasionally anaerobic conditions. Aerobic resistance involves oxygen-scavenging pathways and possibly ferredoxin [63]. Oxygen competition for ferredoxin-bound electrons could decrease the amount of reduced metronidazole. Additionally, metronidazole metabolites can be oxidized back into the prodrug by oxygen and oxygen radicals (known as "futile cycling"), which leads to only limited cell damage [63, 64]. Other mechanisms of resistance involve cytosolic flavin reductase (FR) activity, malate-dependent electron transport, and single nucleotide polymorphisms in nitroreductase genes [64]. Further studies are needed to fully explain differences in cross-resistance of metronidazole and tinidazole.

Emerging nitroimidazole-resistant trichomoniasis is concerning as few alternatives to standard therapy exist. While resistance is not vastly widespread, the existence of treatment failure suggests that relying on metronidazole as a single class of treatment for trichomoniasis may be a risk for development of resistance, and development of novel drug treatments is necessary.

American Trypanosomiasis

American trypanosomiasis (commonly known as Chagas disease) is caused by the parasite, *Trypanosoma cruzi*. The infection is usually passed to humans from triatomine "kissing bugs" through insect feces that pass through skin breaks or mucus membranes and can also be passed through congenital transmission, organ trans-

plantation, and blood transfusions [65]. Chagas disease has become an emerging issue in the Americas, particularly in impoverished and rural areas of Latin America [65]. In the acute phase of infection, symptoms can be nonspecific or mild and may include classic signs such as swelling of the eyelid known as Romaña sign [66]. Chronically, patients may experience cardiac and gastrointestinal complications [66]. In the United States, two treatments are available: benznidazole and nifurtimox. However, both nitroheterocyclic drugs are known to cause toxic side effects, and skin manifestations such as hypersensitivity, dermatitis, and edema are notorious side effects of benznidazole [67]. Concerns in recent years have emerged regarding the development of refractory infections and reports of resistance to treatment [68–70].

Efficacy of *T. cruzi* treatment varies, and treatment failure may be influenced by drug susceptibility differences between strains, host immune system characteristics, incomplete treatment administration, and differences in evaluation methods [71, 72]. Resistance to nifurtimox and benznidazole has been observed in the Americas, and it has been readily induced in studies by culturing *T. cruzi* in the presence of drugs [73–75]. The molecular mechanisms for resistance have recently been studied, and cross-resistance to nifurtimox and benznidazole has been linked to the trypanosome type I nitroreductase (NTR). Loss of this *TcNTR* gene in *T. cruzi* has been found to cause resistance to trypanocidal drugs by reducing or preventing activation of the prodrugs [74, 75]. However, other mechanisms of resistance likely exist given the naturally found variations in sensitivity to drugs. Campos et al. studied *T. cruzi* clones that had been selected for resistance by exposure, and surprisingly, they found that there were significant differences in benznidazole (but not nifurtimox) resistance between clones [76]. This suggested that potentially there are multiple mechanisms involved that cause variability in resistance to benznidazole.

Other processes that may be involved with variations in susceptibility include alternative drug activation enzymes, enhancement of oxidative defense, increased drug efflux, or decreased drug uptake [77]. Another mechanism of resistance that has been proposed involves drug detoxification and trypanosomal cytochrome P450 reductase (TcCPR). Overexpression of TcCPR-B in *T. cruzi* has shown increased resistance to benznidazole and nifurtimox [78]. As the burden of trypanosomiasis continues, the emergence of resistance to established drugs is a crucial issue. Further studies are needed to better understand the mechanisms contributing to resistance in *T. cruzi*. Development of novel treatments for Chagas disease are necessary and dependent on enhanced understanding of mechanisms underlying resistance.

Leishmaniasis

Leishmaniasis, a vector-borne disease, caused by an obligate intracellular protozoan of the genus *Leishmania*, is transmitted by female sand flies. Depending on the species, it may cause a range of clinical manifestations, from self-healing ulcers (cutaneous leishmaniasis) to systemic multiorgan disease (visceral leishmaniasis). Leishmaniasis not only has a myriad of clinical manifestations but also has variability in vectors, diverse causative species from various regions of the world, and different drug susceptibility and drug resistance profiles [79]. It is difficult to define treatment failure in patients with leishmaniasis as persistence of symptoms regularly occurs. In cutaneous leishmaniasis, the ulcer and local inflammation may take up to months to completely heal after completing treatment. A clinical cure in cutaneous cases is complete scarring without inflammatory signs. Defining drug resistance is even more difficult, as host immunity is required for achieving complete cure and differences in individual pharmacokinetics show stratified responses in leishmaniasis. Resistance to the classical drugs for the treatment of leishmaniasis is a real and emerging challenge.

Pentavalent Antimonials

Pentavalent antimonials (Sb^v compounds), including sodium stibogluconate (SSG) and meglumine antimoniate, have been success-fully used for the treatment of leishmaniasis since the early 1900s. Classically known for its narrow therapeutic window, the exact mechanism of action of this drug class is still unclear. In the last few decades, there has been an increase in observed PA resistance in leishmaniasis, which has necessitated the use of other therapeutic drugs, especially in the Indian subcontinent [80].

Extensive research has been done to understand resistance mechanisms to antimonials. While the exact cause is still unclear, multiple possible mechanisms of drug resistance have been uncovered:

1. Diminished biological reduction – Pentavalent antimony (Sb^v) reduction to its trivalent form (SbIII) is necessary for drug activity. In parasites, a thiol-dependent reductase (TDR1) and an arsenate reductase (ACR2) have been identified as possibly responsible [79].
2. Decreased internalization – Sb^v enters the parasite by an unknown transporter, while the SbIII enters the parasite via aquaporin 1 (AQP1) membrane carrier. Its activity is inversely related to resistance, with resistant parasites accumulating less antimony [79].
3. Increased levels of trypanothione – Trypanothione allows for increased thiol redox potential. This mechanism protects the parasite from oxidative stress and also establishes conjugates with SbIII for efflux and sequestration [80].
4. Overexpression of ATP-binding cassette (ABC) transporters – Higher efflux of the drug is associated with increased expression of ATP-binding cassette (ABC) transporters, including MRP1 and P-glycoprotein [81].
5. Parasite immunomodulation – *Leishmania* upregulates the anti-inflammatory interleukin 10 (IL-10) which likely allows for overexpression of the multidrug resistance protein 1 (MDR1) and lowers the total levels of antimony reaching the parasite [79].
6. Genome plasticity – *Leishmania* has a highly plastic genome with potential for aneuploidy, local copy number variations of specific loci,

and extrachromosomal circular or linear amplification of sets of genes [79]. This allows for a large number of transcripts to be made of many given genes and causes genetic diversity. Aneuploidy also causes increases or decreases in gene quantities, and it is not the same among individual cells of a strain. This mosaicism allows for selection of the fittest cells in the given population [82].

With several mechanisms of resistance discovered against antimonials, the overall development of resistance in a particular region is multifactorial. Resistance to pentavalent antimonials in India is widespread, and without a vaccine, this has created challenges in controlling leishmaniasis. Second-line and novel drugs were therefore necessary to employ as resistance to antimonials spread (Fig. 10.3).

Amphotericin B (AmB)

Amphotericin B (AmB) is a polyene antibiotic given as treatment for leishmaniasis in areas with pentavalent antimony (Sb^v) resistance [83]. Clinical AmB resistance is considered low risk, although there are reported treatment failure cases, usually in patients with immunosuppression. In a study in France, sensitivity to AmB was found in promastigote and amastigote forms in the context of multiple relapses [84]. Researchers have found multiple mechanisms that contribute to AmB resistance in *Leishmania* including altered membrane composition, ATP-binding cassette transporters, and an upregulated thiol metabolic pathway [79].

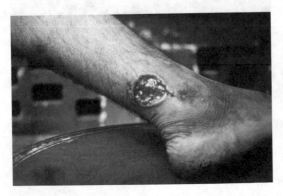

Fig. 10.3 Cutaneous leishmaniasis presenting as an ulcer

Miltefosine

Miltefosine (MIL) is an alkyl phospholipid whose mechanism of action of is not fully understood. The drug interferes with biosynthesis of phospholipids and metabolism of alkyl-lipids. It is known it cause cell shrinkage, nuclear DNA condensation, and DNA fragmentation resulting in apoptosis-like cell death in *L. donovani* [79]. Ten years after the implementation of miltefosine, its efficacy decreased with a relapse rate of 10–20% [79]. Laboratory-based experimentation has shown selection of resistant promastigotes associated with a mechanism of significant reduction in drug internalization due to reduced uptake and increased efflux [79]. Other mechanisms contributing to MIL resistance include inactivating mutations in LMT and LRos3 translocation machinery and overexpression of ABC transporters. Modifications in length and levels of unsaturation of fatty acids, reduction in ergosterol levels, altered expression of genes involved in thiol metabolism, modification in replication machinery, amplified redox potential, as well as increases in metacyclogenesis and infectivity are all correlated with miltefosine-resistant strains of *Leishmania* [79]. Lastly, MIL has a long half-life which can lead to subtherapeutic levels of the drug for some weeks after the standard treatment course, a risk factor for selecting new resistant strains.

Pentamidine

Pentamidine is a drug less often used for leishmaniases that interacts with kinetoplast DNA, inhibits topoisomerase II, and interferes with aerobic glycolysis [82]. Pentamidine resistance protein 1 (PRP1) is an ABC transporter protein associated with resistance by causing an efflux of pentamidine leading to reduced intracellular drug level [80]. Resistance to pentamidine in *Leishmania* is also associated with changes in the intracellular concentration of ornithine and arginine within the cell [80].

Paromomycin

Paromomycin acts on ribosomes causing inhibition of protein synthesis and induces alterations in membrane fluidity; it affects lipid metabolism and mitochondrial activity. There is one paromomycin resistance gene identified in *Leishmania*, and it is a hypothetical protein that encodes a leucine-rich repeat domain [80]. In vitro, paromomycin has shown heterogeneity in susceptibility in different species, but whether these susceptibilities will be seen clinically is yet to be known [79]. As paromomycin use has been limited in the treatment of leishmaniasis, reports of clinical resistance have not been well-defined [79, 85]. Monitoring for resistance is crucial as this drug class begins to be used more often to treat *Leishmania*.

Leishmaniasis Resistance in Combination Therapy

Combination therapy using at least two drugs with separate mechanisms of action is known to be beneficial and can potentially overcome resistance. Combination therapy in *Leishmania* has not been as extensively established as in other diseases such as malaria, AIDS, or tuberculosis. The WHO has recommendations based on regions including India, Sudan, and other East African countries [86]. Efficacy of combination therapy in leishmaniasis is necessary to establish in comparison to monotherapy.

In recent years, studies have shown that *Leishmania* promastigotes are able to develop resistance even to combinations of drugs, in particular, MIL/paromomycin and SSG/paromomycin pairings [79]. Multidrug-resistant *Leishmania* is a possibility related to multiple metabolic pathway changes, activating stress responses with enhanced ability to neutralize drug-induced ROS production, and decreases in membrane fluidity [79]. Drug-combination-resistant parasites are more tolerant of ATP loss, have increased thiol levels, resist depolarization of the mitochondrial membrane, show no DNA fragmentation under drug pressure, and sustain membrane integrity [3, 87]. Overall, current research suggests that it is possible for *Leishmania* to acquire multidrug resistance and combination therapy should be studied closely.

Mechanisms of Drug Resistance in Ectoparasites

Ectoparasites are arthropods that can cause illness directly or act as vectors of viral, bacterial, or other parasitic infections. Two important and prevalent ectoparasites cause the diseases, scabies and pediculosis (lice). Over the years, the diagnoses of scabies and pediculosis have not changed; however, the development of new treatments has occurred. Still, the emergence of treatment-resistant ectoparasites has increased, and mechanisms of resistance are under investigation.

Scabies

Scabies is an infestation of the skin by the ectoparasite, *Sarcoptes scabiei* var. *hominis* [88]. The mite burrows into the upper skin and lays eggs which leads to intense pruritus and erythematous papules (Fig. 10.4). Scabies is found globally in all races, and outbreaks can rapidly spread through skin to skin contact. The WHO included scabies in the list of neglected tropical diseases in 2013.

Multiple treatments for scabies are available including topical treatments of permethrin cream 5%, crotamiton lotion or cream 10%, sulfur ointment 5–10%, and lindane lotion 1%; oral ivermectin is also used particularly in patients who

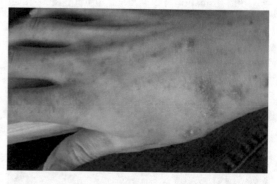

Fig. 10.4 Skin rash caused by scabies. (Source: CDC; https://www.cdc.gov/parasites/scabies/fact_sheet.html)

have failed treatment or cannot tolerate the FDA-approved topical treatment [88]. Although there are multiple treatments, resistance to scabicides have increased throughout the years [89–91]. Although studies support the notion of resistance to scabicides, continued studies to are needed to validate this conclusion for certain drugs such as permethrin. Numerous mechanisms have been studied in recent years that could confer resistance.

One possible mechanism of resistance to permethrin includes mutations in voltage-gated sodium channels. When the channel is in the open or active state, permethrin preferentially binds, preventing the channel from closing. The continuous sodium flow that follows allows axons to continuously fire and eventually causes paralysis and death [92]. Mutations of the sodium channel that favor a closed state therefore prevent binding of the drug, resulting in resistance [93]. Another proposed mechanism of resistance involves increased activity or expression of glutathione S-transferase (GST). The thioester bond formed by GST tags drugs for elimination, and it has been suggested that GST may mediate a cross-resistance to both ivermectin and permethrin [92, 94].

Ivermectin resistance has also been associated with changes in ATP-binding cassette transporters as well as ligand-gated chloride channels. Resistance has been seen with increased expression of multidrug resistance protein (MDRP) or P-glycoprotein, ABC transporters that can increase efflux of drugs [92, 95]. Lastly, ivermectin is known to act on chloride channels by binding and keeping the channels open to cause paralysis and death. Studies have shown that a novel ligand-gated chloride channel, known as SscCl, that exists in scabies is activated by ivermectin and contributes to scabies resistance [96].

Pediculosis

Pediculosis is caused by the ectoparasite commonly known as lice. There are three types of lice that live on humans: *Pediculus humanus capitis* (head louse), *Pediculus humanus corporis* (body louse), and *Pthirus pubis* (pubic louse) [97]. There are numerous treatments available for the different types of lice infections. These include topical permethrin 1% or 5%, lindane, pyrethrins, malathion 0.5%, ivermectin 0.5%, spinosad 0.9%, benzyl alcohol 5%, and oral ivermectin. Resistance to pediculicides continues to emerge, and regional differences are observed [98]. Selection pressure due to the widespread use of medications has led to resistance spread.

As with scabies, there are multiple mechanisms proposed as responsible for drug-resistant lice. Permethrin resistance was thought to be associated with the recessive *kdr* trait due to the point mutations M8151, T9171, and L920F (known as knockdown resistance). However, other studies found that the *kdr* mutant alleles were not correlated with clinical failure, suggesting that this gene's involvement with resistance should be cautiously interpreted [99]. Another mechanism is enhanced drug metabolism due to increased monooxygenase activity, and resistance has been found to be overcome by using a synergistic agent such as piperonyl butoxide [100].

Other possible mechanisms of resistance include accelerated detoxification of insecticides by enzyme-mediated reduction, esterification, and alterations of the binding site (such as altered acetylcholinesterase or altered nerve voltage-gated sodium channel) [99]. Given the continued resistance development in pediculosis, non-insecticidal treatments like dimeticone lotion and mechanical methods such as heated air and suction may be effective alternatives [98, 99]. Further studies are needed to better understand existence and distribution of lice resistance in communities, and additional research into the mechanisms of resistance is warranted to ensure effective treatments.

Conclusion and Recommendations

Parasites are major causes of infection globally and account for a vast number of deaths annually. While efforts at prevention have improved rates of infection in certain populations, there are currently no vaccines against any significant parasites. Reliance on anti-helminthic and anti-protozoan drugs has been the backbone for the treatment of parasitic infections, and these drugs have been used to control spread in community-based prevention programs. Additionally, drug treatments against ectoparasites have played a major role in controlling infection such as scabies and pediculosis. However, the number of effective drugs against parasitic diseases is limited, and in the last few decades, the emergence of resistance has occurred. The resistance seen in livestock is now being increasingly reported in humans. In order to minimize the impact of community-based treatment in the selection of drug-resistant parasites, the following strategies are recommended [3, 87]:

1. Develop a campaign that is justified based on screening of populations. Treatment should be targeted toward communities where parasite infection is overwhelming and benefit outweighs costs of treatment.
2. Incorporate other control measures such as education and sanitation which can lead to long-term improvement, as well as better living conditions.
3. Balance the number of treatments such that they are not too frequent or prolonged. Drug resistance is best delayed by reducing selection pressure.
4. Rather than mass treatment, focus on treating a portion of the population. This protects from indiscriminately exposing the whole parasite population.
5. Guarantee the correct drug dosage to avoid low dosages that would not be therapeutic and may contribute to resistance development. Review pharmacokinetics carefully and dose appropriately.
6. Use different drugs simultaneously in multidrug therapy or in rotation to delay resistance development against a single agent.
7. Develop drug failure monitoring programs and enhanced tracking of the spread of resistance.

Lastly, the potential for multidrug resistance is a concern, particularly with such few effective drugs against parasites. Continued research is necessary to fully understand anti-parasitic drug resistance and further combat the global infection and public health threat posed by these devastating and preventable diseases.

References

1. CDC – Parasites – About Parasites [Internet]. [cited 2020 Aug 8]. Available from: https://www.cdc.gov/parasites/about.html
2. Torgerson PR, Devleesschauwer B, Praet N, Speybroeck N, Willingham AL, Kasuga F, et al. World Health Organization Estimates of the Global and Regional Disease Burden of 11 Foodborne Parasitic Diseases, 2010: A Data Synthesis. PLoS Med [Internet]. 2015 [cited 2020 Aug 8];12(12). Available from: /pmc/articles/PMC4668834/?report=abstract
3. Geerts S, Gryseels B. Drug resistance in human helminths: current situation and lessons from livestock [Internet]. Vol. 13, Clinical Microbiology Reviews. American Society for Microbiology (ASM); 2000 [cited 2020 Aug 7]. p. 207–22. Available from: /pmc/articles/PMC100151/?report=abstract
4. Hodgkinson JE, Kaplan RM, Kenyon F, Morgan ER, Park AW, Paterson S, et al. Refugia and anthelmintic resistance: concepts and challenges. Vol. 10, Int J Parasitol. Elsevier Ltd; 2019. p. 51–7.
5. Vercruysse J, Levecke B, Prichard R. Human soil-transmitted helminths: implications of mass drug administration. [cited 2020 Aug 11]; Available from: www.co-infectiousdiseases.com
6. Furtado LFV, de Paiva Bello ACP, Rabelo ÉML. Benzimidazole resistance in helminths: from problem to diagnosis. Vol. 162, Acta Tropica. Elsevier B.V.; 2016. p. 95–102.
7. Sanchez AL, Gabrie JA, Rueda MM, Mejia RE, Bottazzi ME, Canales M. A scoping review and prevalence analysis of soil-transmitted helminth infections in Honduras. Steinmann P, editor. PLoS Negl Trop Dis [Internet]. 2014 [cited 2020 Aug 8];8(1):e2653. Available from: https://dx.plos.org/10.1371/journal.pntd.0002653
8. Partridge FA, Forman R, Bataille CJR, Wynne GM, Nick M, Russell AJ, et al. Anthelmintic drug discovery: Target identification, screening methods and the role of open science [Internet]. Vol. 16, Beilstein J Organ Chem. Beilstein-Institut Zur Forderung der Chemischen Wissenschaften; 2020 [cited 2020 Aug 8]. p. 1203–24. Available from: /pmc/articles/PMC7277699/?report=abstract
9. Matamoros G, Rueda MM, Rodríguez C, Gabrie JA, Canales M, Fontecha G, et al. High endemicity of soil-transmitted helminths in a population frequently

exposed to albendazole but no evidence of antiparasitic resistance. Trop Med Infect Dis [Internet]. 2019 [cited 2020 Aug 8];4(2). Available from: /pmc/articles/PMC6631243/?report=abstract

10. Hansen TVA, Nejsum P, Olsen A, Thamsborg SM. Genetic variation in codons 167, 198 and 200 of the beta-tubulin gene in whipworms (Trichuris spp.) from a range of domestic animals and wildlife. Vet Parasitol [Internet]. 2013 [cited 2020 Aug 8];193(1–3):141–9. Available from: https://pubmed.ncbi.nlm.nih.gov/23352105/

11. Hansen TV, Thamsborg SM, Olsen A, Prichard RK, Nejsum P. Genetic variations in the beta-tubulin gene and the internal transcribed spacer 2 region of Trichuris species from man and baboons. Parasit Vectors [Internet]. 2013 [cited 2020 Aug 8];6(1):236. Available from: https://parasitesandvectors.biomed-central.com/articles/10.1186/1756-3305-6-236

12. Zuccherato LW, Furtado LF, Medeiros C da S, Pinheiro C da S, Rabelo ÉM. PCR-RFLP screening of polymorphisms associated with benzimidazole resistance in Necator americanus and Ascaris lumbricoides from different geographical regions in Brazil. PLoS Negl Trop Dis [Internet]. 2018 [cited 2020 Aug 8];12(9). Available from: https://pubmed.ncbi.nlm.nih.gov/30222749/

13. Diawara A, Halpenny CM, Churcher TS, Mwandawiro C, Kihara J, Kaplan RM, et al. Association between response to albendazole treatment and β-tubulin genotype frequencies in soil-transmitted helminths. Keiser J, editor. PLoS Negl Trop Dis [Internet]. 2013 [cited 2020 Aug 8];7(5):e2247. Available from: https://dx.plos.org/10.1371/journal.pntd.0002247

14. Diawara A, Drake LJ, Suswillo RR, Kihara J, Bundy DAP, Scott ME, et al. Assays to detect β-tubulin codon 200 polymorphism in Trichuris trichiura and Ascaris lumbricoides. PLoS Negl Trop Dis [Internet]. 2009 [cited 2020 Aug 8];3(3). Available from: https://pubmed.ncbi.nlm.nih.gov/19308251/

15. Beech RN, Skuce P, Bartley DJ, Martin RJ, Prichard RK, Gilleard JS. Anthelmintic resistance: markers for resistance, or susceptibility? [Internet]. Vol. 138, Parasitology; 2011 [cited 2020 Aug 8]. p. 160–74. Available from: https://pubmed.ncbi.nlm.nih.gov/20825689/

16. Fleming JT, Squire MD, Barnes TM, Tornoe C, Matsuda K, Ahnn J, et al. Caenorhabditis elegans levamisole resistance genes lev-1, unc-29, and unc-38 encode functional nicotinic acetylcholine receptor subunits. J Neurosci [Internet]. 1997 [cited 2020 Aug 8];17(15):5843–57. Available from: https://pubmed.ncbi.nlm.nih.gov/9221782/

17. Robertson AP, Bjorn HE, Martin RJ. Resistance to levamisole resolved at the single-channel level. FASEB J [Internet]. 1999 [cited 2020 Aug 8];13(6):749–60. Available from: https://pubmed.ncbi.nlm.nih.gov/10094935/

18. Robertson AP, Bjørn HE, Martin RJ. Pyrantel resistance alters nematode nicotinic acetylcholine recep-tor single-channel properties. Eur J Pharmacol [Internet]. 2000 [cited 2020 Aug 8];394(1):1–8. Available from: https://pubmed.ncbi.nlm.nih.gov/10771027/

19. Prichard R. Drug resistance in nematodes. In: Antimicrobial drug resistance [Internet]. Humana Press; 2009 [cited 2020 Aug 8]. p. 621–8. Available from: https://link.springer.com/chapter/10.1007/978-1-59745-180-2_44

20. Whittaker JH, Carlson SA, Jones DE, Brewer MT. Molecular mechanisms for anthelmintic resistance in strongyle nematode parasites of veterinary importance [Internet]. Vol. 40, J Vet Pharmacol Ther. Blackwell Publishing Ltd; 2017 [cited 2020 Aug 8]. p. 105–15. Available from: https://pubmed.ncbi.nlm.nih.gov/27302747/

21. Osei-Atwenebone MY, Eng JK, Boakye DA, Gyapong JO, Prichard RK. Prevalence and intensity of Onchocerca volvulus infection and efficacy of ivermectin in endemic communities in Ghana: a two-phase epidemiological study. Lancet [Internet]. 2007 [cited 2020 Aug 8];369(9578):2021–9. Available from: https://linkinghub.elsevier.com/retrieve/pii/S0140673607609428

22. Osei-Atweneboana MY, Awadzi K, Attah SK, Boakye DA, Gyapong JO, Prichard RK. Phenotypic evidence of emerging ivermectin resistance in Onchocerca volvulus. Lustigman S, editor. PLoS Negl Trop Dis [Internet]. 2011 [cited 2020 Aug 8];5(3):e998. Available from: https://dx.plos.org/10.1371/journal.pntd.0000998

23. Blagburn BL, Dillon AR, Arther RG, Butler JM, Newton JC. Comparative efficacy of four commercially available heartworm preventive products against the MP3 laboratory strain of Dirofilaria immitis. Vet Parasitol [Internet]. 2011 [cited 2020 Aug 8];176(2–3):189–94. Available from: https://pubmed.ncbi.nlm.nih.gov/21295409/

24. Lespine A, Ménez C, Bourguinat C, Prichard RK. P-glycoproteins and other multidrug resistance transporters in the pharmacology of anthelmintics: prospects for reversing transport-dependent anthelmintic resistance [Internet]. Vol. 2, Int J Parasitol Drugs Drug Resist; 2012 [cited 2020 Aug 8]. p. 58–75. Available from: https://pubmed.ncbi.nlm.nih.gov/24533264/

25. Schinkel AH, Smit JJM, van Tellingen O, Beijnen JH, Wagenaar E, van Deemter L, et al. Disruption of the mouse mdr1a P-glycoprotein gene leads to a deficiency in the blood-brain barrier and to increased sensitivity to drugs. Cell [Internet]. 1994 [cited 2020 Aug 8];77(4):491–502. Available from: https://pubmed.ncbi.nlm.nih.gov/7910522/

26. Awadzi K, Boakye DA, Edwards G, Opoku NO, Attah SK, Osei-Atweneboana MY, et al. An investigation of persistent microfilaridermias despite multiple treatments with ivermectin, in two onchocerciasis-endemic foci in Ghana. Ann Trop Med Parasitol [Internet]. 2004 [cited 2020 Aug

8];98(3):231–49. Available from: https://pubmed.ncbi.nlm.nih.gov/15119969/

27. Kudzi W, Dodoo ANO, Mills JJ. Genetic polymorphisms in MDR1, CYP3A4 and CYP3A5 genes in a Ghanaian population: A plausible explanation for altered metabolism of ivermectin in humans? BMC Med Genet [Internet]. 2010 [cited 2020 Aug 8];11(1). Available from: https://pubmed.ncbi.nlm.nih.gov/20630055/

28. Mottier MDL, Prichard RK. Genetic analysis of a relationship between macrocyclic lactone and benzimidazole anthelmintic selection on Haemonchus contortus. Pharmacogenet Genom [Internet]. 2008 [cited 2020 Aug 8];18(2):129–40. Available from: https://pubmed.ncbi.nlm.nih.gov/18192899/

29. Ardelli BF. Transport proteins of the ABC systems superfamily and their role in drug action and resistance in nematodes [Internet]. Vol. 62, Parasitol Int; 2013 [cited 2020 Aug 8]. p. 639–46. Available from: https://pubmed.ncbi.nlm.nih.gov/23474412/

30. James CE, Hudson AL, Davey MW. Drug resistance mechanisms in helminths: is it survival of the fittest? [Internet]. Vol. 25, Trends Parasitol; 2009 [cited 2020 Aug 8]. p. 328–35. Available from: https://pubmed.ncbi.nlm.nih.gov/19541539/

31. Molento MB, Prichard RK. Effects of the multidrug-resistance-reversing agents verapamil and CL 347,099 on the efficacy of ivermectin or moxidectin against unselected and drug-selected strains of Haemonchus contortus in jirds (Meriones unguiculatus). Parasitol Res [Internet]. 1999 [cited 2020 Aug 8];85(12):1007–11. Available from: https://pubmed.ncbi.nlm.nih.gov/10599924/

32. Prevention C-C for DC and. CDC – Lymphatic Filariasis. 2020;

33. Determinants of parasite drug resistance in human lymphatic filariasis – PubMed [Internet]. [cited 2020 Aug 8]. Available from: https://pubmed.ncbi.nlm.nih.gov/27858056/

34. Is anthelmintic resistance a threat to the program to eliminate lymphatic filariasis? – PubMed [Internet]. [cited 2020 Aug 8]. Available from: https://pubmed.ncbi.nlm.nih.gov/16103580/

35. Evidence of nonsusceptibility to diethylcarbamazine in Wuchereria bancrofti – PubMed [Internet]. [cited 2020 Aug 8]. Available from: https://pubmed.ncbi.nlm.nih.gov/2019765/

36. McManus DP, Dunne DW, Sacko M, Utzinger J, Vennervald BJ, Zhou XN. Schistosomiasis. Natl Rev Dis Prim [Internet]. 2018 [cited 2020 Aug 8];4(1):1–19. Available from: www.nature.com/nrdp

37. CDC – Schistosomiasis [Internet]. [cited 2020 Aug 8]. Available from: https://www.cdc.gov/parasites/schistosomiasis/index.html

38. Stelma FF, Talla I, Sow S, Kongs A, Niang M, Polman K, et al. Efficacy and side effects of praziquantel in an epidemic focus of Schistosoma mansoni. Am J Trop Med Hyg [Internet]. 1995 [cited 2020 Aug 8];53(2):167–70. Available from: https://pubmed.ncbi.nlm.nih.gov/7677219/

39. Ismail M, Metwally A, Farghaly A, Bruce J, Tao LF, Bennett JL. Characterization of isolates of Schistosoma mansoni from Egyptian villagers that tolerate high doses of praziquantel. Am J Trop Med Hyg [Internet]. 1996 [cited 2020 Aug 8];55(2):214–8. Available from: https://pubmed.ncbi.nlm.nih.gov/8780463/

40. Botros S, Sayed H, Amer N, El-Ghannam M, Bennett JL, Day TA. Current status of sensitivity to praziquantel in a focus of potential drug resistance in Egypt. In: International Journal for Parasitology [Internet]. Int J Parasitol; 2005 [cited 2020 Aug 8]. p. 787–91. Available from: https://pubmed.ncbi.nlm.nih.gov/15925597/

41. Greenberg RM. New approaches for understanding mechanisms of drug resistance in schistosomes [Internet]. Vol. 140, Parasitology. NIH Public Access; 2013 [cited 2020 Aug 8]. p. 1534–46. Available from: /pmc/articles/PMC3775338/?report=abstract

42. Vale N, Gouveia MJ, Rinaldi G, Brindley PJ, Gärtner F, da Costa JMC. Praziquantel for schistosomiasis: Single-drug metabolism revisited, mode of action, and resistance [Internet]. Vol. 61, Antimicrobial Agents and Chemotherapy. Am Soc Microbiol; 2017 [cited 2020 Aug 8]. Available from: https://pubmed.ncbi.nlm.nih.gov/28264841/

43. Onchocerciasis [Internet]. [cited 2020 Aug 5]. Available from: https://www.who.int/news-room/fact-sheets/detail/onchocerciasis

44. Ardelli BF, Prichard RK. Identification of variant ABC-transporter genes among Onchocerca volvulus collected from ivermectin-treated and untreated patients in Ghana, West Africa. Ann Trop Med Parasitol [Internet]. 2004 [cited 2020 Aug 8];98(4):371–84. Available from: https://pubmed.ncbi.nlm.nih.gov/15228718/

45. Lustigman S, McCarter JP. Ivermectin resistance in Onchocerca volvulus: toward a genetic basis. PLoS Negl Trop Dis [Internet]. 2007 [cited 2020 Aug 8];1(1). Available from: https://www.ncbi.nlm.nih.gov/pmc/articles/PMC2041823/

46. Malaria [Internet]. 2020 [cited 2020 Aug 5]. Available from: https://www.who.int/news-room/fact-sheets/detail/malaria

47. Achan J, Mwesigwa J, Edwin CP, D'alessandro U. Malaria medicines to address drug resistance and support malaria elimination efforts [Internet]. Vol. 11, Exp Rev Clin Pharmacol. Taylor and Francis Ltd; 2018 [cited 2020 Aug 5]. p. 61–70. Available from: https://www.tandfonline.com/doi/abs/10.1080/17512433.2018.1387773

48. Cui L, Mharakurwa S, Ndiaye D, Rathod PK, Rosenthal PJ. Antimalarial drug resistance: literature review and activities and findings of the ICEMR network. Am J Trop Med Hyg [Internet]. 2015 [cited 2020 Aug 6];93(3 Suppl):57–68. Available from: /pmc/articles/PMC4574275/?report=abstract

49. Moore D V., Lanier JE. Observations on two Plasmodium falciparum infections with an abnor-

mal response to chloroquine. Am J Trop Med Hyg [Internet]. 1961 [cited 2020 Aug 6];10:5–9. Available from: https://pubmed.ncbi.nlm.nih.gov/13772281/

50. Wernsdorfer WH, Payne D. The dynamics of drug resistance in Plasmodium falciparum [Internet]. Vol. 50, Pharmacol Ther; 1991 [cited 2020 Aug 6]. p. 95–121. Available from: https://pubmed.ncbi.nlm.nih.gov/1891480/

51. Dondorp AM, Nosten F, Yi P, Das D, Phyo AP, Tarning J, et al. Artemisinin Resistance in Plasmodium falciparum Malaria. New Engl J Med [Internet]. 2009 [cited 2020 Aug 6];361(5):455–67. Available from: http://www.nejm.org/doi/abs/10.1056/NEJMoa0808859

52. Ariey F, Witkowski B, Amaratunga C, Beghain J, Langlois AC, Khim N, et al. A molecular marker of artemisinin-resistant Plasmodium falciparum malaria. Nature [Internet]. 2014 [cited 2020 Aug 6];505(7481):50–5. Available from: https://pubmed.ncbi.nlm.nih.gov/24352242/

53. Wang ZD, Liu HH, Ma ZX, Ma HY, Li ZY, Yang Z, Bin X, et al. Toxoplasma gondii infection in immunocompromised patients: a systematic review and meta-analysis. Front Microbiol [Internet]. 2017 [cited 2020 Aug 6];8(MAR). Available from: https://pubmed.ncbi.nlm.nih.gov/28337191/

54. Montazeri M, Mehrzadi S, Sharif M, Sarvi S, Tanzifi A, Aghayan SA, et al. Drug Resistance in Toxoplasma gondii. Front Microbiol [Internet]. 2018 [cited 2020 Aug 6];9:2587. Available from: https://www.frontiersin.org/article/10.3389/fmicb.2018.02587/full

55. Reynolds MG, Oh J, Roos DS. In vitro generation of novel pyrimethamine resistance mutations in the Toxoplasma gondii dihydrofolate reductase. Antimicrob Agents Chemother [Internet]. 2001 [cited 2020 Aug 7];45(4):1271–7. Available from: http://aac.asm.org/

56. Donald RGK, Roos DS. Stable molecular transformation of Toxoplasma gondii: a selectable dihydrofolate reductase-thymidylate synthase marker based on drug-resistance mutations in malaria. Proc Natl Acad Sci U S A [Internet]. 1993 [cited 2020 Aug 7];90(24):11703–7. Available from: /pmc/articles/PMC48052/?report=abstract

57. Oliveira CBS, Meurer YSR, Andrade JMA, Costa MESM, Andrade MMC, Silva LA, et al. Pathogenicity and phenotypic sulfadiazine resistance of toxoplasma gondii isolates obtained from livestock in Northeastern Brazil. Memorias do Instituto Oswaldo Cruz [Internet]. 2016 [cited 2020 Aug 7];111(6):391–8. Available from: /pmc/articles/PMC4909038/?report=abstract

58. Silva LA, Reis-Cunha JL, Bartholomeu DC, Vítor RWA. Genetic Polymorphisms and Phenotypic Profiles of Sulfadiazine-Resistant and Sensitive Toxoplasma gondii Isolates Obtained from Newborns with Congenital Toxoplasmosis in Minas Gerais, Brazil. Tanowitz HB, editor. PLOS ONE [Internet]. 2017 [cited 2020 Aug 7];12(1):e0170689. Available from: https://dx.plos.org/10.1371/journal.pone.0170689

59. Sexually transmitted diseases treatment guidelines, 2010 – PubMed [Internet]. [cited 2020 Aug 7]. Available from: https://pubmed.ncbi.nlm.nih.gov/21160459/

60. Robinson SC. Trichomonal vaginitis resistant to metranidazole. Can Med Assoc J [Internet]. 1962 [cited 2020 Aug 7];86(14):665. Available from: http://www.pubmedcentral.nih.gov/articlerender.fcgi?artid=1849337&tool=pmcentrez&rendertype=abstract

61. Kirkcaldy RD, Augostini P, Asbel LE, Bernstein KT, Kerani RP, Mettenbrink CJ, et al. Trichomonas vaginalis antimicrobial drug resistance in 6 US cities, STD surveillance network, 2009–2010. Emerg Infect Dis [Internet]. 2012 [cited 2020 Aug 7];18(6):939–43. Available from: /pmc/articles/PMC3358158/?report=abstract

62. Schwebke JR, Barrientes FJ. Prevalence of Trichomonas vaginalis isolates with resistance to metronidazole and tinidazole. Antimicrob Agents Chemother [Internet]. 2006 [cited 2020 Aug 7];50(12):4209–10. Available from: https://pubmed.ncbi.nlm.nih.gov/17000740/

63. Cudmore SL, Delgaty KL, Hayward-McClelland SF, Petrin DP, Garber GE. Treatment of infections caused by metronidazole-resistant Trichomonas vaginalis [Internet]. Vol. 17, Clinical Microbiology Reviews. American Society for Microbiology (ASM); 2004 [cited 2020 Aug 7]. p. 783–93. Available from: /pmc/articles/PMC523556/?report=abstract

64. Dunne RL, Dunn LA, Upcroft P, O'Donoghue PJ, Upcroft JA. Drug resistance in the sexually transmitted protozoan Trichomonas vaginalis. Cell Res [Internet]. 2003 [cited 2020 Aug 7];13(4):239–49. Available from: http://www.cell-research.com

65. CDC – Chagas Disease – Detailed FAQs [Internet]. [cited 2020 Aug 10]. Available from: https://www.cdc.gov/parasites/chagas/gen_info/detailed.html#intro

66. Kollipara R, Peranteau AJ, Nawas ZY, Tong Y, Woc-Colburn L, Yan AC, et al. Emerging infectious diseases with cutaneous manifestations Fungal, helminthic, protozoan and ectoparasitic infections. Vol. 75, J Am Acad Dermatol. Mosby Inc.; 2016. p. 19–30.

67. Castro JA, de Mecca MM, Bartel LC. Toxic side effects of drugs used to treat Chagas' disease (American trypanosomiasis). Human Exp Toxicol [Internet]. 2006 [cited 2020 Aug 10];25(8):471–9. Available from: https://pubmed.ncbi.nlm.nih.gov/16937919/

68. Filardi LS, Brener Z. Susceptibility and natural resistance of Trypanosoma cruzi strains to drugs used clinically in Chagas disease. Trans Royal Soc Trop Med Hyg [Internet]. 1987 [cited 2020 Aug 10];81(5):755–9. Available from: https://pubmed.ncbi.nlm.nih.gov/3130683/

69. Wilkinson SR, Kelly JM. Trypanocidal drugs: mechanisms, resistance and new targets [Internet]. Vol. 11, Expert Rev Mol Med; 2009 [cited 2020 Aug 10]. Available from: https://pubmed.ncbi.nlm.nih.gov/19863838/

70. Ribeiro V, Dias N, Paiva T, Hagström-Bex L, Nitz N, Pratesi R, et al. Current trends in the pharmacological management of Chagas disease. Vol. 12, Int J Parasitol Drugs Drug Resist. Elsevier Ltd; 2020. p. 7–17.

71. Zingales B, Miles MA, Moraes CB, Luquetti A, Guhl F, Schijman AG, et al. Drug discovery for chagas disease should consider Trypanosoma cruzi strain diversity. Memorias do Instituto Oswaldo Cruz [Internet]. 2014 [cited 2020 Aug 10];109(6):828–33. Available from: /pmc/articles/PMC4238778/?report=abstract

72. Urbina JA. Specific chemotherapy of Chagas disease: relevance, current limitations and new approaches. Acta Trop 2010;115(1–2):55–68.

73. Nozaki T, Engel JC, Dvorak JA. Cellular and molecular biological analyses of nifurtimox resistance in Trypanosoma cruzi. Am J Trop Med Hyg [Internet]. 1996 [cited 2020 Aug 10];55(1):111–7. Available from: https://pubmed.ncbi.nlm.nih.gov/8702014/

74. Mejia AM, Hall BS, Taylor MC, Gómez-Palacio A, Wilkinson SR, Triana-Chávez O, et al. Benznidazole-resistance in trypanosoma cruzi is a readily acquired trait that can arise independently in a single population. J Infect Dis [Internet]. 2012 [cited 2020 Aug 10];206(2):220–8. Available from: /pmc/articles/PMC3379838/?report=abstract

75. Wilkinson SR, Taylor MC, Horn D, Kelly JM, Cheeseman I. A mechanism for cross-resistance to nifurtimox and benznidazole in trypanosomes. Proc the Natl Acad Sci U S A [Internet]. 2008 [cited 2020 Aug 10];105(13):5022–7. Available from: https://www.pnas.org/cgi/doi/10.1073/pnas.0711014105

76. Campos MCO, Leon LL, Taylor MC, Kelly JM. Benznidazole-resistance in Trypanosoma cruzi: evidence that distinct mechanisms can act in concert. Mol Biochem Parasitol [Internet]. 2014 [cited 2020 Aug 10];193(1):17–9. Available from: /pmc/articles/PMC3988956/?report=abstract

77. Francisco AF, Jayawardhana S, Olmo F, Lewis MD, Wilkinson SR, Taylor MC, et al. Challenges in Chagas disease drug development [Internet]. Vol. 25, Molecules. MDPI AG; 2020 [cited 2020 Aug 10]. Available from: /pmc/articles/PMC7355550/?report=abstract

78. Portal P, Villamil SF, Alonso GD, de Vas MG, Flawiá MM, Torres HN, et al. Multiple NADPH-cytochrome P450 reductases from Trypanosoma cruzi. Suggested role on drug resistance. Mol Biochem Parasitol. 2008;160(1):42–51.

79. Ponte-Sucre A, Gamarro F, Dujardin JC, Barrett MP, López-Vélez R, García-Hernández R, et al. Drug resistance and treatment failure in leishmaniasis: a 21st century challenge [Internet]. Vol. 11, PLoS Negl Trop Dis. Public Library of Science; 2017 [cited 2020 Aug 7]. Available from: /pmc/articles/PMC5730103/?report=abstract

80. Uliana SRB, Trinconi CT, Coelho AC. Chemotherapy of leishmaniasis: present challenges [Internet]. Vol. 145, Parasitology. Cambridge University Press; 2018 [cited 2020 Aug 7]. p. 464–80. Available from: https://pubmed.ncbi.nlm.nih.gov/28103966/

81. Mukherjee B, Mukhopadhyay R, Bannerjee B, Chowdhury S, Mukherjee S, Naskar K, et al. Antimony-resistant but not antimony-sensitive Leishmania donovani up-regulates host IL-10 to overexpress multidrug-resistant protein 1. Proc Natl Acad Sci U S A [Internet]. 2013 [cited 2020 Aug 7];110(7):E575–82. Available from: www.pnas.org/lookup/suppl/doi:10.1073/pnas.1213839110/-/DCSupplemental.www.pnas.org/cgi/doi/10.1073/pnas.1213839110

82. Singh K, Garg G, Ali V. Current therapeutics, their problems and thiol metabolism as potential drug targets in leishmaniasis. Curr Drug Metabol [Internet]. 2016 [cited 2020 Aug 7];17(9):897–919. Available from: https://pubmed.ncbi.nlm.nih.gov/27549807/

83. Flow cytometric assessment of amphotericin B susceptibility in Leishmania infantum isolates from patients with visceral leishmaniasis. J Antimicrob Chemother | Oxford Academic [Internet]. [cited 2020 Aug 7]. Available from: https://academic.oup.com/jac/article/44/1/71/750558

84. Purkait B, Kumar A, Nandi N, Sardar AH, Das S, Kumar S, et al. Mechanism of amphotericin B resistance in clinical isolates of Leishmania donovani. Antimicrob Agents Chemother [Internet]. 2012 [cited 2020 Aug 7];56(2):1031–41. Available from: https://pubmed.ncbi.nlm.nih.gov/22123699/

85. Berg M, García-Hernández R, Cuypers B, Vanaerschot M, Manzano JI, Poveda JA, et al. Experimental resistance to drug combinations in leishmania donovani: metabolic and phenotypic adaptations. Antimicrob Agents Chemother [Internet]. 2015 [cited 2020 Aug 7];59(4):2242–55. Available from: https://pubmed.ncbi.nlm.nih.gov/25645828/

86. Evidence of a drug-specific impact of experimentally selected paromomycin and miltefosine resistance on parasite fitness in Leishmania infantum – PubMed [Internet]. [cited 2020 Aug 7]. Available from: https://pubmed.ncbi.nlm.nih.gov/27084919/

87. Ovid: drug resistance in nematodes: a paper tiger or a real problem? [Internet]. [cited 2020 Aug 7]. Available from: https://ovidsp.dc1.ovid.com/ovid-b/ovidweb.cgi?ID=shib%3Adc1%3A0x2813f0a9e3e1415ba78f325d5c2f0c6b&PASSWORD=0x2813f0a9e3e1415ba78f325d5c2f0c6b&T=JS&PAGE=oaklogin

88. Prevention C-C for DC and. CDC – Scabies. 2019;

89. Purvis RS, Tyring SK. An outbreak of lindane-resistant scabies treated successfully with permethrin 5% cream. J Am Acad Dermatol 1991;25(6):1015–6.

90. Currie BJ, Harumal P, McKinnon M, Walton SF. First documentation of in vivo and in vitro ivermectin resistance in Sarcoptes scabiei. Clin Infect Dis [Internet]. 2004 [cited 2020 Aug 11];39(1):e8–12. Available from: https://academic.oup.com/cid/article-lookup/doi/10.1086/421776

91. Meyersburg D, Kaiser A, Bauer JW. Loss of efficacy of topical 5% permethrin for treating scabies: an Austrian single-center study. J Dermatol Treat [Internet]. 2020 [cited 2020 Aug 11];1–4. Available from: https://www.tandfonline.com/doi/full/10.1080/09546634.2020.1774489

92. Khalil S, Abbas O, Kibbi AG, Kurban M. Scabies in the age of increasing drug resistance [Internet]. Vol. 11, PLoS Negl Trop Dis. Public Library of Science; 2017 [cited 2020 Aug 10]. Available from: /pmc/articles/PMC5708620/?report=abstract

93. Davies TGE, Field LM, Usherwood PNR, Williamson MS. DDT, pyrethrins, pyrethroids and insect sodium channels [Internet]. Vol. 59, IUBMB Life; 2007 [cited 2020 Aug 11]. p. 151–62. Available from: https://pubmed.ncbi.nlm.nih.gov/17487686/

94. Mounsey KE, Pasay CJ, Arlian LG, Morgan MS, Holt DC, Currie BJ, et al. Increased transcription of Glutathione S-transferases in acaricide exposed scabies mites. Parasit Vectors [Internet]. 2010 [cited 2020 Aug 11];3(1). Available from: https://pubmed.ncbi.nlm.nih.gov/20482766/

95. Currie BJ, Hengge UR. Scabies. In: Tropical dermatology. 2nd ed: Elsevier; 2016. p. 377–86.

96. Mounsey KE, Dent JA, Holt DC, McCarthy J, Currie BJ, Walton SF. Molecular characterisation of a pH-gated chloride channel from Sarcoptes scabiei. Invert Neurosci [Internet]. 2007 [cited 2020 Aug 11];7(3):149–56. Available from: http://www.cbs.dtu.dk/services/

97. Prevention C-C for DC and. CDC - Lice. 2019;

98. Mumcuoglu KY, Pollack RJ, Reed DL, Barker SC, Gordon S, Toloza AC, et al. International recommendations for an effective control of head louse infestations. Int J Dermatol [Internet]. 2020 [cited 2020 Aug 11];ijd.15096. Available from: https://onlinelibrary.wiley.com/doi/abs/10.1111/ijd.15096

99. Durand R, Bouvresse S, Berdjane Z, Izri A, Chosidow O, Clark JM. Insecticide resistance in head lice: clinical, parasitological and genetic aspects [Internet]. Vol. 18, Clin Microbiol Inf. Blackwell Publishing Ltd; 2012 [cited 2020 Aug 11]. p. 338–44. Available from: http://www.clinicalmicrobiologyandinfection.com/article/S1198743X14614440/fulltext

100. Ko C, Elston DM. Pediculosis. In: Tropical dermatology. 2nd ed: Elsevier; 2016. p. 387–92.

Emerging and Re-emerging Protozoan/Helminth Infections

Fabio Francesconi, Valeska Francesconi, Omar Lupi, and Yasmin Khalfe

Abbreviations

ACL Atypical cutaneous leishmaniasis
CLM Cutaneous larva migrans
DCL Diffuse cutaneous leishmaniasis
DL Disseminated leishmaniasis
GAA Gastro-allergic anisakiasis
GAE Granulomatous amebic encephalitis
IRIS Immune reconstitution inflammatory syndrome
NTDs Neglected tropical diseases
PKDL Post-kala-azar dermal leishmaniasis
VL Visceral leishmaniasis

F. Francesconi
Dermatology Section - Federal University of the State of Amazonas (UFAM), Manaus, Brazil

Dermatologist - Hospital de Medicina Tropical, Manaus, Brazil

V. Francesconi
Dermatology Section - State University of Amazonas, Manaus, Brazil

Dermatologist - Hospital de Medicina Tropical, Manaus, Brazil

O. Lupi
Associate Professor of Dermatology - Federal University of the State of Rio de Janeiro (UNIRIO), Rio de Janeiro, Brazil

Immunology Section - Federal University of Rio de Janeiro (UFRJ), Rio de Janeiro, Brazil

Titular Professor & Chairman - Policlinica Geral do Rio de Janeiro (PGRJ), Rio de Janeiro, Brazil

Ibero Latin American College of Dermatology (CILAD), Buenos Aires, Argentina

International League of Dermatological Societies (ILDS), London, UK

Y. Khalfe (✉)
School of Medicine, Baylor College of Medicine, Houston, TX, USA
e-mail: yasmin.khalfe@bcm.edu

Introduction

Parasites, such as protozoa and helminths, are the cause of some of the most severe health problems in the world today. Some are classified in the World Health Organization's Neglected Tropical Diseases (NTDs) list, such as Chagas disease, cysticercosis, echinococcosis, African trypanosomiasis, schistosomiasis, leishmaniasis, soil-transmitted helminthiasis, lymphatic filariasis, and onchocerciasis [1]. Most of the infections caused by protozoan and helminthic parasites are found in rural areas of low socioeconomic countries and affect millions of people annually. Other parasites, however, are ubiquitous and present all over the world.

Most of the protozoan and helminthic parasites cause skin manifestations, and in some cases, they directly produce specific lesions by infestation and influence of local inflammation. In other situations, the systemic immunologic response against the infectious agent also affects the skin. In the third scenario, the parasite interferes with the

© Springer Nature Switzerland AG 2021
S. K. Tyring et al. (eds.), *Overcoming Antimicrobial Resistance of the Skin*, Updates in Clinical Dermatology, https://doi.org/10.1007/978-3-030-68321-4_11

immune system of the host, producing, amplifying, or reducing some inflammatory reactions and causes allergic or autoinflammatory responses.

It is crucial for the dermatologist not just to recognize the typical dermatological manifestations caused by the multitude of protozoan and helminthic parasites but also to recognize the changing picture of this complicated relationship – the emerging/re-emerging infections. Studies of these infections are being challenged by the evolving and changing geography and epidemiology of these diseases. Such changes can be the result of international travel for leisure, education, and economic reasons as well as increased travel among countries [2]. Immunocompromising diseases such as AIDS, immunosuppressive treatments, and organ/bone marrow transplants have markedly widened the spectrum of opportunistic infections. With this, helminths and protozoans need to be included in the differential diagnoses of opportunistic infections with possible skin manifestations.

The main goal of this chapter is to aid the clinician in making a timely diagnosis of emerging and re-emerging helminthic and protozoan infections based on skin manifestations. Rather than presenting the information based on the taxonomy and parasitology point of view, the classification will prioritize the clinical presentations with a syndromic approach starting with the skin.

Group I: Direct Infestation of the Skin

Many factors influence the clinical presentation of skin diseases caused by direct infestation of a parasite. In some cases, the skin is the target of the infectious agent, while in other cases, an accidental infestation happens. A third scenario is systemic disease that manifests skin conditions.

The host-parasite interaction directly influences the intensity of the skin inflammatory reaction, as well as the type of inflammation. On the parasite side, the parasite load, the substances produced by the infectious agent, and the parasite's metabolic activity must be considered. On the host side, previous contacts with the parasite, the patient's immune status, and any potential coinfection should be reviewed.

Progressive Necrotic Ulcer (Fig. 11.1)

The parasite, *Entamoeba histolytica*, causes necrotic ulcers in five distinct, rare clinic-epidemiological scenarios:

1. Postoperative after abdominal or thoracic surgery
2. Peristomal ulcer
3. Perianal ulcer
4. Sexually transmitted infection with a genital or anal lesion
5. Diaper ulcer (associated diarrhea is a clinical clue)

The ulcer is typically painful and progressive with an outer bright red zone, an inner raised purple margin (sometimes serpiginous), and a central granulomatous floor obscured by necrosis. In the center, the histology is nonspecific with acute or subacute inflammation. Erythrophagocytosis is a

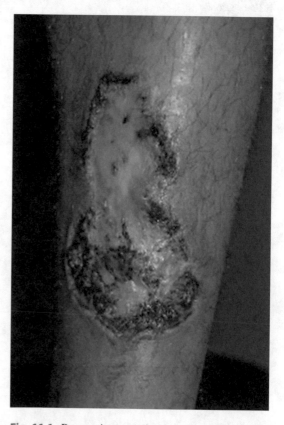

Fig. 11.1 Progressive necrotic ulcer due to *Entamoeba histolytica*. (Source: Dr. Omar Lupi)

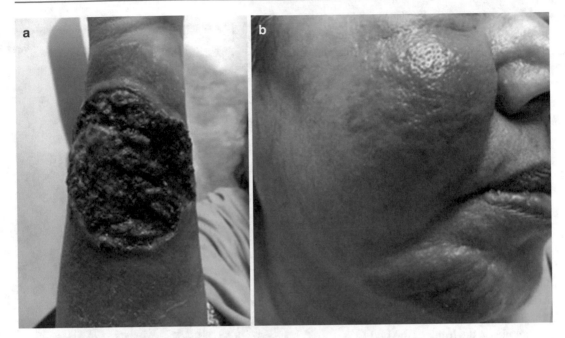

Fig. 11.2 Patient with *L. tropica* lesions on (**a**) arm and (**b**) face. (Source: Dr. Stephen Tyring)

characteristic and diagnostic finding. This clinical presentation is known as cutaneous amebiasis [3].

Acanthamoeba is a free-living amebae species that is a rare cause of a necrotic ulcer. In some cases, local trauma precedes the infection. In others, it is an opportunistic manifestation and epidemiologic history may not be present. The lesion is similar to the ulcer caused by other amebas. Granulomatous necrotic inflammation with amebic trophozoites is typically seen on skin histology. Systemic dissemination to the CNS leading to granulomatous amebic encephalitis (GAE) is the chief cause of death [4].

Balamuthia mandrillaris is another ameba that is a rare cause of the necrotic ulcer, and it usually afflicts extremes of age. Local trauma commonly precedes the clinical presentation by many months to a few years. The ulcer can appear similar to cutaneous amebiasis, or it can present over an infiltrated plaque with small ulcers. Histology reveals a granulomatous inflammatory reaction around the amebic trophozoites. Without treatment, hematogenous dissemination to the central nervous system with a high mortality rate can occur. This clinical presentation is known as *Balamuthia* amebic encephalitis [5].

Dracunculiasis is a disease caused by the parasitic worm, *Dracunculus medinensis* which is endemic in rural and poverty-stricken areas of the world, most commonly in Africa [6]. The disease usually presents a year after infection as patients are initially asymptomatic. The patient may have blistering and the formation of an ulcer, most commonly on the foot. In this case, the ulcer will be accompanied by a worm migrating out of the lesion. This may last for up to 2 months as the worm is fully extracted from the body. In terms of complications, it is possible for abscesses to occur in the lungs, pericardium, and spinal cord if the worm migrates to these sites in the body [6].

Leishmaniasis is a neglected tropical disease, and cutaneous leishmaniasis is the most common form of *Leishmania* infection which presents as ulcers on exposed body parts (Fig. 11.2). The disease can be caused by several species of *Leishmania*. Old World leishmaniasis (in the Eastern hemisphere) is commonly caused by *L. tropica*, *L. major*, and *L. aethiopica*, while New World leishmaniasis (in the Americas) is commonly caused by the *L. mexicana* species complex (*L. mexicana*, *L. amazonensis*, and *L. venezuelensis*) or *Viannia* subgenus (*L. braziliensis*, *L. guyanensis*, *L. panamensis*, and *L. peruviana*) [7]. The cutaneous lesions may appear as papules or plaques that evolve into ulcerative lesions. The ulcers can be granulomatous and crusted with hypertrophic margins [8]. They are usually painless but occasionally may be painful. Scars can commonly form, and they may result in disability or stigma.

Trypanosoma brucei gambiense (West African trypanosomiasis) and *Trypanosoma brucei rhodesiense* (East African trypanosomiasis) are transmitted to humans through the tsetse fly. The disease presents in two stages: a blood and lymphatic stage followed by central nervous system invasion. During the first stage, the bite can develop into an ulcer or chancre [9, 10]. This is more commonly seen in East African trypanosomiasis, and a chancre is commonly the earliest sign of infection within 2 weeks of the bite [11]. After the chancre desquamates, patients may present with erythematous macular rashes most commonly on the trunk of the body.

Inflammatory Plaque (Fig. 11.3)

Leishmaniasis may present with an inflammatory papule or plaque without an ulcer. Dispersed, papulonodular lesions may be due to a subcategory of leishmaniasis, known as diffuse cutaneous leishmaniasis (DCL) [8]. This manifestation is rare and has been reported most commonly in cases caused by *L. aethiopica* of Old World leishmaniasis and *L. mexicana amazonensis* and *L. amazonensis* of New World leishmaniasis [12, 13]. Clinically, the infection appears as multiple, diffuse papular lesions that are non-ulcerative. Parasites grow uncontrollably, and the lesions may be seen on the limbs, buttocks, or face.

The most common presentation of *Balamuthia mandrillaris* is a plaque sometimes with satellite lesions. It commonly has ill-defined raised borders, producing an annular lesion [14]. On the face, particularly the cheek or nose, plaque-like lesions may precede neurological symptom development [15].

Acanthamoeba sp. may present with granulomatous skin infiltration manifested as papules or plaques. While ulcers may occur later in the dis-

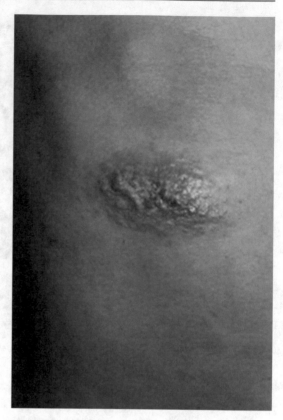

Fig. 11.3 Inflammatory plaque secondary to leishmaniasis. (Source: Dr. Omar Lupi)

ease, acanthamoebiasis may begin as a firm papulonodule. In cases in which the lesions do ulcerate, the patient may have both newer lesions as plaques and older lesions as cutaneous necrotic ulcers [16].

Microsporidia are a group of opportunistic infections associated with advanced AIDS. In infected patients, the most common presentations are protracted and debilitating diarrhea. In recent years, there have been reports of microsporidia presenting with skin manifestations [17, 18]. These have been described as presenting with painful, erythematous, nodular plaques, or papules, and diagnosis can be made by identification of the parasite from the skin [17, 18].

Chagas disease is an infection caused by *Trypanosoma cruzi*. Acute infection with *T. cruzi* may present with an inflammatory reaction at the inoculation site that develops in to a hard, red swollen nodule known as a "chagoma" [19]. It

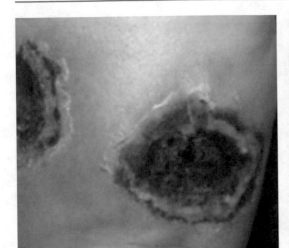

Fig. 11.4 Ulcerated plaques on leg from Chagas pannic-ulitis. Reactivated disease in solid organ transplant recipient. (Source: Dr. Stephen K. Tyring)

may present initially after the bite and persist for weeks. An opportunistic reactivation syndrome due to *T. cruzi* may present with a localized erythematous plaque (Fig. 11.4) [20].

Central Inflammatory Facial Lesion (Fig. 11.5)

All species of the *Viannia* subgenus of *Leishmania* can afflict the upper airway mucosa after hematogenous spread. Mucosal leishmaniasis commonly occurs months to years after presentation of cutaneous leishmaniasis. If untreated, the infection can persist and even lead to nasal septum perforation [7].

Balamuthia mandrillaris typically afflicts the central face, presenting as a painless, skin tone, or dark red plaque that may feel indurated or rubbery [21]. If untreated, the infection can lead to infiltration and deformity. The infection precedes CNS involvement (*Balamuthia* amebic encephalitis). It is thought to spread by direct extension through olfactory nerve structures and vessel walls to the central nervous system [14]. *Acanthamoeba* sp. can lead to a clinical picture similar to *Balamuthia mandrillaris* infection. In

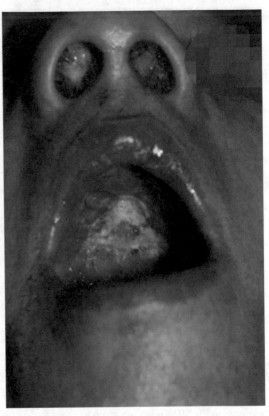

Fig. 11.5 Central inflammatory facial lesion from the *Viannia* subgenus of *Leishmania*. (Source: Dr. Omar Lupi)

immunocompromised patients, *Acanthamoeba* can present with nasal obstruction, crusting, and epistaxis as well as necrosis of bone and cartilage surrounded by erythematous mucosa [22].

Diffuse Papules (Fig. 11.6)

Disseminated leishmaniasis (DL) is defined as ten or more lesions in two or more noncontiguous body parts, and lymphatic spread cannot explain the distribution. *Leishmania V. braziliensis* is the principal etiologic agent of this presentation, although species such as *L.* guyanensis and *L. panamensis* can also cause the disease [23]. Diffuse papules that may ulcerate and acneiform eruptions are the primary lesions. Some patients may have hundreds of lesions throughout the body.

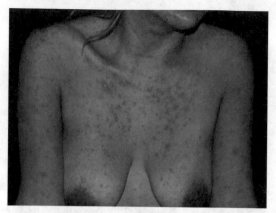

Fig. 11.6 Diffused papules from disseminated leishmaniasis. (Source: Dr. Omar Lupi)

Post-kala-azar dermal leishmaniasis (PKDL) is a complication occasionally seen after treatment of visceral leishmaniasis (VL). The pathogenesis is not fully understood but is likely due to a cell-mediated immune response [24]. Clinical presentation varies based on the geographical location but often appears as macular or maculopapular lesions distributed across the body. In patients with HIV who previously were infected with VL, PKDL has been thought to be a potential presentation of immune reconstitution inflammatory syndrome (IRIS) [24].

Toxoplasma gondii is a parasite that infects humans in utero or through ingestion of contaminated food or water. It is usually asymptomatic; however, reactivation may occur in patients who are posttransplant, in post-chemotherapy for hematological malignancies, and with advanced AIDS. Cutaneous toxoplasmosis only occurs in less than 10% of acquired infections and is more severe in the immunocompromised [25]. While the signs of infection may be variable, the most common appearance is a maculopapular, erythematous rash involving the trunk. Diagnosis is confirmed through PCR and immunohistochemical stain.

Schistosoma haematobium, *S. mansoni*, and rarely *S. japonicum* can cause cutaneous schistosomiasis; however, this type of manifestation is rare. When it does occur, it may present as pruritic erythematous papules or nodules. A late diagnosis and treatment can be consequential as skin lesions have been seen to cause neuroschistosomiasis. The identification of the egg in the dermis is diagnostic [26].

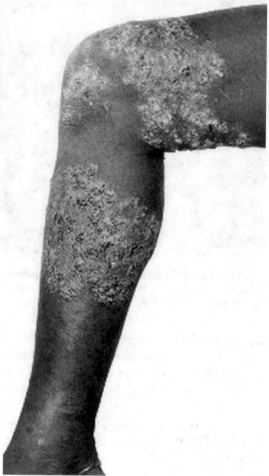

Fig. 11.7 Numerous cutaneous lesions, which were determined to be due to a chronic onchocerciasis infection, caused by *Onchocerca volvulus*. (Source: CDC PHIL)

Onchocerciasis is caused by *Onchocerca volvulus* and has dermatologic, ocular, and systemic symptoms (Fig. 11.7). It is the second most common infectious cause of blindness in the world after trachoma, and 99% of disease burden occurs in Africa [27]. While major strides in the last decade have been made to control the disease, challenges still exist in the implementation of elimination programs. Presentation of cutaneous symptoms vary, but most often patients present with onchodermatitis featuring a maculopapular rash anywhere on the body that is commonly pruritic [28]. Chronic papular onchodermatitis involves flat-topped pruritic papules, often symmetrically distributed over buttocks, waist, and shoulders. Post-inflammatory hyperpigmentation and lichenification are common complications [28]. Reactive onchodermatitis is known as *sowda*, which means black in Arabic. This is in reference to the hyperpigmentation that occurs in this condition, and it is a concerning issue that has emerged in countries such as Yemen and Sudan [29].

Subcutaneous Nodules

Toxoplasma gondii has been reported in certain instances as causing a cutaneous disease consisting of nodules. Although rare, toxoplasmosis should be considered in patients presenting with nodular lesions [30]. Another parasitic disease that presents with subcutaneous nodules is dirofilariasis, a nematode genus that infects carnivorous hosts. This infection can cause either pulmonary or subcutaneous dirofilariasis. Multiple species in the *Dirofilaria* subspecies, *Nochtiella*, can cause subcutaneous infections most commonly on exposed body parts that lead to tender nodules that can be granulomatous [31].

Rarely, infection with the *Echinococcus* sp. can cause extrahepatic hydatidosis of the skin. Clinically, it can appear as a painless, slow-growing, subcutaneous mass. The overlying skin is usually normal in appearance but can be erythematous [32]. On imaging, it appears as a cyst [14]. Although rare, *Echinococcus* should be on a differential for soft tissue masses and subcutaneous nodules.

Fascioliasis is caused by *Fasciola hepatica*, a liver fluke that is found usually in patients who have eaten raw vegetables, such as watercress contaminated with the parasite. Rarely, the flukes can migrate to other locations in the body including the skin. Clinically, cutaneous fascioliasis can be seen as subcutaneous nodules [33].

There have recently been increasing numbers of reports of infection with the parasite, *Gnathostoma spinigerum*, in non-endemic countries. The cutaneous symptoms may begin 3–4 weeks after initial larvae infection. The lesion presents as a solitary, fixed nodule that is hard or lumpy nodules and can also be painful or itchy. Signs that the nodule may be gnathostomiasis are an elongated infiltration pattern and a *peau d'orange* finding on the overlaying erythematous skin [34].

Cutaneous cysticercosis is caused by the larva of *Taenia solium*, known as cysticercus cellulosae

cutis. The disease is due to ingestion of eggs from the tapeworm and can be localized or disseminated. Other organs that can be involved are the central nervous system (neurocysticercosis), muscle (myalgic type, nodular type, or pseudohypertrophy), and eyes. The cyst is identified in histology specimen or with imaging techniques [35]. Lastly, *Wuchereria bancrofti*, the cause of lymphatic filariasis, rarely causes a subcutaneous nodule when microfilariae mature in the skin and subcutaneous tissue. In this case, the nodule will contain the parasite [36].

Vasculitic and Purpuric (Fig. 11.8)

Disseminated strongyloidiasis is an opportunistic manifestation of *Strongyloides stercoralis*. In *Strongyloides* infection, lungs or skin may be possibly infected organs. Purpura is the most common primary lesion caused by the destruction or obstruction of the skin vasculature by the nematode. Abdominal wall lesions, especially with periumbilical gathering and gluteal lesions, are the typical distribution. In more advanced stages of *Strongyloides*, the periumbilical thumbprint parasitic purpura sign predicts a poor prognostic [37].

Rare cases of rheumatoid purpura have been reported to be associated with toxocariasis. This parasitic infection is caused by the roundworm, *Toxocara canis* in dogs and *Toxocara cati*. The association between toxocariasis and manifestations of vasculitis is uncommon, and the mechanism is poorly understood but likely involves an immune-mediated inflammatory response to larva [38]. While vasculitis is a rare presentation of toxocariasis, patients with purpura should be

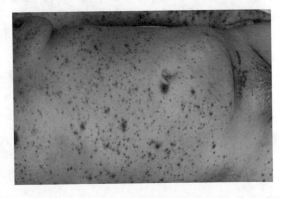

Fig. 11.8 Vasculitic and purpuric lesions due to disseminated strongyloidiasis. (Source: Dr. Omar Lupi)

investigated for *Toxocara* if the clinical history and laboratory findings suggest risk factors of infection.

Creeping Eruption (Fig. 11.9)

Larva currens is the migratory lesion caused by *Strongyloides stercoralis*. Although *S. stercoralis* is usually a gastrointestinal or pulmonary disorder, larvae are sometimes able to migrate out of the body and affect the perirectal skin. Larva currens is characterized by a serpiginous, erythematous eruption that can extend to the buttocks, thighs, and abdomen. In the setting of disseminated infection, the larva can migrate at speeds up to 5–15 cm per hour, which is specific to strongyloidiasis. The condition can be a manifestation of chronic strongyloidiasis. Hyperinfection can occur in immunocompromised patients which leads to rapid eruption [39].

Unlike larva currens caused by *Strongyloides*, cutaneous larva migrans (CLM) does not demonstrate the characteristic fast movement through the skin. CLM is caused by hookworms such as *Ancylostoma* species. The parasite burrows into the skin, often after walking barefoot on a beach or infested soil. Infection presents as a classically serpiginous rash following that is pruritic and migrates slower at up to 2 cm per day [40]. The disease is self-limited as the hookworms die

before reproducing; however, migration can continue for months. *Gnathostoma spinigerum* can occasionally present very superficially in an identical way to cutaneous larva migrans (CLM); however, it can be distinguished from CLM by location, including thoracic and breast areas which are uncommon in CLM [34].

Dirofilaria repens may appear as a creeping eruption in the subcutaneous type, which can lead to pain and burning. Other presentations reported include palpebral creeping eruption, and worms can be found on the conjunctiva [31, 41]. *Fasciola hepatica* is another cause of migratory lesions. The first case of creeping eruption was reported in 2010 in which the infection appeared in a migratory vesicular track [42]. The presentation occurs with crusts and nodules leaving a serpentine track, and the parasite is at the end of the eruption.

Loa loa is a parasite endemic to Central and West Africa that is often asymptomatic. It can present as episodic angioedema (Calabar swellings) and subconjunctival migration of the worm. In some cases, it may cause a serpiginous palpebral lesion, and worms can migrate through the subcutaneous tissue. The diagnosis is sometimes made by finding microfilariae in the peripheral blood or adult worms in Calabar swellings or in the eye [43].

Lastly, capillariasis is a rare infection in humans that is caused by *Capillaria hepatica* or *Capillaria philippinensis*. Infection most commonly presents as acute/subacute hepatitis. It has been reported as a cause of cutaneous creeping eruption as well [44].

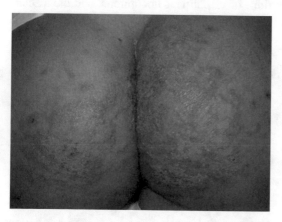

Fig. 11.9 Creeping eruption from *Strongyloides stercoralis*. (Source: Dr. Omar Lupi)

Skin Fistulization

In rare instances, *Echinococcus* sp. can cause skin fistulas from hepatic lesions, abdominal lesions, or alveolar lesions [45]. *T. vaginalis* has also been associated with a case of multiple urethral fistulas of the glans penis, showing that *T. vaginalis* can lead to tissue destruction and fibrotic healing [46].

Folliculitis

Pelodera strongyloides (*Rhabditis*) dermatitis is a rare disorder seen in animals more often than in humans. The parasite can penetrate the skin through the follicle aperture after contact with contaminated soil. Skin scraping identifies the rhabditiform larvae. The nodular lesion is predominantly follicular and can be superficial or deep [47].

Folliculitis can also be caused by parasites in the cases of demodicosis or scabies. The *Demodex* mite lives in or near hair follicles of mammals and is more commonly found on the face [48]. Scabies can provoke folliculitis, and the rash can become infected with bacteria.

Verrucous Lesions (Fig. 11.10)

Atypical cutaneous leishmaniasis (ACL) can present as verrucous lesions. These lesions are uncommonly reported in the literature, but it is important to consider in the differential diagnoses of verrucous carcinoma [49].

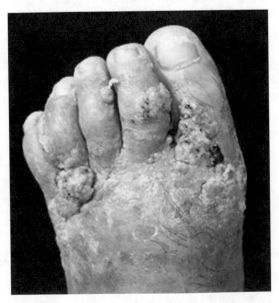

Fig. 11.10 Verrucous lesions of atypical cutaneous leishmaniasis. (Source: Dr. Omar Lupi)

Perianal and Genital Ulcers

T. vaginalis has been associated with chronic ulcer [46]. The ulcers are usually painful with associated discharge. Cultures are usually positive, and resolution of the lesion occurs after metronidazole. *Entamoeba histolytica* causes amebic vaginitis or cervicitis that can be confused with carcinoma. It presents with necrosis and ulcers; in these cases the parasite is considered a cause of STI with genital or perianal involvement [50].

Group II: Systemic Inflammatory Reaction

The skin may be distressed by a systemic inflammatory reaction elicited by a parasite. In some cases, the inflammatory response is specific to the parasite, while in others it is not necessarily a specific connection.

Urticaria

Urticaria can be a reaction to many parasitic infections. Certain mechanisms of type I reactions include interactions between parasite-specific IgE and high-affinity IgE receptors, products released by helminths, and tissue damage that causes alarmin production with mastocyte degranulation and eosinophil recruitment to the skin.

Anisakiasis is a parasitic infection that is transmitted to humans by consuming raw or undercooked fish. It presents with abdominal pain, nausea, vomiting, and diarrhea. Patients with anisakiasis can be affected by urticaria in three scenarios. The first is gastrointestinal anisakiasis characterized by severe gastric symptoms and occasional urticaria. In this case, there is a penetration of *A. simplex* in the intestinal wall and production of specific IgE against the helminth. The second clinical picture is gastro-allergic anisakiasis (GAA) caused by acute parasitism manifested by penetration of the *A.*

simplex in the gastric mucosa and production of IgE. Acute urticaria that rarely exceeds 48 hours is the main clinical presentation. Angioedema can also occur. Prolonged acute urticaria and chronic urticaria are also caused by *A. simplex*. In both cases, there is a history of exposure to raw fish, and a positive prick test against *A. simplex* helps to confirm the diagnosis [51].

Toxocariasis caused by *T. cati* and *T. canis* can manifest as urticaria. Chronic urticaria is one of the most common cutaneous signs of infection, and there are few reports of acute urticaria [52]. There have also been studies that have shown a positive association between urticaria and positive serology for *Toxocara* [53]. Drug therapy with albendazole is the treatment of choice.

Ascaris infection can lead to high IgE levels and allergic manifestations, including asthma, urticaria, and atopic dermatitis [54]. This is due to cross-reactivity between worm proteins and highly similar molecules in dust mites. It has been shown that helminth infections play a role in the production of Th2 cytokines and IL-10 which affect hypersensitivity reaction in skin [54].

The clinical symptoms of *Blastocystis* are varied from gastrointestinal symptoms and pain to urticaria and other pruritic skin lesions. While the mechanisms of *Blastocystis*-induced cutaneous lesions are not fully understood, the process is likely due to immune responses or gut microbiota modifications. In one review, the rate of urticaria reached 22.5%, and the link between *Blastocystis* and urticaria was supported by the resolution of lesions following parasite treatment [55]. Therefore, researchers have suggested that screening for *Blastocystis hominis* should be considered in patients with urticaria [55].

Giardia intestinalis is considered a protozoa that can cause urticaria. Evidence that links this infection with the allergy includes the presence of a specific serum anti-Giardia IgE in symptomatic giardiasis patients with allergic symptoms. Researchers have concluded a causal connection due to the finding that therapy with metronidazole or tinidazole successfully resolves skin lesions [56].

Other, less frequent, parasitic causes of urticaria include *Enterobius vermicularis*, *T. vaginalis*, and *Trichinella spiralis* [57–59].

Acute Inflammatory Reactions

Katayama fever is the name of an acute reaction to the first exposure to *Schistosoma*. After a period of 2 weeks to 12 months, the patient can develop an acute inflammatory reaction with fever, pulmonary infiltration, and rash. This is thought to be caused by an immune complex phenomenon in response to egg-laying by newly matured adult female schistosomes. This reaction is usually seen in travelers to endemic regions [60].

Cercarial dermatitis, also called swimmer's itch, is a seasonal inflammatory skin reaction to cercaria (larvae) of avian schistosomes. Clinical manifestations occur with the penetration of the cercariae and include fever, cough, and a rash [61]. In some cases, a type I reaction predominates with wheals and occasional vesicles. In others, a type IV reaction with eosinophils will be the major immunological mechanism manifested by hard erythematous papules or nodules. Usually, the parasite dies in the skin. Rarely human schistosomiasis may cause cercarial dermatitis, especially in individuals visiting an endemic region.

T. cruzi rarely causes schizotrypanides, a generalized morbilliform eruption that occurs weeks after acute inoculation [20]. In African trypanosomiasis, it presents as an evanescent macular rash of the upper trunk, sometimes with a polycyclic configuration, and it can be missed in black skin. It is a lymphocytic inflammatory dermatosis associated with edema.

Miscellaneous Inflammatory Skin Reactions (Table 11.1)

Table 11.1 Miscellaneous inflammatory skin reactions

Organism	Inflammatory skin reaction
Toxoplasma gondii	Can cause erythema multiforme and sweet syndrome [62]
Babesia microti	Rarely causes skin rash similar to necrolytic migratory erythema or with mottled skin [63]
Enterobius vermicularis	Intestinal infection is associated with sweet syndrome and eosinophilic dermatitis [64] An increased risk of atopic dermatitis and allergic rhinitis [65]
Fasciola hepatica	Associated with nodular vasculitis; subsides with fascioliasis treatment [66]
Giardia intestinalis	Causes erythema nodosum, Well's syndrome, and chronic urticaria [67]
Trypanosoma cruzi	Reactivation in HIV coinfected patients may produce subcutaneous involvement reminiscent of erythema nodosum [68]
Onchocerca volvulus	Mazzotti reaction is caused by the killing of the microfilaria after treatment with diethylcarbamazine. Papular or urticarial rash, ocular inflammation associated with viral and cardiovascular symptoms can all occur [69]

Group III: Immunomodulation and Indirect Associations

Immunomodulation of Inflammatory Skin Conditions

Numerous studies have asked whether a correlation exists between infectious diseases and the decreased incidence of allergic diseases and chronic inflammatory disorders. It is hypothesized that repetitive or constant infection induces the host to develop an immunological tolerance in order to establish a long-lasting relationship. Medical knowledge today recognizes that some infections may influence the human immune system and modulate the inflammatory response of a well-established disease, while in others, an inflammatory reaction occurs.

Toxoplasma gondii chronic infection in murine studies causes less Th2 response in atopic rats and diminishes the clinical symptoms of atopic dermatitis. An epidemiological study in

Brazil showed a relationship between atopic dermatitis and negative toxoplasma serology [70]. Similarly, maternal hookworm (Ancylostoma sp.) infestation was inversely associated with atopic dermatitis development in the first 5 years of the child. The same scenario was found to occur in cases of childhood infestation by Trichuris trichiura or hookworm [71].

Intestinal helminth infections also influence skin test reactivity, both in early and later childhood. Ascaris lumbricoides heavy infections in later childhood, at the time of allergen skin tests, have been found to be inversely correlated with skin test reactivity. The same is found with T. trichiura heavy infestation. Similarly, schistosomiasis infection has been associated with reduced risk for allergic reactivity [72]. Conversely, Clonorchis sinensis is positively associated with atopic sensitization to common aeroallergens and total serum IgE levels [73]. It has no association with wheezing, airway hyperresponsiveness, asthma, or allergic rhinitis. Lastly, the number of malaria infections in the first 5 years of life has been found to be inversely associated with infantile eczema [71].

Indirect Associations

In most reports, the connection between the skin manifestation and the parasite infestation occurs after symptom relief with anti-parasitic treatment. In some cases, there are indirect associations, and infections are seen to be associated with certain dermatologic conditions (Table 11.2).

Skin as the Parasite Reservoir

In some cases, there is no clinical manifestation of the infestation, even with the infectious agent within the skin. In African trypanosomiasis, the protozoan localized in the skin is asymptomatic and considered an essential source of transmission to the tsetse flies. It has been found that when flies feed on skin but not blood, they can become infected, thus skin-dwelling parasites contribute to disease transmission. With this, skin can be

Table 11.2 Indirect associations between infections and dermatologic conditions

Dermatomyositis and *Toxoplasma gondii*	Rare reports connect dermatomyositis and toxoplasmosis, with symptom relief after the anti-parasitic treatment [74]
Chronic prurigo and *Toxoplasma gondii*	Presentation associated in 22% of cases in one study [74]
Palmoplantar pruritus and *Blastocystis hominis*	Initially pruritus can be localized, manifested intermittently, and predominantly at night [55]
Echinococcus granulosus and acute generalized exanthematous pustulosis	Association in one case suggested immunocomplex formation may be related to development of AGEP [75]
Enterobius vermicularis and photodermatitis-like papular eruption	Plaques and papules caused by proven enterobiasis presented in one case of UV-exposed skin [76]
Giardia intestinalis and Interface dermatitis	Granuloma annulare-like lesions have been attributed to *Giardia intestinalis* [67]
Trichomonas vaginalis	Vaginitis treatment found to resolve eczema, pruritic dermatoses of the limbs, extragenital pruritus, and oral aphthous ulcer [77]
Angiostrongylus cantonensis	Skin paresthesia (up to 80% of the patients) can be the clinical manifestation [78]

considered an anatomical reservoir for infection [79, 80].

Additionally, *Onchocerca volvulus* and *Mansonella streptocerca* microfilaria are located within the skin of carriers and are used as the source of diagnosis in asymptomatic individuals [79, 80]. A skin snip can be positive in up to 90% of the adults living in an endemic area. Overall, these organisms primarily use the skin as a reservoir.

Conclusion

Parasites cause some of the world's most severe health problems and include many of the World Health Organization's Neglected Tropical Diseases (NTDs) list, including Chagas disease, cysticercosis, echinococcosis, African trypanosomiasis, schistosomiasis, leishmaniasis, soil-transmitted helminthiasis, lymphatic filariasis, and onchocerciasis. Parasitic infections commonly present with a myriad of cutaneous manifestations and immunologic reactions. With this, it is important for dermatologists to be aware of the emergence of parasitic infections of the skin, particularly as the world development continues to ease international travel amongst countries. As many parasitic diseases can have dire consequences, it is important for dermatologists to have the necessary knowledge to identify and diagnose emerging and re-emerging skin manifestations of parasitic diseases.

References

1. Mitra AK, Mawson AR. Neglected tropical diseases: epidemiology and global burden [Internet]. Vol. 2, Trop Med Infect Dis. MDPI AG; 2017 [cited 2020 Aug 14]. Available from: /pmc/articles/PMC6082091/?report=abstract
2. Atehmengo NL, Nnagbo CS. Emerging animal parasitic diseases: a global overview and appropriate strategies for their monitoring and surveillance in Nigeria. Open Microbiol J [Internet]. 2014 [cited 2020 Aug 14];8(1):87–94. Available from: /pmc/articles/PMC4200699/?report=abstract
3. Parshad S, Grover PS, Sharma A, Verma DK, Sharma A. Primary cutaneous amoebiasis: case report with review of the literature. In: International Journal of Dermatology [Internet]. Int J Dermatol; 2002 [cited 2020 Aug 15]. p. 676–80. Available from: https://pubmed.ncbi.nlm.nih.gov/12390191/
4. Khan NA. Acanthamoeba: biology and increasing importance in human health [Internet]. Vol. 30, FEMS Microbiol Rev. Oxford Academic; 2006 [cited 2020 Aug 15]. p. 564–95. Available from: http://www.ncbi.nlm.nih.
5. Francisco AF, Jayawardhana S, Olmo F, Lewis MD, Wilkinson SR, Taylor MC, et al. Challenges in Chagas Disease Drug Development [Internet]. Vol. 25, Molecules. MDPI AG; 2020 [cited 2020 Aug 10]. Available from: /pmc/articles/PMC7355550/?report=abstract
6. Parenti DM. Dracunculiasis. In: Medical parasitology [Internet]. CRC Press; 2009 [cited 2020 Aug 15]. p. 58–62. Available from: https://www.ncbi.nlm.nih.gov/books/NBK538231/
7. Prevention C-C for DC and. CDC - Leishmaniasis - Resources for Health Professionals. 2020;
8. Choi CM, Lerner EA. Leishmaniasis as an emerging infection. J Invest Dermatol Symp Proc [Internet].

2001 [cited 2020 Aug 15];6(3):175–82. Available from: https://pubmed.ncbi.nlm.nih.gov/11924824/

9. CDC – African Trypanosomiasis – General Information – East African Trypanosomiasis FAQs [Internet]. [cited 2020 Aug 15]. Available from: https://www.cdc.gov/parasites/sleepingsickness/gen_info/faqs.html

10. Ponte-Sucre A. An overview of trypanosoma brucei infections: an intense host-parasite interaction [Internet]. Vol. 7, Front Microbiol. Frontiers Media S.A.; 2016 [cited 2020 Aug 15]. Available from: /pmc/articles/PMC5183608/?report=abstract

11. Mcgovern TW, Williams W, Fitzpatrick JE, Cetron MS, Hepburn BC, Gentry RH. Cutaneous manifestations of African trypanosomiasis. Arch Dermatol [Internet]. 1995 [cited 2020 Aug 15];131(10):1178–82. Available from: https://jamanetwork.com/

12. Khandelwal K, Bumb RA, Mehta RD, Kaushal H, Lezama-Davila C, Salotra P, et al. Case report: a patient presenting with Diffuse Cutaneous Leishmaniasis (DCL) as a first indicator of HIV infection in India. Am J Trop Med Hyg [Internet]. 2011 [cited 2020 Aug 15];85(1):64–5. Available from: /pmc/articles/PMC3122345/?report=abstract

13. Hashiguchi Y, Gomez EL, Kato H, Martini LR, Velez LN, Uezato H. Diffuse and disseminated cutaneous leishmaniasis: clinical cases experienced in Ecuador and a brief review [Internet]. Vol. 44, Trop Med Health. BioMed Central Ltd.; 2016 [cited 2020 Aug 16]. Available from: /pmc/articles/PMC4934146/?report=abstract

14. Bravo FG, Seas C. Balamuthia mandrillaris amoebic encephalitis: an emerging parasitic infection. Curr Infect Dis Rep [Internet]. 2012 [cited 2020 Aug 15];14(4):391–6. Available from: https://link.springer.com/article/10.1007/s11908-012-0266-4

15. CDC – Free Living Amebic Infections [Internet]. [cited 2020 Aug 15]. Available from: https://www.cdc.gov/dpdx/freelivingamebic/index.html

16. Marciano-Cabral F, Cabral G. Acanthamoeba spp. as agents of disease in humans [Internet]. Vol. 16, Clin Microbiol Rev. American Society for Microbiology (ASM); 2003 [cited 2020 Aug 15]. p. 273–307. Available from: /pmc/articles/PMC153146/?report=abstract

17. Nadelman DA, Bradt AR, Qvarnstrom Y, Goldsmith CS, Zaki SR, Wang F, et al. Cutaneous microsporidiosis in an immunosuppressed patient. J Cutan Pathol [Internet]. 2020 [cited 2020 Aug 15];47(7):659–63. Available from: https://onlinelibrary.wiley.com/doi/abs/10.1111/cup.13674

18. Kester KE, Turiansky GW, McEvoy PL. Nodular cutaneous microsporidiosis in a patient with AIDS and successful treatment with long-term oral clindamycin therapy. Ann Int Med [Internet]. 1998 [cited 2020 Aug 15];128(11):911–4. Available from: http://www.acponline.org.

19. Patel S, Sethi A. Imported tropical diseases. Dermatol Ther [Internet]. 2009 [cited 2020 Aug 15];22(6):538–49. Available from: http://doi.wiley.com/10.1111/j.1529-8019.2009.01275.x

20. Hemmige V, Tanowitz H, Sethi A. Trypanosoma cruzi infection: a review with emphasis on cutaneous manifestations [Internet]. Vol. 51, Int J Dermatol. NIH Public Access; 2012 [cited 2020 Aug 15]. p. 501–8. Available from: /pmc/articles/PMC3552304/?report=abstract

21. Bravo FG, Gotuzzo E. Cutaneous manifestations of infection by free-living Amebas. In: Tyring S, editor. Tropical dermatology. 2nd ed: Elsevier Inc.; 2016. p. 50–5.

22. Dickson JM, Zetler PJ, Walker B, Javer AR. Acanthamoeba rhinosinusitis. J Otolaryngol. 2009;38(3):E87–90.

23. Machado GU, Prates FV, Machado PRL. Disseminated leishmaniasis: clinical, pathogenic, and therapeutic aspects. An Bras Dermatol [Internet]. 2019 [cited 2020 Aug 16];94(1):9–16. Available from: /pmc/articles/PMC6360961/?report=abstract

24. Farooq U, Choudhary S, Chacon AH, Lebrun E, Shiman MI, Hernandez J, et al. Post-kala-azar dermal leishmaniasis in HIV-infected patients with AIDS: a report of two cases diagnosed in the USA. Int J Dermatol [Internet]. 2013 [cited 2020 Aug 16];52(9):1098–104. Available from: http://doi.wiley.com/10.1111/ijd.12139

25. Rand AJ, Buck AB, Love PB, Prose NS, Angelica SM. Cutaneous acquired toxoplasmosis in a child: a case report and review of the literature. Am J Dermatopathol. 2015;37(4):305–10.

26. de Mota LS, de Almeida FC, Teixeira RDL, de Silva SF, de Mesquita LSU, Soares AM. Ectopic cutaneous schistosomiasis – case report. An Bras Dermatol [Internet]. 2014 [cited 2020 Aug 16];89(4):646–8. Available from: /pmc/articles/PMC4148281/?report=abstract

27. Gebrezgabiher G, Mekonnen Z, Yewhalaw D, Hailu A. Reaching the last mile: Main challenges relating to and recommendations to accelerate onchocerciasis elimination in Africa [Internet]. Vol. 8, Infect Dis Poverty. BioMed Central Ltd.; 2019 [cited 2020 Aug 29]. p. 1–20. Available from: https://doi.org/10.1186/s40249-019-0567-z

28. Okulicz JF, Stibich AS, Elston DM, Schwartz RA. Cutaneous onchocercoma. Int J Dermatol [Internet]. 2004 [cited 2020 Aug 16];43(3):170–2. Available from: http://doi.wiley.com/10.1111/j.1365-4632.2004.02279.x

29. Al-Kubati AS, Mackenzie CD, Boakye D, Al-Qubati Y, Al-Samie AR, Awad IE, et al. Onchocerciasis in Yemen: moving forward towards an elimination program [Internet]. Vol. 10, Int Health. Oxford University Press; 2018 [cited 2020 Aug 16]. p. i89–96. Available from: https://academic.oup.com/inthealth/article/10/suppl_1/i89/4868662

30. Marina S, Broshtilova V, Botev I, Guleva D, Hadzhiivancheva M, Nikolova A, et al. Cutaneous manifestations of toxoplasmosis: a case report.

Serbian J Dermatol Venereol [Internet]. 2015 [cited 2020 Aug 16];6(3):113–9. Available from: https://content.sciendo.com/view/journals/sjdv/6/3/article-p113.xml

31. CDC – DPDx – Dirofilariasis [Internet]. [cited 2020 Aug 16]. Available from: https://www.cdc.gov/dpdx/dirofilariasis/index.html

32. Kayaalp C, Dirican A, Aydin C. Primary subcutaneous hydatid cysts: a review of 22 cases. Vol. 9, Int J Surg. Elsevier; 2011. p. 117–21.

33. Yi-Zhu X, Zhi-Bang Y. A case of ectopic fascioliasis in the skin. Tropical doctor [Internet]. 2010 [cited 2020 Aug 16];40(4):253–4. Available from: http://www.ncbi.nlm.nih.gov/pubmed/20846990.

34. Bravo F, Gontijo B. Gnathostomiasis: a emerging infectious disease relevant to all dermatologists. An Bras Dermatol [Internet]. 2018 [cited 2020 Aug 16];93(2):172–80. Available from: /pmc/articles/PMC5916386/?report=abstract

35. Bandyopadhyay D, Sen S. Disseminated cysticercosis with huge muscle hypertrophy. Indian J Dermatol [Internet]. 2009 [cited 2020 Aug 16];54(1):49–51. Available from: /pmc/articles/PMC2800871/?report=abstract

36. Filarial Nematodes – Medical Microbiology – NCBI Bookshelf [Internet]. [cited 2020 Aug 16]. Available from: https://www.ncbi.nlm.nih.gov/books/NBK7844/

37. Periumbilical thumbprint parasitic purpura: a highly fatal sign in disseminated Strongyloides infection that may mimic vasculitis clinically. J Am Acad Dermatol. 2015;72(5):AB129.

38. Bellanger A-P, Bamoulid J, Millon L, Chalopin J-M, Humbert P. Rheumatoid purpura associated with toxocariasis. Can Fam Phys Med [Internet]. 2011 [cited 2020 Aug 17];57(12):1413–4. Available from: http://www.ncbi.nlm.nih.gov/pubmed/22170196.

39. Lupi O, Downing C, Lee M, Pino L, Bravo F, Giglio P, et al. Mucocutaneous manifestations of helminth infections: nematodes. Vol. 73, J Am Acad Dermatol. Mosby Inc.; 2015. p. 929–44.

40. Cutaneous Larva Migrans – StatPearls – NCBI Bookshelf [Internet]. [cited 2020 Aug 20]. Available from: https://www.ncbi.nlm.nih.gov/books/NBK507706/

41. Lindner AK, Tappe D, Gertler M, Equihua Martinez G, Richter J. A live worm emerging from the eyelid. J Travel Med [Internet]. 2018 [cited 2020 Aug 20];25(1):1–2. Available from: www.blast.ncbi.nlm.nih.gov

42. Cutaneous fascioliasis: a case report in Vietnam – PubMed [Internet]. [cited 2020 Aug 20]. Available from: https://pubmed.ncbi.nlm.nih.gov/15891121/

43. Rakita RM, White AC, Kielhofner MA. Loa loa infection as a cause of migratory angioedema: report of three cases from the texas medical center. Clin Infect Dis [Internet]. 1993 [cited 2020 Aug 20];17(4):691–4. Available from: https://pubmed.ncbi.nlm.nih.gov/8268351/

44. Morishita K, Tani T. A case of capillaria infection causing cutaneous creeping eruption in man. J Parasitol [Internet]. 1960 [cited 2020 Aug 20];46(1):79. Available from: https://www.jstor.org/stable/3275338?origin=crossref

45. Schmoldt S, Bruns CJ, Rentsch M, Siegert S, Nikolaou K, Hogardt M, et al. Skin fistulization associated with extensive alveolar echinococcosis. Ann Trop Med Parasitol [Internet]. 2010 [cited 2020 Aug 20];104(2):175–80. Available from: https://www.tandfonline.com/action/journalInformation?journalCode=ypgh20

46. Gosnell BI, Costiniuk CT, Mathaba E, Moosa MYS. Case report: trichomonas vaginalis associated with chronic penile ulcers and multiple urethral fistulas. Am J Trop Med Hyg [Internet]. 2015 [cited 2020 Aug 20];92(5):943–4. Available from: /pmc/articles/PMC4426582/?report=abstract

47. Ginsburg B, Beaver PC, Wilson ER, Whitky RJ. Dermatitis Due to Larvae of a Soil Nematode, Pelodera strongyloides. Pediatr Dermatol [Internet]. 1984 [cited 2020 Aug 20];2(1):33–7. Available from: https://pubmed.ncbi.nlm.nih.gov/6542207/

48. Rather PA, Hassan I. Human demodex mite: the versatile mite of dermatological importance. Indian J Dermatol [Internet]. 2014 [cited 2020 Aug 20];59(1):60–6. Available from: /pmc/articles/PMC3884930/?report=abstract

49. Salman A, Yucelten A, Seckin D, Ergun T, Demircay Z. Cutaneous leishmaniasis mimicking verrucous carcinoma: a case with an unusual clinical course [Internet]. Vol. 81, Indian J Dermatol Venereol Leprol. Medknow Publications; 2015 [cited 2020 Aug 20]. p. 392–4. Available from: https://pubmed.ncbi.nlm.nih.gov/25994897/

50. Musthyala N, Indulkar S, Palwai V, Babaiah M, Ali M, Marriapam P. Amebic infection of the female genital tract: a report of three cases. J Mid Life Health [Internet]. 2019 [cited 2020 Aug 20];10(2):96–8. Available from: /pmc/articles/PMC6643709/?report=abstract

51. Daschner A, de Frutos C, Valls A, Vega F. Anisakis simplex sensitization-associated urticaria: short-lived immediate type or prolonged acute urticaria. Arch Dermatol Res [Internet]. 2010 [cited 2020 Aug 22];302(8):625–9. Available from: https://link.springer.com/article/10.1007/s00403-010-1069-9

52. Kim MH, Jung JW, Kwon JW, Kim TW, Kim SH, Cho SH, et al. A case of recurrent toxocariasis presenting with urticaria. Allergy Asthma Immunol Res [Internet]. 2010 [cited 2020 Aug 25];2(4):267–70. Available from: /pmc/articles/PMC2946705/?report=abstract

53. Fialho PMM, Correa CRS, Lescano SZ. Seroprevalence of toxocariasis in children with urticaria: a population-based study. J Trop Pediatr [Internet]. 2017 [cited 2020 Aug 25];63(5):352–7. Available from: https://pubmed.ncbi.nlm.nih.gov/28077610/

54. Qualizza R, Losappio LM, Furci F. A case of atopic dermatitis caused by Ascaris lumbricoides infection.

Clin Mol Allergy [Internet]. 2018 [cited 2020 Aug 27];16(1):10. Available from: https://clinicalmolecularallergy.biomedcentral.com/articles/10.1186/s12948-018-0088-5

55. Bahrami F, Babaei E, Badirzadeh A, Riabi TR, Abdoli A. Blastocystis, urticaria, and skin disorders: review of the current evidences [Internet]. Vol. 39, Eur J Clin Microbiol Infect Dis. Springer; 2020 [cited 2020 Aug 27]. p. 1027–42. Available from: https://doi.org/10.1007/s10096-019-03793-8.

56. Nenoff P, Domula E, Willing U, Herrmann J. Giardia lamblia. Ursache von urtikaria und pruritus oder zufällige assoziation? Hautarzt [Internet]. 2006 [cited 2020 Aug 27];57(6):518–22. Available from: https://pubmed.ncbi.nlm.nih.gov/15875147/

57. Clark RF. Localized urticaria due to enterobius vermicularis. Arch Dermatol [Internet]. 1961 [cited 2020 Aug 27];84(6):1026. Available from: https://jamanetwork.com/journals/jamadermatology/fullarticle/527175

58. Renner R, Fleck A, Schubert S, Baerwald C, Beer J, Schober R, et al. Chronic urticaria and angioedema with concomitant eosinophilic vasculitis due to trichinella infection [12] [Internet]. Vol. 88, Acta Derm Venereol; 2008 [cited 2020 Aug 27]. p. 78–9. Available from: https://pubmed.ncbi.nlm.nih.gov/18176764/

59. F Purello-D'Ambrosio, S Gangemi, L Ricciardi, A Marcazzò, NC Levanti. Urticaria from Trichomonas vaginalis infection – PubMed. [cited 2020 Aug 27]; Available from: https://pubmed.ncbi.nlm.nih.gov/10353101/

60. Logan S, Armstrong M, Moore E, Nebbia G, Jarvis J, Suvari M, et al. Short report: acute schistosomiasis in travelers: 14 Years' experience at the hospital for tropical diseases, London. Am J Trop Med Hyg [Internet]. 2013 [cited 2020 Aug 27];88(6):1032–4. Available from: /pmc/articles/PMC3752798/?report=abstract

61. Horák P, Mikeš L, Lichtenbergová L, Skála V, Soldánová M, Brant SV. Avian schistosomes and outbreaks of cercarial dermatitis. Clin Microbiol Rev [Internet]. 2015 [cited 2020 Aug 27];28(1):165–90. Available from: /pmc/articles/PMC4284296/?report=abstract

62. Delfino M, Suppa F, de Luca F, Lembo G. Sweet's syndrome and toxoplasmosis: a coincidental association? Dermatology [Internet]. 1985 [cited 2020 Aug 27];171(2):102–5. Available from: https://pubmed.ncbi.nlm.nih.gov/4043468/

63. Moreno Gimenez J, Jimenez Puya R, Galan Gutierrez M, Ortega Salas R, Duenas Jurado J. Erythema figuratum in septic babesiosis. J Eur Acad Dermatol Venereol [Internet]. 2006 [cited 2020 Aug 27];20(6):726–8. Available from: http://doi.wiley.com/10.1111/j.1468-3083.2006.01492.x

64. Sulk M, Ehrchen J. Sweet syndrome in association with enterobiasis. J Dermatol [Internet]. 2019 [cited 2020 Aug 27];46(3):e106–7. Available from: http://doi.wiley.com/10.1111/1346-8138.14615

65. Bøås H, Tapia G, Rasmussen T, Rønningen KS. Enterobius vermicularis and allergic conditions in Norwegian children. Epidemiol Infect [Internet]. 2014 [cited 2020 Aug 27];142(10):2114–20. Available from: https://pubmed.ncbi.nlm.nih.gov/24331127/

66. Taghipour A, Zaki L, Rostami A, Foroutan M, Ghaffarifar F, Fathi A, et al. Highlights of human ectopic fascioliasis: a systematic review. Vol. 51, Infect Dis. Taylor and Francis Ltd.; 2019. p. 785–92.

67. Humbert P, Guichard A, Bennani I, Chiheb S. Giardia duodenalis et son implication dans diverses dermatoses. Ann Dermatol Vénéréol [Internet]. 2017 [cited 2020 Aug 27];144(11):676–84. Available from: https://linkinghub.elsevier.com/retrieve/pii/S0151963817303113

68. Lattes R, Lasala MB. Chagas disease in the immunosuppressed patient. Vol. 20, Clin Microbiol Infect. Blackwell Publishing Ltd; 2014. p. 300–9.

69. Ackerman SJ, Kephart GM, Francis H, Awadzi K, Gleich GJ, Ottesen EA. Eosinophil degranulation. An immunologic determinant in the pathogenesis of the Mazzotti reaction in human onchocerciasis. J Immunol. 1990;144(10)

70. Fernandes JFC, Taketomi EA, Mineo JR, Miranda DO, Alves R, Resende RO, et al. Antibody and cytokine responses to house dust mite allergens and Toxoplasma gondii antigens in atopic and non-atopic Brazilian subjects. Clin Immunol [Internet]. 2010 [cited 2020 Aug 27];136(1):148–56. Available from: /pmc/articles/PMC3039445/?report=abstract

71. Mpairwe H, Ndibazza J, Webb EL, Nampijja M, Muhangi L, Apule B, et al. Maternal hookworm modifies risk factors for childhood eczema: results from a birth cohort in Uganda. Pediatr Allergy Immunol [Internet]. 2014 [cited 2020 Aug 27];25(5):481–8. Available from: /pmc/articles/PMC4312885/?report=abstract

72. Cooper PJ. Interactions between helminth parasites and allergy [Internet]. Vol. 9, Curr Opin Allergy Clin Immunol. Europe PMC Funders; 2009 [cited 2020 Aug 27]. p. 29–37. Available from: /pmc/articles/PMC2680069/?report=abstract

73. Choi M-H, Chang Y-S, Lim MK, Bae YM, Hong S-T, Oh J-K, et al. Clonorchis sinensis infection is positively associated with atopy in endemic area. Clin Exp Allergy [Internet]. 2011 [cited 2020 Aug 27];41(5):697–705. Available from: http://doi.wiley.com/10.1111/j.1365-2222.2011.03746.x

74. Topi G, D'Alessandro Gandolfo L, Giacalone B, Griso D, Zardi O, Argiroffo A. Acquired cutaneous toxoplasmosis. Dermatologica [Internet]. 1983 [cited 2020 Aug 27];167(1):24–32. Available from: https://pubmed.ncbi.nlm.nih.gov/6628795/

75. Cannistraci C, Parola ILL, RiganO R, Bassetti F, Ortona E, Santucci B, et al. Acute generalized exanthematous pustulosis in cystic echinococcosis: immunological characterization. Br J Dermatol [Internet]. 2003 [cited 2020 Aug 27];148(6):1245–9. Available from: http://doi.wiley.com/10.1046/j.1365-2133.2003.05346.x

76. Zorko MS, Horvat AT. Papular eruption on UV-exposed skin in a 7-year-old boy caused by Enterobius vermicularis infection. Acta Dermatovenerol Alp Pannonica Adriat. 2019;28(4):179–81.

77. Bachmann LH, Hobbs MM, Seña AC, Sobel JD, Schwebke JR, Krieger JN, et al. Trichomonas vaginalis genital infections: progress and challenges [Internet]. Vol. 53, Clin Infect Dis. Oxford University Press; 2011 [cited 2020 Aug 27]. p. S160. Available from: /pmc/articles/PMC3897282/?report=abstract

78. [Clinical observation on 25 cases of severe angiostrongyliasis cantonensis] – PubMed [Internet]. [cited 2020 Aug 27]. Available from: https://pubmed.ncbi.nlm.nih.gov/18038807/

79. Puente S, Ramirez-Olivencia G, Lago M, Subirats M, Perez-Blazquez E, Bru F, et al. Dermatological manifestations in onchocerciasis: a retrospective study of 400 imported cases. Enferm Infecc Microbiol Clin [Internet]. 2018 [cited 2020 Aug 27];36(10):633–9. Available from: https://pubmed.ncbi.nlm.nih.gov/29275076/

80. Ta-Tang T-H, Crainey J, Post RJ, Luz SLB, Rubio J. Mansonellosis: current perspectives. Res Rep Trop Med [Internet]. 2018 [cited 2020 Aug 27];9:9–24. Available from: /pmc/articles/PMC6047625/?report=abstract

Part V

Innovative Therapies on the Forefront

Phage Therapy

12

Stephen Andrew Moore and Angela Yen Moore

Abbreviations

ESKAPE *Enterococcus faecium, Staphylococcus aureus, Klebsiella pneumoniae, Acinetobacter baumannii, Pseudomonas aeruginosa, and Enterobacter sp.*

MRSA Methicillin-resistant *Staphylococcus aureus*

Introduction and History

Dermatologists are always seeking new and innovative methods for treating bacterial infections as antibiotic resistance continues to increase. The development of phage therapy, or the use of bacteriophages to treat bacterial infections, was developed as early as 1915, but it was not until the middle of the twentieth century that phage therapy had more significant research [1, 2]. Due to the advent of innovative antibiotics, the development of bacteriophages was throttled in the United States, while the Soviet Union continued research after World War II [1]. However, as bacterial infections have become resistant to antibiotics, renewed interest exists in nontraditional approaches.

Bacteriophages are currently used to treat battle wounds primarily in Eastern Europe since they are not yet cleared for treatment in either the United States or the European Union. Bacteriophage therapy succeeds over antibiotics because of the immense number of bacteriophages available even if a bacterium becomes resistant to a particular bacteriophage [3]. Treatment with bacteriophages is not limited to such infections as methicillin-resistant *Staphylococcus aureus* (MRSA), however, but covers all conditions that may be secondarily infected, including atopic dermatitis, folliculitis, furuncles, and carbuncles.

Mechanism of Action

Bacteriophages infect bacterium in a species- or strain-specific manner, and 96% are classified in the order of *Caudovirales* (tailed, double-stranded DNA) (see Fig. 12.1) and further classified in the families of *Siphoviridae*, *Myoviridae*, and *Podoviridae* [4]. Isolated, characterized, and genetically sequenced prior to therapeutic uses [1, 5], bacteriophages are then selected based on specificity, efficacy, and side effect profile [6]. This high

The original version of this chapter was revised. The correction to this chapter can be found at https://doi.org/10.1007/978-3-030-68321-4_17.

S. A. Moore
Arlington Center for Dermatology, Arlington, TX, USA

Arlington Research Center, Arlington, TX, USA

A. Y. Moore (✉)
Division of Dermatology, Baylor University Medical Center, Dallas, TX, USA

Arlington Center for Dermatology, Arlington, TX, USA

Arlington Research Center, Arlington, TX, USA

© Springer Nature Switzerland AG 2021, corrected publication 2022
S. K. Tyring et al. (eds.), *Overcoming Antimicrobial Resistance of the Skin*, Updates in Clinical Dermatology, https://doi.org/10.1007/978-3-030-68321-4_12

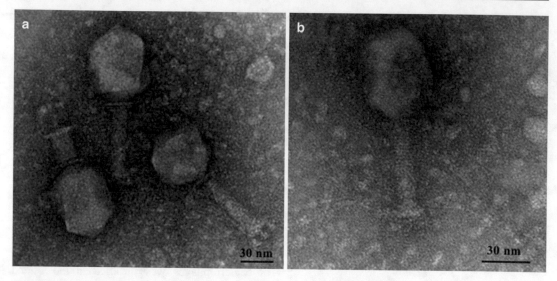

Fig. 12.1 (**a**) and (**b**) Electron micrograph of phage vB_Kpn_F48 negatively stained with uranyl acetate. The bars indicate 30 nm

specificity has greatly limited antibiotic resistance [7] and minimized impact on normal gut microflora [8]. Inappropriate selection of bacteriophages and inadequate preparation or storage has contributed to the occasional failure of phage therapy [6, 9]. In one study on the combined effect of the antibacterial peptide nisin with two lytic phages against *S. aureus*, nisin resistance confers resistance to the two phages, while loss of nisin resistance restores phage susceptibility [10].

Bacteriophages are classified as lytic or temperate. Only lytic bacteriophages should be used to treat infections instead of temperate bacteriophages, since temperate phages may propagate antibiotic resistance and transduce undesirable genes [11]. Mostly associated with temperate rather than lytic bacteriophages, safety concerns of bacteriophage therapy include possible destruction of human tissue and nontarget microbiota, possible expression of virulence genes, transduction of DNA between bacteria, and induction of immunological reactions [11, 12]. As an example, a recent in vitro study isolated two novel lytic bacteriophages called Max and Zip, to treat antibiotic-resistant *Enterococcus faecium* and *Enterococcus faecalis* [13]. This

investigation also highlighted the short latent periods and efficient replication cycles of the bacteriophages [13] (see Fig. 12.2).

In order to successfully reduce bacteria populations, current estimates suggest that 108 bacteriophages/ml are required excluding the phage replication in the infection site [14]. Consequently, enteral administration of bacteriophages is the most effective, although phages can also be administered topically, orally, or intramuscularly [15]. According to a literature review by Speck and Smithyman, bacteriophages administered intravenously have been found safe, without any anaphylaxis [16]. Local administration of sera results in greater antiphage activity than the oral route [17]. Interestingly, while antiphage antibodies inactivate many phages [17], this high rate of inactivation does not necessarily result in treatment failure [18].

Genetic engineering of bacteriophages is also being attempted to create sequence-specific antimicrobials [19, 20], to enhance antibiotic activity [21, 22], or to reverse antibiotic resistance [23]. Genetically engineered bacteriophages are being designed to sensitize bacterial populations on skin microbiota of hospital personnel or surfaces to prevent transmission of infection [24, 25].

Fig. 12.2 Lytic bacteriophage life cycle

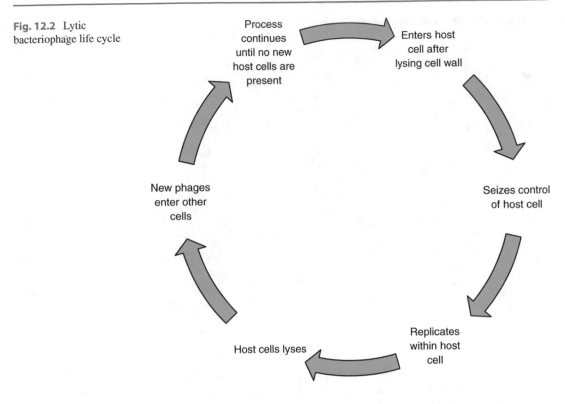

Animal Model Studies

In 2017, the WHO created a list of the most frequent bacteria causing severe hospital-acquired infections, especially in those critically ill [26, 27]. Under the pneumonic, "ESKAPE," these bacteria include *E. faecium*, *S. aureus*, *Klebsiella pneumoniae*, *Acinetobacter baumannii*, *Pseudomonas aeruginosa*, and *Enterobacter sp.* [26]. Phage therapy has shown efficacy in mice infected with vancomycin-resistant *E. faecium* and vancomycin-resistant *E. faecalis* [28]. Similarly, bacteriophage therapy against MRSA in a rabbit study protects against abscess formation [29]. In another study in rabbits, MRSA count decreased by 99% with *S. Aureus*-specific bacteriophage Sb-1 treatment only when combined with debridement [30]. In a similar study on mice with MRSA, treatment with phage therapy eliminated the MRSA [31]. In other mice infected with imipenem-resistant *P. aeruginosa*, Wang et al. intraperitoneally injected phages to cure the mice successfully, even when injections were delayed for up to 3 hours [32]. Similarly, topical bacteriophage applications in *A. baumannii* wound infection models in mice were successful [33] and two topical phage applications in a murine burn wound model successfully treated *K. pneumoniae*, as reported by Kumari et al. [33, 34]

Clinical Applications

Treatment of Wounds and Burns

Phage therapies for burns and wounds have been heavily investigated even before the advent of antibiotics [1, 7]. Bacteriophage cocktails are utilized for burns and wounds because of the mixed flora and frequent colonization by bacterial biofilms which are tolerant to antibiotics. In a case

Table 12.1 Human studies with phage therapy

Study	Case study/ trial phase	Target bacterium	Condition	Carrier (IV/ oral/topical)	References
Polish case studies	I/II	Several multidrug-resistant bacteria	Burns and wounds	Topical	[35]
Phagoburn project	I/II	*Escherichia coli*; *Pseudomonas aeruginosa*	Burns and wounds	Topical	[36]
BFC-1 Belgium study	Case study	*Pseudomonas aeruginosa* and *Staphylococcus aureus*	Burns and wounds	Topical	[37]
WPP-201 cocktail of bacteriophages	I	*Escherichia coli*; *Staphylococcus aureus*; *Pseudomonas aeruginosa*	Venous leg ulcers	Topical	[38]
Eliava BioPreparations Georgian case study with Sb-1	Case study	Methicillin-sensitive *Staphylococcus aureus* (MSSA), with methicillin-resistant *Staphylococcus aureus* (MRSA)	Diabetic leg ulcers	Topical	[39]
AmpliPhi biosciences corporation trial	I/II	*Staphylococcus aureus*	Secondary infections of those using ventricular assist devices	Intravenous	[40]

series of patients with recalcitrant infections from the Phage Therapy Unit in the Hirszfeld Institute, Wroclaw, Poland, between 2008 and 2010, a 40% response rate to phage therapy was observed. Morozova et al. conducted a research study detailing the methodology behind his approach to treat diabetic foot ulcers based on his practice in Russia [35] (see Table 12.1 for a list of all human studies). First, all diabetic foot ulcers are cultured and sensitivities to a battery of bacteriophages are determined. After debridement and rinsing, the wound is covered with gauze soaked with the specified bacteriophage solution diluted with sterile 0.9% saline (1:2–1:10) and wrapped after 10–15 minutes [35]. This dressing is repeated up to four times per day and the wound cultured every 5–6 days to confirm that titers are decreasing by 3–4 orders of magnitude until the infection has cleared [35].

A multicenter trial in France, Belgium, and Switzerland investigated the efficacy and tolerability of a cocktail of bacteriophages to treat burn wounds infected by *P. aeruginosa and E. coli* [36]. This phase I/II study compared application of 1% sulfadiazine silver emulsion cream and a cocktail of 12 lytic anti-*P. aeruginosa* bacteriophages in 27 burn patients [36]. Phage therapy at

higher concentration markedly reduced the spread of infection and may be a promising future option in treating burn sites [36]. Another experimental study investigated the phage cocktail BFC-1 to treat burn patients infected with *P. aeruginosa* and *S. aureus* in Europe with less promising results [37]. Of the ten burn wounds treated with BFC-1 spray, the bacterial load did not change significantly. Nevertheless, they believe that the issue was penetration into the wound by the spray and that the phages may work better if a different carrier is utilized [37].

Phase I trials have begun in Lubbock to analyze the effect of chronic venous leg ulcers after the treatment of a wide cocktail of phages designed to treat *P. aeruginosa*, *S. aureus*, and *E. coli* [38]. Forty-two patients with chronic venous leg ulcers were treated for 12 weeks with either a saline control or bacteriophages targeted against *P. aeruginosa*, *S. aureus*, and *E. coli* without any safety issues [38].

Treatment of *Staphylococcus aureus*

As successes have been seen with bacteriophage cocktails, targeted bacteriophages have been developed against various organisms, with Sb-1 being the most widely used bacteriophage against *S. aureus* [41, 42]. Treatment with bacteriophages of *S. aureus*, especially novel treatments for MRSA, has been widely studied [30]. They are often applied concomitantly with such topical treatments commonly used for burns as silver cream, honey, or bioelectric dressings [1]. Fish et al. demonstrated drastic improvement with topical application of a commercially available Georgian staphylococcal phage preparation in a case series of nine patients with recalcitrant diabetic foot ulcers with MRSA and methicillin-sensitive *S. Aureus* [43].

Kutateladze and Adamia highlight 70% and 55% response rates of an anti-staphylococcal phage preparation in the treatment of staphylococcal infections and staphylococcal sepsis, respectively, in Georgian clinical trials [39].

Another human study investigated the use of staphylococcal phage Sb-1 to treat diabetic leg ulcers that had been infected with MRSA [41, 42]. It demonstrated remarkable success even in treatment areas of poor vascularity and antibiotic failure [42]. However, larger clinical trials are needed to verify these findings [42].

In February, 2019, the FDA announced the approval of the first study of intravenous phage therapy for *S. Aureus* [40]. This study is investigating the efficacy of phage therapy through intravenous methods in order to prevent biofilm in patients with ventricular assist devices [40]. This research may be a viable future treatment option for intravenous phage therapy for *S. Aureus*.

Treatment of Acne

In the face of increasing antimicrobial resistance to antibiotics for acne treatment (primarily antibiotics targeting *Cutibacterium acnes* (formerly *Propionibacterium acnes*)), novel approaches are always significant [9]. Currently, these investigations are primarily still in early in vitro phases, so much more research is needed

to determine their status in vivo [9]. These studies display great initial promise, especially since many bacteriophages are found naturally on the skin's biosphere, although often in limited quantities [30]. Furthermore, the resistance of certain bacteria to antibiotics has shown to have no significant impact on the effectiveness of the bacteriophages [44]. Unlike bacteriophages for most conditions, however, many of the bacteriophages utilized to treat acne vulgaris have had more widespread effectiveness and diversity [45]. However, this could be a potential risk in the future as it may lead to mutations and resistance, although no data thus far supports this [44]. Currently, each cocktail of bacteriophages is concocted individually for a specific bacterium (not in bulk) so that it may be several years before any bacteriophages are commercially sustainable.

A later investigation into the most effective application of phages to treat acne finds that a semisolid preparation could be applied to acne and that potentially other semisolid preparations that could be preserved for 90 days [46].

Common Misconceptions

The more common idea of bacteriophages is that they are carriers of antibiotic resistance from one bacterium to another. Along the same lines, these bacteriophages could pass along proteins genetically engineered to kill bacteria. Although some speculate that bacteriophages would be used independently of antibiotics, antibiotics will still continue to be used in order to achieve better efficacy rates [41].

Conclusion

Bacteriophages rise in importance in the age of antibiotic resistance, but they should be administered carefully in order to prevent further microbial resistance. Continued research is necessary to confirm the proposed treatment options.

References

1. Karinja SJ, Spector JA. Treatment of infected wounds in the age of antimicrobial resistance: contemporary alternative therapeutic options. Plast Reconstr Surg. 2018;142(4):1082–92.
2. Lin DM, Koskella B, Lin HC. Phage therapy: an alternative to antibiotics in the age of multi-drug resistance. World J Gastrointest Pharmacol Ther. 2017;8(3):162–73.
3. Geoghegan JA, Irvine AD, Foster TJ. Staphylococcus aureus and atopic dermatitis: a complex and evolving relationship. Trends Microbiol. 2018;26(6):484–97.
4. Sharp R. Bacteriophages: biology and history. J Chem Technol Biotechnol. 2001;76(7):667–72.
5. Gill JJ, Hyman P. Phage choice, isolation, and preparation for phage therapy. Curr Pharm Biotechnol. 2010;11(1):2–14.
6. Weber-Dąbrowska B, Jończyk-Matysiak E, Żaczek M, Łobocka M, Łusiak-Szelachowska M, Górski A. Bacteriophage procurement for therapeutic purposes. Front Microbiol. 2016;7:1177.
7. Gelman D, Eisenkraft A, Chanishvili N, Nachman D, Coppenhagem Glazer S, Hazan R. The history and promising future of phage therapy in the military service. J Trauma Acute Care Surg. 2018;85(1S Suppl 2):S18–26.
8. Loc-Carrillo C, Abedon ST. Pros and cons of phage therapy. Bacteriophage. 2011;1(2):111–4.
9. Jończyk-Matysiak E, Weber-Dąbrowska B, Żaczek M, Międzybrodzki R, Letkiewicz S, Łusiak-Szelchowska M, et al. Prospects of phage application in the treatment of acne caused by. Front Microbiol. 2017;8:164.
10. Martínez B, Obeso JM, Rodríguez A, García P. Nisin-bacteriophage crossresistance in Staphylococcus aureus. Int J Food Microbiol. 2008;122(3):253–8.
11. Abedon ST. Bacteriophage clinical use as antibacterial "drugs": utility and precedent. Microbiol Spectr. 2017;5(4)
12. Abedon ST, Kuhl SJ, Blasdel BG, Kutter EM. Phage treatment of human infections. Bacteriophage. 2011;1(2):66–85.
13. Melo LDR, Ferreira R, Costa AR, Oliveira H, Azeredo J. Efficacy and safety assessment of two enterococci phages in an in vitro biofilm wound model. Sci Rep. 2019;9(1):6643.
14. Abedon ST. Phage therapy: various perspectives on how to improve the art. Methods Mol Biol. 1734;2018:113–27.
15. Abedon ST, Thomas-Abedon C. Phage therapy pharmacology. Curr Pharm Biotechnol. 2010;11(1):28–47.
16. Speck P, Smithyman A. Safety and efficacy of phage therapy via the intravenous route. FEMS Microbiol Lett. 2016;363(3)
17. Łusiak-Szelachowska M, Zaczek M, Weber-Dąbrowska B, Międzybrodzki R, Kłak M, Fortuna W, et al. Phage neutralization by sera of patients receiving phage therapy. Viral Immunol. 2014;27(6):295–304.
18. Żaczek M, Łusiak-Szelachowska M, Jończyk-Matysiak E, Weber-Dąbrowska B, Międzybrodzki R, Owczarek B, et al. Antibody production in response to staphylococcal MS-1 phage cocktail in patients undergoing phage therapy. Front Microbiol. 2016;7:1681.
19. Citorik RJ, Mimee M, Lu TK. Sequence-specific antimicrobials using efficiently delivered RNA-guided nucleases. Nat Biotechnol. 2014;32(11):1141–5.
20. Bikard D, Euler CW, Jiang W, Nussenzweig PM, Goldberg GW, Duportet X, et al. Exploiting CRISPR-Cas nucleases to produce sequence-specific antimicrobials. Nat Biotechnol. 2014;32(11):1146–50.
21. Pires DP, Cleto S, Sillankorva S, Azeredo J, Lu TK. Genetically engineered phages: a review of advances over the last decade. Microbiol Mol Biol Rev. 2016;80(3):523–43.
22. Lu TK, Collins JJ. Engineered bacteriophage targeting gene networks as adjuvants for antibiotic therapy. Proc Natl Acad Sci U S A. 2009;106(12):4629–34.
23. Edgar R, Friedman N, Molshanski-Mor S, Qimron U. Reversing bacterial resistance to antibiotics by phage-mediated delivery of dominant sensitive genes. Appl Environ Microbiol. 2012;78(3):744–51.
24. Yosef I, Manor M, Kiro R, Qimron U. Temperate and lytic bacteriophages programmed to sensitize and kill antibiotic-resistant bacteria. Proc Natl Acad Sci U S A. 2015;112(23):7267–72.
25. Viertel TM, Ritter K, Horz HP. Viruses versus bacteria-novel approaches to phage therapy as a tool against multidrug-resistant pathogens. J Antimicrob Chemother. 2014;69(9):2326–36.
26. Esposito S, De Simone G. Update on the main MDR pathogens: prevalence and treatment options. Infez Med. 2017;25(4):301–10.
27. WHO publishes list of bacteria for which new antibiotics are urgently needed [press release]. WHO Newsroom; 2017.
28. Cheng M, Liang J, Zhang Y, Hu L, Gong P, Cai R, et al. The bacteriophage EF-P29 efficiently protects against lethal vancomycin-resistant Enterococcus faecalis and alleviates gut microbiota imbalance in a murine bacteremia model. Front Microbiol. 2017;8(837)
29. Wills QF, Kerrigan C, Soothill JS. Experimental bacteriophage protection against Staphylococcus aureus abscesses in a rabbit model. Antimicrob Agents Chemother. 2005;49(3):1220–1.
30. Seth AK, Geringer MR, Nguyen KT, Agnew SP, Dumanian Z, Galiano RD, et al. Bacteriophage therapy for Staphylococcus aureus biofilm-infected wounds: a new approach to chronic wound care. Plast Reconstr Surg. 2013;131(2):225–34.
31. Oduor JM, Onkoba N, Maloba F, Arodi WO, Nyachieo A. Efficacy of lytic Staphylococcus aureus bacteriophage against multidrug-resistant Staphylococcus aureus in mice. J Infect Dev Ctries. 2016;10(11):1208–13.
32. Wang J, Hu B, Xu M, Yan Q, Liu S, Zhu X, et al. Use of bacteriophage in the treatment of experimental animal bacteremia from imipenem-resistant Pseudomonas aeruginosa. Int J Mol Med. 2006;17(2):309–17.

33. Kusradze I, Karumidze N, Rigvava S, Dvalidze T, Katsitadze M, Amiranashvili I, et al. Characterization and testing the efficiency of acinetobacter baumannii phage vB-GEC_Ab-M-G7 as an antibacterial agent. Front Microbiol. 2016;7(1590)

34. Kumari S, Harjai K, Chhibber S. Bacteriophage versus antimicrobial agents for the treatment of murine burn wound infection caused by Klebsiella pneumoniae B5055. J Med Microbiol. 2011;60(Pt 2):205–10.

35. Morozova VV, Kozlova YN, Ganichev DA, Tikunova NV. Bacteriophage treatment of infected diabetic foot ulcers. Methods Mol Biol. 1693;2018:151–8.

36. Jault P, Leclerc T, Jennes S, Pirnay JP, Que YA, Resch G, et al. Efficacy and tolerability of a cocktail of bacteriophages to treat burn wounds infected by Pseudomonas aeruginosa (PhagoBurn): a randomised, controlled, double-blind phase 1/2 trial. Lancet Infect Dis. 2019;19(1):35–45.

37. Rose T, Verbeken G, Vos DD, Merabishvili M, Vaneechoutte M, Lavigne R, et al. Experimental phage therapy of burn wound infection: difficult first steps. Int J Burns Trauma. 2014;4(2):66–73.

38. Rhoads DD, Wolcott RD, Kuskowski MA, Wolcott BM, Ward LS, Sulakvelidze A. Bacteriophage therapy of venous leg ulcers in humans: results of a phase I safety trial. J Wound Care. 2009;18(6):237–8. 40–3

39. Kutateladze M, Adamia R. Phage therapy experience at the Eliava Institute. Med Mal Infect. 2008;38(8):426–30.

40. Voelker R. FDA approves bacteriophage trial. JAMA. 2019;321(7):638.

41. Morozova VV, Vlassov VV, Tikunova NV. Applications of bacteriophages in the treatment of localized infections in humans. Front Microbiol. 2018;9:1696.

42. Fish R, Kutter E, Wheat G, Blasdel B, Kutateladze M, Kuhl S. Bacteriophage treatment of intransigent diabetic toe ulcers: a case series. J Wound Care. 2016;25(Sup7):S27–33.

43. Fish R, Kutter E, Wheat G, Blasdel B, Kutateladze M, Kuhl S. Compassionate use of bacteriophage therapy for foot ulcer treatment as an effective step for moving toward clinical trials. Methods Mol Biol. 1693;2018:159–70.

44. Liu J, Yan R, Zhong Q, Ngo S, Bangayan NJ, Nguyen L, et al. The diversity and host interactions of Propionibacterium acnes bacteriophages on human skin. ISME J. 2015;9(9):2078–93.

45. Marinelli LJ, Fitz-Gibbon S, Hayes C, Bowman C, Inkeles M, Loncaric A, et al. Propionibacterium acnes bacteriophages display limited genetic diversity and broad killing activity against bacterial skin isolates. MBio. 2012;3(5)

46. Brown TL, Petrovski S, Dyson ZA, Seviour R, Tucci J. The formulation of bacteriophage in a semi solid preparation for control of Propionibacterium acnes growth. PLoS One. 2016;11(3):e0151184.

The Role of Biofilms and the Microbiome

13

Stephen Andrew Moore and Angela Yen Moore

Abbreviations

AD	Atopic Dermatitis
HS	Hidradenitis Suppurativa
PDT	Photodynamic Therapy
PEF	Pulsed Electric Fields
VLU	Venous Leg Ulcers
ΦT	Phage Therapy

Introduction on Biofilms and the Microbiome

Biofilms are a diverse and complex collection of microorganisms, including bacteria, protein, and DNA, either embedded or attached to a living or nonliving surface, which form an extracellular polysaccharide [1–5]. While the composition of each biofilm varies greatly, the general formation is similar [5]. The bacteria adhere excessively to one another in addition to the wound site, piling up on one another [1, 2, 5]. These collections of bacteria pose a significant threat because white blood cells cannot pass through multiple layers of bacteria [1, 2].

Biofilms were first reported in the early 1990s on animals [6]. While they were initially quite neglected as a potential threat, biofilms have subsequently been more widely studied and addressed [6]. Antibiotics cannot kill the bacteria as easily due to the slow-growing and anaerobic nature of the bacteria conglomerates [1, 2]. Instead of the normal growth phase for bacteria, biofilms often grow slowly due to a lack of nutrients, specifically reduced glucose and oxygen [7]. Additionally, many of these bacteria often enter metabolic dormancy, surviving the antibiotics, and later repopulate the biofilm [7]. Furthermore, these biofilms also become resistant to topical antibiotic treatment after surviving bacteria repopulate the entire region [8].

Original research suggested surgical removal of the biofilm layer [9]. However, novel approaches to treat biofilm are being discovered, including weak organic acids such as vinegar, phage therapy (ΦT) (see Chap. 12), and photodynamic therapy (PDT) [3, 7]. One in vitro study examined the use of low concentrations of acetic and formic acids with pulsed electric fields (PEF) to treat *Staphylococcus aureus* and *Pseudomonas aeruginosa* [10]. They determined that these organic acids significantly increased the efficacy of the known treatment of PEF [10]. ΦT works by using bacterium-killing viruses to destroy the bacteria in the area when

S. A. Moore
Arlington Center for Dermatology, Arlington, TX, USA
Arlington Research Center, Arlington, TX, USA

A. Y. Moore (✉)
Division of Dermatology, Baylor University Medical Center, Dallas, TX, USA
Arlington Center for Dermatology, Arlington, TX, USA
Arlington Research Center, Arlington, TX, USA

© Springer Nature Switzerland AG 2021
S. K. Tyring et al. (eds.), *Overcoming Antimicrobial Resistance of the Skin*, Updates in Clinical Dermatology, https://doi.org/10.1007/978-3-030-68321-4_13

applied directly on the wound site. PDT works through directly damaging the infection by activating a dye to release toxic reactive oxygen against the targeted organism [11, 12]. Other treatments focus on interfering with the extracellular polymeric substances by enzymes [13].

While biofilm formation is seen to negatively affect cell growth and slow healing, microbiomes seem to positively benefit the skin [14]. This healthy, normal flora of bacteria and other microbes have been researched for their role in the natural recovery process [14]. However, the enormous variety of niches and great diversity of this microbiome proves burdensome to fully grasp [14]. Therefore, more research is necessary to examine the exact response and relationship between the skin's biofilm and microbiome [14].

Normal Microbiome of Glabrous Skin

Due to the difficulty in culturing bacteria in a laboratory, scientists have historically underestimated the relative abundance of the microbiome [15]. The skin microbiome has four major regions: sebaceous skin (glabella), moist skin (antecubital fossa), dry skin (volar forearm), and feet (toe web space) [15]. These four divisions represent the major microenvironments of the skin [15]. *Cutibacterium acnes* (formerly *Propionibacterium acnes*) dominated the sebaceous sites, and *Staphylococcus* and *Corynebacterium* species were found most commonly in moist areas [15] (Table 13.1). Additionally, *Cutibacterium acnes* and *Corynebacterium* spp. were found on dry skin along with *Staphylococcus epidermidis*, *Staphylococcus aureus*, *Micrococcaceae*, *Bacteroidetes*, and *Cyanobacteria* in lesser amounts in each section [15, 16]. Fungi of the genus *Malassezia* spp., *Aspergillus* spp., *Cryptococcus* spp., *Rhodotorula* spp., *Epicoccum* spp., and others were unique to the foot in addition to the other bacteria in a relatively lower abundance [15]. Due to the nature of antibiotics and the similarity in these positive microflora with their pathogenic cousins, antibiotics often kill the positive bacteria with the pathogenic ones [15, 16].

Normal Microbiome of Vaginal Mucosa

The *Lactobacillus genus*, including *L. crispatus*, *L. iners*, *L. gasseri*, and *L. jensenii*, is traditionally thought to be part of the microflora of healthy vagina [17]. They are thought to protect the

Table 13.1 Microbiome species sorted by relative abundance[a] and region

Dry	Moist	Sebaceous	Foot
Bacteria			
Cutibacterium acnes	Corynebacterium tuberculostearicum	Cutibacterium acnes	Corynebacterium tuberculostearicum
Corynebacterium tuberculostearicum	Staphylococcus hominis	Staphylococcus epidermidis	Staphylococcus hominis
Streptococcus mitis	Cutibacterium acnes	Corynebacterium tuberculostearicum	Staphylococcus warneri
Streptococcus oralis	Staphylococcus epidermidis	Staphylococcus capitis	Staphylococcus epidermidis
Streptococcus pseudopneumoniae	Staphylococcus capitis	Corynebacterium simulans	Staphylococcus capitis
Fungi			
Malassezia restricta	Malassezia globosa	Malassezia restricta	Malassezia restricta
Malassezia globosa	Malassezia restricta	Malassezia globosa	Trichophyton rubrum
Aspergillus tubingensis	Tilletia walkeri	Malassezia sympodialis	Malassezia globosa
Candida parapsilosis	Malassezia sympodialis	Aureoumbra lagunensis	Pyramimonas parkeae
Zymoseptoria tritici	Pyramimonas parkeae	Tilletia walkeri	Trichophyton mentagrophytes

[a]Listed from highest population density to lowest by region

vagina by producing lactic acid to lower the pH to 3.5–4.5 [17]. Interestingly, up to 40% of Black and Hispanic women have microbiota of the genera *Atopobium, Corynebacterium, Anaerococcus, Peptoniphilus, Prevotella, Gardnerella, Sneathia, Eggerthella, Mobiluncus,* and *Finegoldia* [17]. Even members from the *Atopobium, Streptococcus, Staphylococcus, Megasphaera,* and *Leptotrichia* genera seem capable of homolactic or heterolactic acid fermentations. Therefore, the exact concept of a "normal" microflora is still being investigated [17].

Normal Microbiome of the Gastrointestinal Tract

A normal gastrointestinal tract's microbiome as determined from biopsy samples shows increased *Lactobacillus* (*Firmicutes*), *Veillonella* (*Firmicutes*), and *Helicobacter* (*Proteobacteria*) in the proximal gut, whereas *Bacilli* (*Firmicutes*), *Streptococcaceae* (*Firmicutes*), *Actinomycinaeae,* and *Corynebacteriaceae* (both *Actinobacteria*) are abundant in the duodenum, the jejunum, and the ileum [18]. Increased proportions of *Lachnospiraceae* (*Firmicutes*) and *Bacteroidetes* are found in the colon [18]. Additionally, fungal communities consist primarily the phyla *Ascomycota, Basidiomycota,* and *Zygomycota* with *Penicillium, Candida,* and *Saccharomyces* as the most common genera [19].

Gut-Skin Axis Possibility and Impact of Antibiotics

Broad-spectrum antibiotics have long been touted as a miraculous invention of the twentieth century [20]. However, recent research has demonstrated that while these broad-spectrum antibiotics killed the negative pathogens, they also eliminated many of the healthy gram-negative flora naturally found in the gut microbiome [20, 21]. This may explain why broad-spectrum antibiotics like clindamycin have frequent gastrointestinal side effects [20]. These negative flora also stimulated the rate of antibi-

otic resistance, stress response, phage genes, and resistance genes [21]. Also, third-generation cephalosporins also eradicate *Pseudomonas* spp. and *Candida albicans* microflora [22]. Another hypothesis is that vulvovaginal candidiasis, from *Candida albicans*, results from the disruption of the microbiome [23]. More thorough, blinded clinical trials are necessary to verify these case study findings.

A high prevalence of *Actinobacteria/Cutibacterium* correlated with a high cheek sebum level, while increased forehead hydration correlated with low prevalence of *Actinobacteria/Cutibacterium* [24]. However, cheek hydration and forehead sebum did not impact the microbiome [24].

Acne

In acne vulgaris, *Cutibacterium acnes* can form a glue-like comedonal biofilm that prevents effective treatment [25]. Jahns et al. found that biofilms had formed in 47% of patient samples compared to only 21% of control samples, thereby linking biofilms with *C. acnes* [25, 26]. Even though Coenye et al. explored 119 plant extracts and identified 3 active compounds capable of destroying *C. acnes* biofilm, the primary breakthrough solution found to remove *C. acnes* biofilms and enhance efficacy of antibiotics in acne is *Myrtus communis* (Mediterranean myrtle extract) extract along with ursolic acid [27, 28]. Brackman et al. found that in vitro thiazolidinedione derivatives blocked biofilm-forming compounds but had no direct effect on the *C. acnes* bacterium unless combined with conventional formulations [29]. Others such as Sivasankar et al. achieved 80–91% inhibition in vivo by treating with ellagic acid in combination with tetracycline [30] (Table 13.2).

Jung et al. designed a study in 2013 to assess whether addition of probiotics affects efficacy and reduces the side effects of systemic antibiotics utilized to treat acne [31]. 45 Patients were divided into arms of only probiotic supplementation, only minocycline, and combination treatment with probiotics and minocycline [31]. Combination therapy significantly decreased total lesion counts in acne versus monotherapy with probiotics or minocycline [31]. Additionally, patients with the probiotic supplementation reported lower side effect rates than those with only minocycline [31]. Thus, employing probiotics to restore the microbiome may reduce the side effects; however, larger, blinded studies are needed to verify these findings [31].

The disruption of the skin's microbiome has been thought to play a role in the cause of acne, especially through the disruption of the healthy *C. acnes* found naturally on the skin [32]. Specifically, *C. acnes* has been divided into three types. Type I has been associated more with acne

vulgaris than type II [32], while type III has been found in 20% of isolates but not in acne lesions. It is plausible that some type II and type III *C. acnes* are associated with healthy skin, while type I and some of type II are associated with acne vulgaris [32].

In 2019, narrow-spectrum oral sarecycline was FDA approved for acne. Its narrow spectrum targets *C. acnes* but not gram-negative flora nor candidiasis. Maintenance of the natural microbiome of the skin, gastrointestinal tract, and vagina may account for the low incidence of adverse events with this narrow spectrum antibiotic [32, 33].

Table 13.2 Studies on biofilm treatments

Condition	Bacteria	Mechanism of action	Phase of project	Reference
Acne vulgaris	*Cutibacterium acnes*	Ellagic acid with tetracycline	In vivo	[30]
Atopic dermatitis	*Staphylococcus aureus*	0.02% farnesol and 5% xylitol	Double-blind, controlled case study	[37]
Impetigo	*Staphylococcus aureus*	Acetic acid	In vitro	[40]
Impetigo	*Staphylococcus aureus*	Phage therapy with kayvirus S25-3	Case study	[41]
Candidiasis	*Candida albicans*	Echinocandins and liposomal amphotericin B	In vitro	[39, 48]
Onychomycosis	*Trichophyton rubrum, Trichophyton mentagrophytes, and Microsporum gypseum*	Enzymatic debridement	In vitro	[50]
Onychomycosis	*Trichophyton rubrum, Trichophyton mentagrophytes, and Microsporum gypseum*	Deoxyribonuclease I, α-amylase, lyase, lactic acid, chitosan, terpinen-4-ol-loaded lipid nanoparticles, and povidone-iodine	In vitro	[50]
Onychomycosis	*Trichophyton rubrum, Trichophyton mentagrophytes, and Microsporum gypseum*	Combination therapy of above list and standard antibiotics	In vitro	[50]
Onychomycosis	*Trichophyton rubrum, Trichophyton mentagrophytes, and Microsporum gypseum*	Photodynamic therapy to activate methylene blue	In vitro	[51, 52]
Wounds	Various	Debridement	Used historically	[6]
Wounds	*Pseudomonas aeruginosa* or *Staphylococcus aureus*	Larval debridement therapy	In vitro	[54]
Wounds	*P. aeruginosa*	Lactoferrin	In vitro	[55]
Wounds	Various	Xylitol, dispersin B, and honey	Various	[55, 56]
Wounds	*Staphylococcal* bacteria	*Hamamelis virginiana*	In vivo	[13]
Wounds	*P. aeruginosa*	Gallium	In vitro	[55]
Wounds	*Methicillin-resistant staphylococcal aureus*	5% tea tree oil	In vitro	[3, 7]

Table 13.2 (continued)

Condition	Bacteria	Mechanism of action	Phase of project	Reference
Wounds	Various	Polyhexanide-containing biocellulose dressing Suprasorb X + PHMB	Case study	[57]
Wounds	*P. aeruginosa*	Pressure wound in combination with silver foam for 2 weeks	In vivo	[58]
Venous leg ulcers	Various	Determined simple mechanical desloughing as most effective vs. autolytic debridement, larvae (maggot) therapy, hydro-surgical debridement, mechanical debridement, sharp debridement, and surgical debridement, ultrasonic debridement	Analysis of numerous case studies	[60]
Venous leg ulcers	Various	Next-generation antimicrobial dressing (NGAD; AQUACEL Ag + EXTRA dressing)	Case study	[61]
Diabetic foot ulcers	*Corynebacterium* spp., *Streptococcus, Serratia, Staphylococcus* and *Enterococcus* spp.	Phage therapy, probiotics, and antimicrobial peptides	In vitro and in vivo	[62–64]
Diabetic foot ulcers	Various	Octenidine-based solution and octenilin wound gel	Case study	[65]
Fillers	Various	Intense protocol, including mupirocin locally and prophylactic antimicrobial oral therapy	Retrospective/anecdotal data	[68]
Fillers	Various	Hyaluronidase	Retrospective/anecdotal data	[66]
Fillers	Various	5-fluorouracil with low doses of triamcinolone	Retrospective/anecdotal data	[66]
Fillers	Various	Clarithromycin 500 mg plus moxifloxacin 400 mg twice daily for 10 days, or ciprofloxacin 500–750 mg twice daily for 2–4 weeks, or minocycline 100 mg once daily for 6 months	Retrospective/anecdotal data	[66]
Fillers	Various	Prophylactic treatment with broad-spectrum antibiotics	Retrospective/anecdotal data	[67]

Atopic Dermatitis

Why biofilms are often formed on patients with *S. aureus*-associated atopic dermatitis (AD) is not completely understood, but one hypothesis is the occlusion of sweat ducts by the buildup of *S. aureus* biofilm [34, 35]. In one study, strong correlation was observed between biofilm production and AD extent since 43.0% were classified as high biofilm producers, 41.0% as moderate producers, and 16.0% as weak producers [34]. Of those with severe AD, 60.0% of patients were colonized by high biofilm producers, 35.0% by moderate biofilm producers, and only 5.0% by weak biofilm producers [34]. This relationship

suggests a strong correlation between the extent and severity of AD and biofilm presence [34].

More research is needed to explore the effect of the *S. aureus* biofilm on AD itself, but Katsuyama et al. concluded that xylitol helped in vitro to destroy the biofilm's fibrin fiber and glycocalyx without negatively impacting *Staphylococcus epidermidis*, the healthy microflora naturally found on human skin protecting the skin from pathogenic bacteria [36]. Katsuyama et al. later performed a randomized double-blind placebo-controlled right and left in vivo comparison study where they examined 17 patients with AD treated with 0.02% farnesol and 5% xylitol applied simultaneously for 1 week to remove the biofilm [37]. This study found that, after 1 week, the cream significantly decreased the ratio of *S. aureus* compared to the placebo sites and confirms the hypothesis that removing the *S. aureus* biofilm alone in patients with AD may lead to improvement [37].

Since *Staphylococcus aureus* is often associated with atopic dermatitis (AD) and antibiotics often serve as effective treatments of AD, it is likely the microbiome plays a vital role in its pathogenesis [38]. Additionally, Foolad et al. found that prebiotic supplementation and black currant seed oil effectively reduced AD development [38].

Impetigo

Some research indicates that the colonization and adherence of biofilms to damaged skin may result from *S. aureus* glycocalyx [39]. Besides antibiotics, one of the first approaches to treating *S. aureus* biofilms in impetigo was acetic acid application on immature biofilms [40]. A recent novel treatment of impetigo by Imanishi et al. consists of using ΦT to treat impetigo on a dozen patients successfully with the endolysin derived from the kayvirus S25-3 [41].

Hidradenitis Suppurativa

Chronic nonhealing abscesses or draining sinuses of hidradenitis suppurativa (HS) often involve biofilms, possibly along the luminal surfaces of sinuses, with resulting anatomical changes and new places for biofilm growth [42, 43]. In the study by Ring et al., 75% of perilesional samples from patients had biofilms as well as 67% of chronic lesion samples. Research is needed to identify specific options against HS biofilms besides antibiotics [3, 44].

Miliaria

It has been conjectured that biofilms may contribute to the blocking of the eccrine glands in miliaria [35, 45]. Mowad et al. identified an accumulation of periodic acid-Schiff, possibly from a biofilm, that blocked the sweat ducts in miliaria [46]. Further research is needed to identify specific treatments for biofilms in miliaria [35, 45].

Candidiasis

Since *Candida albicans* is primarily found on mucocutaneous surfaces in occlusive regions, biofilms form fairly often [47]. These biofilms have significantly increased resistance to many common drugs, even up to 2000-fold [47]. However, Kuhn et al. recently discovered that echinocandins and liposomal amphotericin B are effective in vitro and are exploring other experimental therapies [39, 48].

Onychomycosis

Since onychomycosis is caused by a fungus, the presence of a biofilm can pose a significant threat to treatment when antifungal medications cannot penetrate the extracellular matrix of the biofilm [49]. Some research also suggests that biofilms may be the etiology of recalcitrance to traditional antifungal treatment [50].

Enzymatic debridement and other successful treatments of biofilms have included deoxyribonuclease I, α-amylase, lyase, lactic acid, chitosan, terpinen-4-ol-loaded lipid nanoparticles, and povidone-iodine, all with efficacies well over 90% [50]. Most promising success is seen in combination treatments, however, with almost 95% success in combination with standard antibiotics [50]. After disrupting the biofilm, PDT demonstrated a reduction greater than $6–7 \log_{10}$ [50]. One novel approach for removing the biofilm examines the use of antimicrobial PDT [50, 51]. An LED light was used to activate methylene blue as a photosensitizing agent against *Trichophyton rubrum*, *Trichophyton mentagrophytes*, and *Microsporum gypseum* to reduce the biofilm formation significantly [51, 52].

In another study exploring bacterial urinary tract infections, low-frequency surface acoustic waves reduced bacterial biofilms of *Escherichia coli, S. epidermidis*, and *P. aeruginosa* by over 85% when used in conjunction with standard antibiotics [9, 53].

Wounds

Chronic wounds are notorious for being very difficult to treat, likely due to biofilm formation [6]. In fact, disruption of the microbiome in wounds is synonymous with formation of a biofilm. (See earlier in this chapter for more details about the role of the biofilm.) In contrast, only 6% of acute wounds form biofilms [6]. Due to the wide variety of biofilms and the disparity in wounds, research is being done to identify unique characteristics of biofilms in wounds in order to design targeted treatment for particular biofilms [6]. Attinger and Wolcott used polymerase chain reaction to identify the bacteria and fungi in certain biofilms in order to increase the efficacy of debridement [6]. Originally, debridement of wounds was widely employed so that healing could occur as an acute wound instead of a chronic wound [6]. For example, Cowan et al. explored using larval debridement therapy to debride the wound naturally by only removing dead tissue, and not affecting healthy skin [54]. Additionally, such topicals as lactoferrin, xylitol, dispersin B, and even honey have been identified as interfering with bacterial growth within a biofilm [55, 56]. *Hamamelis virginiana* (witch hazel) has been observed to prevent staphylococcal bacteria from gluing together to form a strong biofilm [13].

Other novel methods have been investigated to attack biofilm formation. Kamiya et al. found that gallium disrupts in vitro biofilm formation of *P. aeruginosa* by inhibiting the ability of the pathogen to metabolize iron [55]. Exposure to 5% tea tree oil for 1 hour completely destroyed a biofilm formed by methicillin-resistant SA [3]. The polyhexanide-containing biocellulose dressing Suprasorb X + PHMB demonstrated complete epithelialization without drainage in 75% of patients by week 24 [57]. Of those without closed wounds, a 61% mean wound area had been observed by week 24 [57]. Ngo et al. reported a significant decrease in the number of *P. aerugi-*

nosa biofilm bacteria after using negative pressure wound therapy in combination with silver foam for 2 weeks [58].

Venous Leg Ulcers

Venous leg ulcers (VLU) were first intensively researched by Wolcott et al. [59]. They explored the bacteria diversity within individual VLU through bacterial tag-encoded FLX and titanium amplicon pyrosequencing [59]. After exploring various methods of desloughing, including autolytic debridement, larvae (maggot) therapy, hydro-surgical debridement, mechanical debridement, sharp debridement, and surgical debridement, ultrasonic debridement, and mechanical desloughing, Percival and Suleman concluded that simple mechanical desloughing is most effective [60]. A new, next-generation antimicrobial dressing (NGAD; AQUACEL Ag + EXTRA dressing) was tested in the UK and Ireland where they found that 90% of wounds became smaller and 34% of wounds completely healed, with a median improvement time of 4.5 weeks [61].

Diabetic Foot Ulcers

One school of thought is that mechanical debridement is crucial for treatment of diabetic foot ulcers, even with a confirmed presence of biofilm [62]. Since the most common bacterium associated with diabetic foot ulcers is *Corynebacterium* spp. in addition to obligate anaerobes, including *Bacteroides*, *Peptoniphilus*, *Fingoldia*, *Anaerococcus*, and *Peptostreptococcus* spp., as well as other more common bacteria such as *Streptococcus*, *Serratia*, *Staphylococcus*, and *Enterococcus* spp., specific therapies targeting the biofilms of these organisms have been explored as alternative options specific for diabetic foot ulcers [62–64]. These specialized treatment options include phage therapy, probiotics, and antimicrobial peptides [63]. In contrast to relying on viruses to destroy the biofilm as in bacteriophages, bacteriotherapy relies on bacteria to attack and decimate other bacterial populations [63].

In a case study in Great Britain, after 4 weeks of treatment with povidone-iodine without response, an octenidine-based solution and octenilin wound gel, which contains the surfactant ethylhexylglycerin to loosen the biofilm's devitalized tissue, was applied. After 1 week, the crust was removable [65]. By week 3, clear progress in epithelialization was noticed, and, by week 7, the wound was nearly closed [65].

Fillers

Recent data has even linked filler reactions to biofilm formation [66]. However, the exact role of biofilms in inflammation is still debated [66]. As Alhede and Bjarnsholt have suggested, many of the adverse events of tissue fillers are not immediate but often delayed years after the injection, similar to the delayed symptoms witnessed in biofilm infections [67].

Sadashivaiah and Mysore sought to prevent the possible formation of biofilm completely through a protocol that included thoroughly cleaning the site with an antiseptic, locally applying mupirocin, informing the patient to report any tenderness, and prophylactic antimicrobial oral therapy [68]. However, the exact role of the broad-spectrum antibiotic in preventing biofilm has been questioned [68].

While all injection filler reactions were previously deemed allergic in nature, Dumitrascu and Georgescu now recommend that patients avoid systemic steroids, antihistamines, and nonsteroidal anti-inflammatory drugs for biofilm-like reactions, since these medications fail and simply complicate the local situation [69].

Galvez et al. did find that hyaluronidase could be employed but cautioned against the spread of infection into adjacent tissues if cellulitis occurs [66]. Additionally, but for unknown reasons, mixing 5-fluorouracil with low doses of triamcinolone injected at regular intervals also seemed to treat the biofilm [66].

More conventional antibiotic treatments have been utilized, but combination or long-term therapy appears more successful [66]. One report

recommended clarithromycin 500 mg plus moxifloxacin 400 mg twice daily for 10 days, or ciprofloxacin 500–750 mg twice daily for 2–4 weeks, or minocycline 100 mg once daily for 6 months [66]. Alhede et al. believes that only prophylactic treatment with broad-spectrum antibiotics substantially treat biofilm-related adverse events postinjection [67]. More complete and thorough prospective studies are needed to better explain the connection between biofilms and injection site reactions [69].

Pemphigus Foliaceus

Akiyama et al. detected *Staphylococcus* biofilms in pemphigus foliaceus, but it has not since been studied further [39, 70].

Conclusion

While the role of biofilms in the pathogenesis of most diseases is unclear, their presence in many dermatological conditions is unquestioned [3]. Besides debridement, specific regimens and combination therapy seem promising [3]. Further studies are needed to examine specific bacterial biofilms [3]. Researchers have now noticed a direct relationship between the microbiome and various skin disorders, but more research is necessary to confirm these findings.

References

1. Percival SL, Hill KE, Williams DW, Hooper SJ, Thomas DW, Costerton JW. A review of the scientific evidence for biofilms in wounds. Wound Repair Regen. 2012;20(5):647–57.
2. Chan L. Bacterial biofilm. 2015. https://doi.org/10.1111/j.1524-475X.2012.00836.x.
3. Kravvas G, Veitch D, Al-Niaimi F. The increasing relevance of biofilms in common dermatological conditions. J Dermatolog Treat. 2018;29(2):202–7.
4. Nusbaum AG, Kirsner RS, Charles CA. Biofilms in dermatology. Skin Therapy Lett. 2012;17(7):1–5.
5. Donlan RM. Biofilm formation: a clinically relevant microbiological process. Clin Infect Dis. 2001;33(8):1387–92.

6. Attinger C, Wolcott R. Clinically addressing biofilm in chronic wounds. Adv Wound Care (New Rochelle). 2012;1(3):127–32.

7. Hughes G, Webber MA. Novel approaches to the treatment of bacterial biofilm infections. Br J Pharmacol. 2017;174(14):2237–46.

8. Bowler PG. Antibiotic resistance and biofilm tolerance: a combined threat in the treatment of chronic infections. J Wound Care. 2018;27(5):273–7.

9. Costerton JW, Lewandowski Z, Caldwell DE, Korber DR, Lappin-Scott HM. Microbial biofilms. Annu Rev Microbiol. 1995;49:711–45.

10. Novickij V, Lastauskienė E, Staigvila G, Girkontaitė I, Zinkevičienė A, Švedienė J, et al. Low concentrations of acetic and formic acids enhance the inactivation of Staphylococcus aureus and Pseudomonas aeruginosa with pulsed electric fields. BMC Microbiol. 2019;19(1):73.

11. de Melo WCMA, Avci P, de Oliveira MN, Gupta A, Vecchio D, Sadasivam M, et al. Photodynamic inactivation of biofilm: taking a lightly colored approach to stubborn infection. Expert Rev Anti-Infect Ther. 2013;11(7):669–93.

12. Fila G, Krychowiak M, Rychlowski M, Bielawski KP, Grinholc M. Antimicrobial blue light photoinactivation of Pseudomonas aeruginosa: quorum sensing signaling molecules, biofilm formation and pathogenicity. J Biophotonics. 2018;11(11):e201800079.

13. Kiran MD, Adikesavan NV, Cirioni O, Giacometti A, Silvestri C, Scalise G, et al. Discovery of a quorum-sensing inhibitor of drug-resistant staphylococcal infections by structure-based virtual screening. Mol Pharmacol. 2008;73(5):1578–86.

14. Brandwein M, Steinberg D, Meshner S. Microbial biofilms and the human skin microbiome. NPJ Biofilms Microbiomes. 2016;2:3.

15. Byrd AL, Belkaid Y, Segre JA. The human skin microbiome. Nat Rev Microbiol. 2018;16(3):143–55.

16. Grice EA, Segre JA. The skin microbiome. Nat Rev Microbiol. 2011;9(4):244–53.

17. Ma B, Forney LJ, Ravel J. Vaginal microbiome: rethinking health and disease. Annu Rev Microbiol. 2012;66:371–89.

18. Dieterich W, Schink M, Zopf Y. Microbiota in the gastrointestinal tract. Med Sci (Basel). 2018;6(4):116.

19. Sam QH, Chang MW, Chai LY. The fungal mycobiome and its interaction with gut bacteria in the host. Int J Mol Sci. 2017;18(2):330.

20. Salem I, Ramser A, Isham N, Ghannoum MA. The gut microbiome as a major regulator of the gut-skin axis. Front Microbiol. 2018;9:1459.

21. Langdon A, Crook N, Dantas G. The effects of antibiotics on the microbiome throughout development and alternative approaches for therapeutic modulation. Genome Med. 2016;8(1):39.

22. Zhang S, Chen DC. Facing a new challenge: the adverse effects of antibiotics on gut microbiota and host immunity. Chin Med J. 2019;132(10):1135–8.

23. Pericolini E, Gabrielli E, Ballet N, Sabbatini S, Roselletti E, Cayzeele Decherf A, et al. Therapeutic activity of a Saccharomyces cerevisiae-based probiotic and inactivated whole yeast on vaginal candidiasis. Virulence. 2017;8(1):74–90.

24. Mukherjee S, Mitra R, Maitra A, Gupta S, Kumaran S, Chakrabortty A, et al. Sebum and hydration levels in specific regions of human face significantly predict the nature and diversity of facial skin microbiome. Sci Rep. 2016;6(1):36062.

25. Gowda A, Burkhart C. Virulent acne biofilms offer insight into novel therapeutic options. Open Dermatol J. 2018;12:80–5.

26. Jahns AC, Lundskog B, Ganceviciene R, Palmer RH, Golovleva I, Zouboulis CC, et al. An increased incidence of Propionibacterium acnes biofilms in acne vulgaris: a case-control study. Br J Dermatol. 2012;167(1):50–8.

27. Feuillolay C, Pecastaings S, Le Gac C, Fiorini-Puybaret C, Luc J, Joulia P, et al. A Myrtus communis extract enriched in myrtucummulones and ursolic acid reduces resistance of Propionibacterium acnes biofilms to antibiotics used in acne vulgaris. Phytomedicine. 2016;23(3):307–15.

28. Coenye T, Brackman G, Rigole P, De Witte E, Honraet K, Rossel B, et al. Eradication of Propionibacterium acnes biofilms by plant extracts and putative identification of icariin, resveratrol and salidroside as active compounds. Phytomedicine. 2012;19(5):409–12.

29. Brackman G, Forier K, Al Quntar AA, De Canck E, Enk CD, Srebnik M, et al. Thiazolidinedione derivatives as novel agents against Propionibacterium acnes biofilms. J Appl Microbiol. 2014;116(3):492–501.

30. Sivasankar C, Maruthupandiyan S, Balamurugan K, James PB, Krishnan V, Pandian SK. A combination of ellagic acid and tetracycline inhibits biofilm formation and the associated virulence of Propionibacterium acnes in vitro and in vivo. Biofouling. 2016;32(4):397–410.

31. Jung GW, Tse JE, Guiha I, Rao J. Prospective, randomized, open-label trial comparing the safety, efficacy, and tolerability of an acne treatment regimen with and without a probiotic supplement and minocycline in subjects with mild to moderate acne. J Cutan Med Surg. 2013;17(2):114–22.

32. Yu Y. The role of the microbiome in acne. Dermatol. 2020;28(3):2.

33. Zeichner J. Efficacy and safety of newly approved oral sarecycline for acne practical dermatology. 2019. Available from: https://practicaldermatology. com/articles/2019-apr/efficacy-and-safety-of-newly-approved-oral-sarecycline-for-acne.

34. Di Domenico EG, Cavallo I, Bordignon V, Prignano G, Sperduti I, Gurtner A, et al. Inflammatory cytokines and biofilm production sustain Staphylococcus aureus outgrowth and persistence: a pivotal interplay in the pathogenesis of Atopic Dermatitis. Sci Rep. 2018;8(1):9573.

35. Allen HB, Vaze ND, Choi C, Hailu T, Tulbert BH, Cusack CA, et al. The presence and impact of biofilm-producing staphylococci in atopic dermatitis. JAMA Dermatol. 2014;150(3):260–5.

36. Katsuyama M, Ichikawa H, Ogawa S, Ikezawa Z. A novel method to control the balance of skin microflora. Part 1. Attack on biofilm of Staphylococcus aureus without antibiotics. J Dermatol Sci. 2005;38(3):197–205.

37. Katsuyama M, Masako K, Kobayashi Y, Yusuke K, Ichikawa H, Hideyuki I, et al. A novel method to control the balance of skin microflora Part 2. A study to assess the effect of a cream containing farnesol and xylitol on atopic dry skin. J Dermatol Sci. 2005;38(3):207–13.

38. Grice EA. The skin microbiome: potential for novel diagnostic and therapeutic approaches to cutaneous disease. Semin Cutan Med Surg. 2014;33(2):98–103.

39. Akiyama H, Huh WK, Yamasaki O, Oono T, Iwatsuki K. Confocal laser scanning microscopic observation of glycocalyx production by Staphylococcus aureus in mouse skin: does S. aureus generally produce a biofilm on damaged skin? Br J Dermatol. 2002;147(5):879–85.

40. Akiyama H, Yamasaki O, Tada J, Arata J. Effects of acetic acid on biofilms formed by Staphylococcus aureus. Arch Dermatol Res. 1999;291(10):570–3.

41. Imanishi I, Uchiyama J, Tsukui T, Hisatsune J, Ide K, Matsuzaki S, et al. Therapeutic potential of an endolysin derived from kayvirus S25-3 for staphylococcal impetigo. Viruses. 2019;11(9):769.

42. Ring HC, Bay L, Nilsson M, Kallenbach K, Miller IM, Saunte DM, et al. Bacterial biofilm in chronic lesions of hidradenitis suppurativa. Br J Dermatol. 2017;176(4):993–1000.

43. Kathju S, Lasko LA, Stoodley P. Considering hidradenitis suppurativa as a bacterial biofilm disease. FEMS Immunol Med Microbiol. 2012;65(2):385–9.

44. Hessam S, Sand M, Georgas D, Anders A, Bechara FG. Microbial profile and antimicrobial susceptibility of bacteria found in inflammatory hidradenitis suppurativa lesions. Skin Pharmacol Physiol. 2016;29(3):161–7.

45. Haque MS, Hailu T, Pritchett E, Cusack CA, Allen HB. The oldest new finding in atopic dermatitis: subclinical miliaria as an origin. JAMA Dermatol. 2013;149(4):436–8.

46. Mowad CM, McGinley KJ, Foglia A, Leyden JJ. The role of extracellular polysaccharide substance produced by Staphylococcus epidermidis in miliaria. J Am Acad Dermatol. 1995;33(5 Pt 1):729–33.

47. Vaishnavi KV, Safar L, Devi K. Biofilm in dermatology. J Skin Sex Transm Dis. 2019;1:3–7.

48. Kuhn DM, George T, Chandra J, Mukherjee PK, Ghannoum MA. Antifungal susceptibility of Candida biofilms: unique efficacy of amphotericin B lipid formulations and echinocandins. Antimicrob Agents Chemother. 2002;46(6):1773–80.

49. Gupta AK, Foley KA. Evidence for biofilms in onychomycosis. G Ital Dermatol Venereol. 2019;154(1):50–5.

50. Gupta AK, Carviel J, Shear NH. Antibiofilm treatment for onychomycosis and chronic fungal infections. Skin Appendage Disord. 2018;4(3):136–40.

51. Chen B, Sun Y, Zhang J, Chen R, Zhong X, Wu X, et al. Evaluation of photodynamic effects against biofilms of dermatophytes involved in onychomycosis. Front Microbiol. 2019;10:1228.

52. Biel MA, Sievert C, Usacheva M, Teichert M, Wedell E, Loebel N, et al. Reduction of endotracheal tube biofilms using antimicrobial photodynamic therapy. Lasers Surg Med. 2011;43(7):586–90.

53. Kopel M, Degtyar E, Banin E. Surface acoustic waves increase the susceptibility of Pseudomonas aeruginosa biofilms to antibiotic treatment. Biofouling. 2011;27(7):701–10.

54. Cowan LJ, Stechmiller JK, Phillips P, Yang Q, Schultz G. Chronic ulcers: updating epidemiology, physiopathology, and therapies. Chronic wounds, biofilms and use of medicinal larvae. Ulcers. 2013;2013:7.

55. Kamiya H, Ehara T, Matsumoto T. Inhibitory effects of lactoferrin on biofilm formation in clinical isolates of Pseudomonas aeruginosa. J Infect Chemother. 2012;18(1):47–52.

56. McGuire J, D'Alessandro J. Combating biofilms in the chronic wound. Podiatry Today. 2016;29(8):32–40.

57. Lenselink E, Andriessen A. A cohort study on the efficacy of a polyhexanide-containing biocellulose dressing in the treatment of biofilms in wounds. J Wound Care. 2011;20(11):534, 6–9.

58. Wei D, Zhu XM, Chen YY, Li XY, Chen YP, Liu HY, et al. Chronic wound biofilms: diagnosis and therapeutic strategies. Chin Med J. 2019;132(22):2737–44.

59. Wolcott RD, Gontcharova V, Sun Y, Dowd SE. Evaluation of the bacterial diversity among and within individual venous leg ulcers using bacterial tag-encoded FLX and titanium amplicon pyrosequencing and metagenomic approaches. BMC Microbiol. 2009;9:226.

60. Percival SL, Suleman L. Slough and biofilm: removal of barriers to wound healing by desloughing. J Wound Care. 2015;24(11):498, 500–3, 6–10.

61. Metcalf D, Parsons D, Bowler P. A next-generation antimicrobial wound dressing: a real-life clinical evaluation in the UK and Ireland. J Wound Care. 2016;25(3):132, 4–8

62. Lavery LA, Bhavan K, Wukich DK. Biofilm and diabetic foot ulcer healing: all hat and no cattle. Ann Transl Med. 2019;7(7):159.

63. Santos R, Veiga A, Tavares L, Castanho M, Oliveira M. Bacterial biofilms in diabetic foot ulcers: potential alternative therapeutics. In: Microbial biofilms – importance and applications. Croatia: InTech; 2016.

64. Dowd SE, Wolcott RD, Sun Y, McKeehan T, Smith E, Rhoads D. Polymicrobial nature of chronic diabetic foot ulcer biofilm infections determined using bacterial tag encoded FLX amplicon pyrosequencing (bTE-FAP). PLoS One. 2008;3(10):e3326.

65. Bowen G, Richardson N. Biofilm management in chronic wounds and diabetic foot ulcers. Diabet Foot J. 2016;19:198–204.

66. Urdiales-Gálvez F, Delgado NE, Figueiredo V, Lajo-Plaza JV, Mira M, Moreno A, et al. Treatment of soft tissue filler complications: expert consensus recommendations. Aesthet Plast Surg. 2018;42(2):498–510.

67. Alhede M, Er Ö, Eickhardt S, Kragh K, Alhede M, Christensen LD, et al. Bacterial biofilm formation and treatment in soft tissue fillers. Pathog Dis. 2014;70(3):339–46.

68. Sadashivaiah AB, Mysore V. Biofilms: their role in dermal fillers. J Cutan Aesthet Surg. 2010;3(1):20–2.

69. Dumitraşcu DI, Georgescu AV. The management of biofilm formation after hyaluronic acid gel filler injections: a review. Clujul Med (1957). 2013;86(3):192–5.

70. Nadelmann E, Czernik A. Wound care in immunobullous disease. In: Autoimmune bullous diseases. London: IntechOpen; 2018.

New Classes of Broad-Spectrum Antibiotics and New Mechanisms of Delivery

14

Stephen Andrew Moore, Stephen K. Tyring, and Angela Yen Moore

Abbreviations

aaRS	Aminoacyl-tRNA synthetase
AMP	Antimicrobial peptides
BLI	Non-β-lactam β-lactamase inhibitors
CSA	Cationic steroid antibiotics
FabI	Enoyl-ACP reductase
MRSA	Methicillin-resistant *Staphylococcus aureus*
MSSA	Methicillin-sensitive *S. aureus*
PDF	Peptide deformylase
ROS	Reactive oxygen species

Introduction

In the twentieth century, antibiotics revolutionized medicine [1]. Shortly after Fleming's discovery of penicillin in 1939, beta-lactams, glycopeptides, aminoglycosides, macrolides, tetracyclines, trimethoprim, metronidazole, quinolones, carbapenems, oxazolidinones, macrolides, and several others were discovered or synthesized [1]. However, after these discoveries, approximately 40 years passed before a new antibiotic class – linezolid – was discovered [1]. With the rising number of antibiotic-resistant bacteria in the twenty-first century, new classes of bacteria are now desperately needed [1]. This review articles chronicles the discovery of new classes of antibiotics.

Peptidomimetics

In 2019, Nicolas et al. used the natural *Staphylococcus aureus* peptide toxin PepA1 to manufacture a new family of peptidomimetics or cyclic heptapseudopeptides [2]. Of the four synthesized biomimetics, three of them, containing the aza-β3-amino acid analogs that enhance antimicrobial activity, had higher bactericidal activities than vancomycin [2]. These compounds did not form resistance for 2 weeks after serial passages and 4 or 6 days after mice exposure [2]. Pep 16 and Pep 19, which effectively treat both methicillin-resistant *S. aureus and Pseudomonas aeruginosa,* are the top two candidates [2]. Further research and clinical trials are still needed to confirm these findings [2] (see Fig. 14.1).

S. A. Moore
Arlington Center for Dermatology, Arlington, TX, USA

Arlington Research Center, Arlington, TX, USA

S. K. Tyring (✉)
Department of Dermatology, University of Texas Health Science Center, Houston, TX, USA

Center for Clinical Studies, Houston, TX, USA
e-mail: styring@ccstexas.com

A. Y. Moore (✉)
Division of Dermatology, Baylor University Medical Center, Dallas, TX, USA

Arlington Center for Dermatology, Arlington, TX, USA

Arlington Research Center, Arlington, TX, USA

© Springer Nature Switzerland AG 2021
S. K. Tyring et al. (eds.), *Overcoming Antimicrobial Resistance of the Skin*, Updates in Clinical Dermatology, https://doi.org/10.1007/978-3-030-68321-4_14

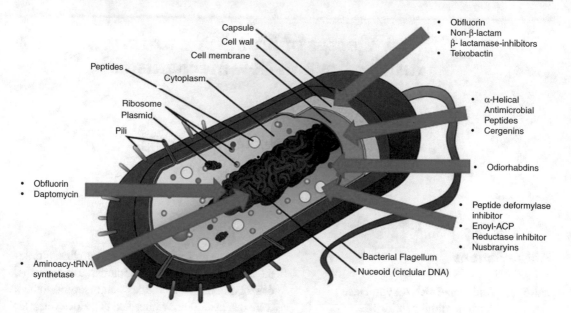

Fig. 14.1 Mechanism of action for novel broad-spectrum antibiotics

α-Helical Antimicrobial Peptides

In 2015, Xiong et al. explored the design of a class of cationic, helical homo-polypeptide antimicrobials [3]. Since most antimicrobial peptides (AMP) are hydrophobic, their team shielded the core with a charged exterior shell to protect the backbone from proteolytic degradation [3]. Like typical AMPs, this process works by disrupting the cell membrane of the bacteria, whether gram-positive or gram-negative [3]. Yang et al. designed the Sushi-replacement peptide (SRP)-2 AMP to demonstrate both gram-negative and gram-positive bactericidal activity as well as against methicillin-resistant *S. aureus* and multidrug-resistant *Acinetobacter baumannii* [4]. However, the greatest potential usage of this class of antibiotic seems to be in combination therapy with traditional, broad-spectrum antibiotics to pierce through the outer bacterial cell membrane [3].

Obafluorin/Daptomycin

In 2019, Kreitler et al. explored the use of nonribosomal peptide synthetases, which rely on neighboring catalytic domains to modify and form new bonds [5]. Specifically, they found that the unique structure of nonribosomal peptide synthetase ObiF, or obafluorin, could generate several obafluorin analogues [5]. However, earlier in 2003, the natural soil lipopeptide daptomycin was approved by the FDA. Despite these significant findings, analogues still need to be created and clinical trials performed to confirm these findings [5].

Pleuromutilin

Since pleuromutilin was discussed in great detail in Chap. 1, it will only be briefly mentioned in this chapter.

Researches and practitioners have debated whether or not to classify pleuromutilin as a novel class of antibiotics [6]. While it was discovered in 1950, no pleuromutilins were approved for human use until 2007 [6]. For dermatologists, the addition of retapamulin, was significant for use in gram-positive and fastidious gram-negative infections, including methicillin-resistant *S. aureus* (MRSA), vancomycin-resistant *S. aureus*, streptococcal species (e.g., penicillin-resistant *Streptococcus pneumoniae*, multidrug-resistant *S.*

pneumoniae), and *Enterococcus faecium* (particularly vancomycin-resistant strains), as well as activity against gram-negative bacteria like *Haemophilus* spp., *Moraxella catarrhalis*, *Neisseria* spp., and *Legionella pneumophila* [6, 7]. However, for many physicians, its use was limited since it was only available topically [6]. In 2010, new pleuromutilins entered clinical trials, and lefamulin (Xenleta™) was approved by the FDA in August 2019 [8, 9].

Peptide Deformylase Inhibitor

In 2005, Jain et al. reviewed many different peptide deformylase (PDF) inhibitors that had been investigated in the last several years [10]. Since PDF is required for bacterial growth but unnecessary for mammalian cells, this antibiotic inhibits this metalloenzyme [10]. While several companies began studies, none have progressed beyond phase I [10, 11].

In 2014, the PDF inhibitor GSK1322322 completed a head-to-head trial against linezolid in bacterial infections caused by MRSA [12]. This study found that treatment with either drug resulted in comparable reductions in the mean lesion area [12]. Additionally, GSK1322322 had a higher incidence of adverse events, e.g., nausea, vomiting, and diarrhea, while those with linezolid had a higher incidence in flatulence, skin infection, pyrexia, and increased blood creatine phosphokinase level [12]. While GSK1322322 demonstrates substantial success over the original PDF inhibitors and linezolid, phase III and IV trials are still pending [12].

Enoyl-ACP Reductase Inhibitor

The enoyl-ACP reductase (FabI) enzyme is well-known and researched as an anti-staphylococcal drug [13]. However, as noted by Yao and Rock, since the FabI enzyme is a single-target inhibitor,

resistance to the drug occurs frequently [14]. They propose that a multi-action antibiotic would decrease resistance since it is more difficult for bacteria to mutate several times in quick succession [13, 14].

In 2016, Hafkin et al. examined the results of a 2012 phase II clinical trial with AFN-1252, which selectively inhibited *S. aureus* [15]. They reported that eradication was 91% for MRSA and 92% for methicillin-sensitive *S. aureus* (MSSA) by day 3 with most drug-related adverse events being mild or moderate, consisting of headache (26%) or nausea (21%) [15]. In 2013, Zheng et al. proposed meleagrin as a possible candidate since it was found to have at least one additional mode of action when compared to triclosan [16]. In 2016, Mistry et al. explored the possibility of benzimidazole-based FabI inhibitors based on their structure [13]. More research and blinded clinical trials are needed to find the optimal analogs [13].

Aminoacyl-tRNA Synthetase Inhibitor

In 2004, Pohlmann and Brötz-Oesterhelt found that aminoacyl-tRNA synthetase (aaRS) could be a new class of antibiotics by leading to protein synthesis inhibition and cell growth arrest [17]. Since this time, more research has been done with varying results and differing conclusions, including research on the many derivations of aaRSs inhibitors [17–20]. In Francklyn and Mullen's 2019 overall assessment of these novel treatments, they found that single aminoacyl-tRNA synthetase inhibition had a relatively high frequency of resistance [21]. However, as Randall et al. observed, even though these antibiotics have entered clinical trials, rapid resistance and frequent mutations will limit their clinical utility [22]. Therefore, for effective clinical application, simultaneous targeting of several different aaRS enzyme inhibitors will likely be required [21].

Non-β-Lactam β-Lactamase Inhibitor

Similar to penicillin which focuses on inhibiting the peptidoglycan layer of the bacterial cell wall, non-β-lactam β-lactamase inhibitors (BLI) seek similar outcomes with less resistance [23, 24]. Earlier research has demonstrated that combining a β-lactamase inhibitor with a β-lactam inhibitor will greatly reduce the rate of resistance [23]. However, this proves cumbersome since over 1300 unique β-lactamase inhibitors have been identified [23].

As a result, Ehmann et al. found avibactam as the first non-β-lactam β-lactamase inhibitor [25]. This results in a BLI that possesses a broader spectrum of activity than other antibiotics [25]. The EU approved a ceftazidime-avibactam combination for complicated urinary tract infections, complicated intra-abdominal infections, hospital-acquired pneumonia, and other infections caused by aerobic gram-negative organisms in 2015 after completing dozens of clinical trials, including many head-to-head trials [26]. More research is needed to confirm efficacy in other conditions [23].

Nusbiarylins

In 2019, Qiu et al. researched a serious of compounds that target the NusB-NusE interaction necessary for bacterial ribosomal RNA synthesis [27]. By inhibiting the NusB protein, it demonstrated excellent success against MRSA strains while the derivative nusbiarylin 23 reduced rRNA production and exhibited excellent pharmacokinetic properties [27]. More clinical trials are needed to verify these findings [27].

Odilorhabdins

Odilorhabdins are a promising new class of ribosome-targeting antibiotics that induce a high rate of miscoding by increasing the affinity for tRNA to attach to the ribosome [28, 29]. Pantel et al. found that, in animal models, odilorhabdins could eradicate both gram-positive and gram-negative pathogens [28]. Specifically, the first member of the family, NOSO-95C, has been explored structurally while demonstrating promise both in vitro and in vivo against *Enterobacteriaceae* [30]. While this biodiversity and unique approach demonstrates great promise, much more research is still needed as well as randomized, blinded clinical trials [28–30].

Arylomycin

In 2012, Smith and Romesberg found that arylomycin could be adapted as an antibiotic by inhibiting bacterial type I signal peptidase [31]. Then, in 2018, Smith et al. obtained G0775, which has potent, broad-spectrum activity against gram-negative bacteria [32]. The results are very promising, since G0775 is effective against multidrug-resistant bacteria, has a low rate of resistance, binds incredibly well, easily penetrates the cell membrane, and demonstrates potent bactericidal activity against *E. faecium*, *S. aureus*, *Klebsiella pneumoniae*, *Acinetobacter baumannii*, *P. aeruginosa*, and *Enterobacter* species pathogens [32]. However, clinical trials are needed [31, 32].

Teixobactin

In 2015, Ling et al. found that teixobactin works by inhibiting the cell wall similar to penicillin [33]. However, unlike penicillin, teixobactin binds lipid II, a precursor of peptidoglycan, and lipid III, a precursor of cell wall teichoic acid, so that the cell wall cannot be properly synthesized [33]. Interestingly, this novel therapy was isolated with the iChip, a novel tool that isolates and identifies microorganisms [34]. More research and clinical trials are necessary to verify these findings [33, 34].

Ceragenins

Originally described in 1993, squalamine is considered the first representative of the ceragenin, or cationic steroid antibiotics (CSA), class of antibiotics, further divided into polymyxin and its mimics, and squalamine and it mimics [35]. Due to the vast amount of research done in this class of antibiotics, this section is further being divided into the two respective sections: polymyxin derivatives and squalamine derivatives.

Polymyxin Mimics

These cholic acid derivatives are active against both gram-positive and gram-negative organisms, including many drug-resistant bacteria [36, 37]. In early trials, these ceragenins have also been researched for their anticancer properties [35]. However, CSA-13 demonstrated greater antibiotic success in an animal model than the human cathelicidin peptide LL-37 [38]. When Bozkurt-Guzel et al. researched CSA-13 in combination with colistin (sulfate), tobramycin, and ciprofloxacin to treat *A. baumannii*, no antagonism was observed [39]. Other solitary and combination therapies, including second-generation ceragenics, had similar bactericidal and fungicidal results [35, 39–43]. More recently, Birteksoz-Tan et al. examined the activity of ceragenins against *L. pneumophila*, finding that CSA-8 and CSA-13 were not only very effective but also displayed broad-spectrum activity [44]. However, clinical trials are needed to verify these findings [36, 37, 44].

Squalamine Derivatives

Squalamine was originally isolated from dogfish shark tissue (*Squalus acanthias*) and the sea lamprey (*Petromyzon marinus*), exhibiting broad-spectrum antiviral activity against human pathogens both in vitro and in vivo, against both RNA and DNA-viruses [45]. Furthermore, Sills et al. first researched squalamine in 1998 for its ability to inhibit angiogenic activity and halt tumor growth by preventing neovascularization [46, 47]. Additionally, since squalamine has exhibited very little systemic toxicity, its anticancer potency has also been studied [47, 48]. In 2017, Perni et al. found that squalamine inhibited the aggregation process of α-synuclein, which leads to Parkinson's disease [49].

Due to the ability of squalamine, a cationic amphipathic sterol, to neutralize the intracellular membrane's electrostatic surface charge, it hinders the cell's viral replication [45, 50]. In 2008, Salmi et al. found that squalamine demonstrated efficacy toward not only such bacterial strains as *E. coli* and *P. aeruginosa* but also fungal strains [51]. Additionally, Hraiech et al. discovered that squalamine significantly reduced the lung bacterial load when inhaled in vivo to treat chronic *P. aeruginosa* pneumonia [52]. While promising, significant more research in vivo and on humans is needed, including phase II and III clinical trials [45, 50, 53].

In 2015, Qin et al. tested the synthesized polyaminosteroid derivative claramine, a synthesized version of squalamine, selectively inhibiting PTP1B in both gram-negative and gram-positive bacteria [54]. Unlike trodusquemine, however, claramine is much more easily synthesized [54]. While polyaminosteroids were initially investigated in the search for a cancer cure and also for diabetes, squalamine and its analogue BSQ-1 were later found to successfully treat mupirocin-resistant *S. aureus* strains in vitro [55]. Adèle et al. found no emergence of resistant bacteria even with repeated exposure of squalamine and BSQ-q to a *S. aureus* strain [55]. Further studies are being done, and much more research is needed to determine the efficacy of polyaminosteroid derivatives in vivo [3, 54, 55] (see Table 14.1).

Table 14.1 Novel classes of broad-spectrum antibiotics

Name of class	Product	Mechanism of action	In vitro/ in vivo	Study phase	Company (licensor)
Peptidomimetics	Pep16 and Pep19	Cell walls and cell membranes deflated by heptapseudopeptides	In vivo	None	None
α-Helical antimicrobial peptides	Sushi-replacement peptide-2	Disrupting cell membrane	In vivo	None	None
Nonribosomal peptide synthetases	ObiF1	Likely disrupts the cell membrane	In vivo	None	None
Nonribosomal peptide synthetases	Daptomycin	Disrupts the cell membrane	In vivo	Completed phase III	Cubicin
Pleuromutilin	Lefamulin	Inhibit bacterial translation	In vivo	Completed phase III	Xenleta
Peptide deformylase inhibitor	GSK1322322	Inhibit the peptide deformylase	In vivo	Completed phase II	GlaxoSmithKline
FabI inhibitor	AFN-1252	Inhibits enoyl-ACP reductase	In vivo	Currently in phase II	Affinium
Aminoacyl-tRNA synthetase inhibitor	Mupirocin (Bactroban®)	Inhibits aminoacyl-tRNA synthetase (helps in protein biosynthesis)	In vivo	Completed phase III	Pfizer
Non-β-lactam β-lactamase inhibitor	Ceftazidime Avibactam	Inhibits the β-lactamase enzyme	In vivo	Completed phase III	AstraZeneca/ Pfizer
Nusbiarylins	Nusbiarylin 23	Interfere with the NusB-NusE interaction	In vitro	None	None
Odilorhabdins	NOSO-502	Inhibit bacterial translation by binding to ribosomal subunit	In vivo	None	None
Arylomycin	G0775	Inhibit type I signal peptidase which helps secretion	In vivo	None	None
Teixobactin	Teixobactin	Inhibits cell wall synthesis by interrupting the production of lipid II and lipid III	In vivo	None	NovoBiotic
Ceragenins: Polymyxin mimics	CSA-13	Depolarization of bacterial membranes	In vivo	None	None
Ceragenins: Squalamine derivates	Claramine	Disrupt the cell membrane	In vivo	None	None

Nanoparticle Technology

Nanoparticles are an emerging approach that includes nano-antibiotic conjugates, small molecules capped nanoparticles, polymers stabilized nanoparticles, and biomolecules functionalized nanoparticles [56]. Their small volume allows them to move freely through the blood stream and cross-biological barriers and effectively deliver drugs for controlled release of the target drug [56].

The two main methods for nanoparticle drug release are local chemical stimulation or external stimulation [56]. Locally chemical stimulated drugs are released through diffusion, enzymatic activities, hydrolysis, and pH [56]. Oftentimes, these nanoparticles may contain toxins, albeit at a lower concentration than the systemic dose, minimizing side effects [57]. These nanoparticles are delivered to the site with some kind of protection, which in a study by Wang et al. consisted of a reactive oxygen species (ROS)-responsive material, i.e., 4-(hydroxymethyl) phenylboronic acid pinacol ester-modified α-cyclodextrin (Oxi-αCD) [58].

In 2000, research suggested that using nanoparticles increased drug concentration while reducing drug toxicity [59]. Specifically, nanoparticles can be designed to target a specific infection site while carrying multiple drugs or antimicrobials within the same nanoparticle [60]. However, preliminary research recently demonstrated that aluminum nanoparticles may disseminate multidrug resistance [60].

Nanoparticles are able to ensure entry to the metabolic pathway through van der Waals forces, electrostatic attractions, 86 receptor-ligand hydrogen bond formations, hydrophobic interactions, oxidative stress, metal ion release, and non-oxidative mechanisms. Consequently, quite a few upcoming studies involve metal ions.

In a 2017 study by Salem et al., antibacterial activity of silver and zinc nanoparticles against *Vibrio cholerae* and enterotoxic *Escherichia coli* increased efficacy but unfortunately also increased biofilm formation of *V. cholerae* [61]. This hypothetically results from the chain reaction of adenylyl cyclase activity inhibition decreasing the second messenger porin, which then decreasing inhibition of biofilm formation [61].

Other metal ion nanoparticles include gold nanoparticles, silver nanoparticles, zinc oxide nanoparticles, copper nanoparticles, titanium dioxide nanoparticles, and magnesium oxide nanoparticles [62]. Other nanoparticles are carbon-based, including fullerenes and carbon nanotubes, while others are semiconductors, polymeric, or even lipid-based [63].

Phase I clinical trials with topical silver nanoparticles after reduction with trisodium citrate have begun. Although testing will occur for various infections, greater activity against fungal infections is anticipated [66, 67]. NanoViricides is developing several antiviral drugs with a polymer-based nanoparticle [64, 65].

Conclusion

While the number of potential new antibiotics is promising, few have advanced to clinical trials [66]. Fortunately, historic data suggests that most antibiotics enter the market after successfully completing phase I clinical trials [66, 67].

Similarly, although significant progress has been made in vitro and in vivo, the lack of studies entering human-phased clinical trials is disappointing. More thorough and comprehensive research is needed to determine if nanoparticles are truly effective in humans, despite their initial promise in 2010 [68].

References

1. Rajeev L. Antibiotic discovery. Mater Meth. 2018;8:2671.
2. Nicolas I, Bordeau V, Bondon A, Baudy-Floc'h M, Felden B. Novel antibiotics effective against gram-positive and -negative multi-resistant bacteria with limited resistance. PLoS Biol. 2019;17(7):e3000337.
3. Xiong M, Lee MW, Mansbach RA, Song Z, Bao Y, Peek RM, et al. Helical antimicrobial polypeptides with radial amphiphilicity. Proc Natl Acad Sci U S A. 2015;112(43):13155–60.
4. Yang C-H, Chen Y-C, Peng S-Y, Tsai AP-Y, Lee TJ-F, Yen J-H, et al. An engineered arginine-rich α-helical antimicrobial peptide exhibits broad-spectrum bactericidal activity against pathogenic bacteria and reduces bacterial infections in mice. Sci Rep. 2018;8(1):14602.
5. Kreitler DF, Gemmell EM, Schaffer JE, Wencewicz TA, Gulick AM. The structural basis of N-acyl-α-amino-β-lactone formation catalyzed by a non-ribosomal peptide synthetase. Nat Commun. 2019;10(1):3432.
6. Novak R, Shlaes DM. The pleuromutilin antibiotics: a new class for human use. Curr Opin Investig Drugs. 2010;11(2):182–91.
7. Paukner S, Riedl R. Pleuromutilins: potent drugs for resistant bugs-mode of action and resistance. Cold Spring Harb Perspect Med. 2017;7(1):a027110.
8. File TM, Goldberg L, Das A, Sweeney C, Saviski J, Gelone SP, et al. Efficacy and safety of intravenous-to-oral lefamulin, a pleuromutilin antibiotic, for the treatment of community-acquired bacterial pneumonia: the phase III lefamulin evaluation against pneumonia (LEAP 1) trial. Clin Infect Dis. 2019;69(11):1856–67.
9. Goethe O, Heuer A, Ma X, Wang Z, Herzon SB. Antibacterial properties and clinical potential of pleuromutilins. Nat Prod Rep. 2019;36(1):220–47.
10. Jain R, Chen D, White RJ, Patel DV, Yuan Z. Bacterial peptide deformylase inhibitors: a new class of antibacterial agents. Curr Med Chem. 2005;12(14):1607–21.
11. Fonseca-Aten M, Salvatore CM, Mejias A, Rios AM, Chavez-Bueno S, Katz K, et al. Evaluation of LBM415 (NVP PDF-713), a novel peptide deformylase inhibitor, for treatment of experimental mycoplasma pneumoniae pneumonia. Antimicrob Agents Chemother. 2005;49(10):4128–36.

12. Corey R, Naderer OJ, O'Riordan WD, Dumont E, Jones LS, Kurtinecz M, et al. Safety, tolerability, and efficacy of GSK1322322 in the treatment of acute bacterial skin and skin structure infections. Antimicrob Agents Chemother. 2014;58(11):6518–27.

13. Mistry TL, Truong L, Ghosh AK, Johnson ME, Mehboob S. Benzimidazole-based FabI inhibitors: a promising novel scaffold for anti-staphylococcal drug development. ACS Infect Dis. 2017;3(1):54–61.

14. Yao J, Rock CO. Resistance mechanisms and the future of bacterial enoyl-acyl carrier protein reductase (FabI) antibiotics. Cold Spring Harb Perspect Med. 2016;6(3):a027045.

15. Hafkin B, Kaplan N, Murphy B. Efficacy and safety of AFN-1252, the first staphylococcus-specific antibacterial agent, in the treatment of acute bacterial skin and skin structure infections, including those in patients with significant comorbidities. Antimicrob Agents Chemother. 2015;60(3):1695–701.

16. Zheng CJ, Sohn MJ, Lee S, Kim WG. Meleagrin, a new FabI inhibitor from Penicillium chryosogenum with at least one additional mode of action. PLoS One. 2013;8(11):e78922.

17. Pohlmann J, Brotz-Oesterhelt H. New aminoacyl-tRNA synthetase inhibitors as antibacterial agents. Curr Drug Targets Infect Disord. 2004;4(4):261–72.

18. Zhang P, Ma S. Recent development of leucyl-tRNA synthetase inhibitors as antimicrobial agents. MedChemComm. 2019;10(8):1329–41.

19. Vondenhoff GH, Van Aerschot A. Aminoacyl-tRNA synthetase inhibitors as potential antibiotics. Eur J Med Chem. 2011;46(11):5227–36.

20. Agarwal V, Nair SK. Aminoacyl tRNA synthetases as targets for antibiotic development. MedChemComm. 2012;3(8):887–98.

21. Francklyn CS, Mullen P. Progress and challenges in aminoacyl-tRNA synthetase-based therapeutics. J Biol Chem. 2019;294(14):5365–85.

22. Randall CP, Rasina D, Jirgensons A, O'Neill AJ. Targeting multiple aminoacyl-tRNA synthetases overcomes the resistance liabilities associated with antibacterial inhibitors acting on a single such enzyme. Antimicrob Agents Chemother. 2016;60(10):6359–61.

23. Grigorenko VG, Andreeva IP, Rubtsova MY, Deygen IM, Antipin RL, Majouga AG, et al. Novel non-beta-lactam inhibitor of beta-lactamase TEM-171 based on acylated phenoxyaniline. Biochimie. 2017;132:45–53.

24. Tehrani K, Martin NI. β-lactam/β-lactamase inhibitor combinations: an update. Medchemcomm. 2018;9(9):1439–56.

25. Ehmann DE, Jahic H, Ross PL, Gu RF, Hu J, Durand-Reville TF, et al. Kinetics of avibactam inhibition against Class A, C, and D beta-lactamases. J Biol Chem. 2013;288(39):27960–71.

26. Shirley M. Ceftazidime-Avibactam: a review in the treatment of serious gram-negative bacterial infections. Drugs. 2018;78(6):675–92.

27. Qiu Y, Chan ST, Lin L, Shek TL, Tsang TF, Zhang Y, et al. Nusbiarylins, a new class of antimicrobial agents: rational design of bacterial transcription inhibitors targeting the interaction between the NusB and NusE proteins. Bioorg Chem. 2019;92:103203.

28. Pantel L, Florin T, Dobosz-Bartoszek M, Racine E, Sarciaux M, Serri M, et al. Odilorhabdins, antibacterial agents that cause miscoding by binding at a new ribosomal site. Mol Cell. 2018;70(1):83–94.e7.

29. Sarciaux M, Pantel L, Midrier C, Serri M, Gerber C, Marcia de Figueiredo R, et al. Total synthesis and structure–activity relationships study of odilorhabdins, a new class of peptides showing potent antibacterial activity. J Med Chem. 2018;61(17):7814–26.

30. Racine E, Gualtieri M. From worms to drug candidate: the story of odilorhabdins, a new class of antimicrobial agents. Front Microbiol. 2019;10:2893.

31. Smith PA, Romesberg FE. Mechanism of action of the arylomycin antibiotics and effects of signal peptidase I inhibition. Antimicrob Agents Chemother. 2012;56(10):5054–60.

32. Smith PA, Koehler MFT, Girgis HS, Yan D, Chen Y, Crawford JJ, et al. Optimized arylomycins are a new class of Gram-negative antibiotics. Nature. 2018;561(7722):189–94.

33. Ling LL, Schneider T, Peoples AJ, Spoering AL, Engels I, Conlon BP, et al. A new antibiotic kills pathogens without detectable resistance. Nature. 2015;517(7535):455–9.

34. Piddock LJV. Teixobactin, the first of a new class of antibiotics discovered by iChip technology? J Antimicrob Chemother. 2015;70(10):2679–80.

35. Surel U, Niemirowicz K, Marzec M, Savage PB, Bucki R. Ceragenins – a new weapon to fight multidrug resistant bacterial infections. Med Stud (Studia Medyczne). 2014;30(3):207–13.

36. Lai X-Z, Feng Y, Pollard J, Chin JN, Rybak MJ, Bucki R, et al. Ceragenins: cholic acid-based mimics of antimicrobial peptides. Acc Chem Res. 2008;41(10):1233–40.

37. Epand RM, Epand RF, Savage PB. Ceragenins (cationic steroid compounds), a novel class of antimicrobial agents. Drug News Perspect. 2008;21(6):307–11.

38. Bucki R, Niemirowicz K, Wnorowska U, Byfield FJ, Piktel E, Watek M, et al. Bactericidal activity of ceragenin CSA-13 in cell culture and in an animal model of peritoneal infection. Antimicrob Agents Chemother. 2015;59(10):6274–82.

39. Bozkurt-Guzel C, Savage PB, Akcali A, Ozbek-Celik B. Potential synergy activity of the novel ceragenin, CSA-13, against carbapenem-resistant Acinetobacter baumannii strains isolated from bacteremia patients. Biomed Res Int. 2014;2014:710273.

40. Ozbek-Celik B, Damar-Celik D, Mataraci-Kara E, Bozkurt-Guzel C, Savage PB. Comparative in vitro activities of first and second-generation ceragenins alone and in combination with antibiotics against multidrug-resistant Klebsiella pneumoniae strains. Antibiotics (Basel). 2019;8(3):130.

41. Durnaś B, Wnorowska U, Pogoda K, Deptuła P, Wątek M, Piktel E, et al. Candidacidal activity of

selected ceragenins and human cathelicidin LL-37 in experimental settings mimicking infection sites. PLoS One. 2016;11(6):e0157242.

42. Olekson MA, You T, Savage PB, Leung KP. Antimicrobial ceragenins inhibit biofilms and affect mammalian cell viability and migration in vitro. FEBS Open Biol. 2017;7(7):953–67.

43. Wnorowska U, Piktel E, Durnaś B, Fiedoruk K, Savage PB, Bucki R. Use of ceragenins as a potential treatment for urinary tract infections. BMC Infect Dis. 2019;19(1):369.

44. Birteksoz-Tan AS, Zeybek Z, Hacioglu M, Savage PB, Bozkurt-Guzel C. In vitro activities of antimicrobial peptides and ceragenins against Legionella pneumophila. J Antibiot. 2019;72(5):291–7.

45. Zasloff M, Adams AP, Beckerman B, Campbell A, Han Z, Luijten E, et al. Squalamine as a broad-spectrum systemic antiviral agent with therapeutic potential. Proc Natl Acad Sci U S A. 2011;108(38):15978–83.

46. Sills AK Jr, Williams JI, Tyler BM, Epstein DS, Sipos EP, Davis JD, et al. Squalamine inhibits angiogenesis and solid tumor growth in vivo and perturbs embryonic vasculature. Cancer Res. 1998;58(13):2784–92.

47. Pietras RJ, Weinberg OK. Antiangiogenic steroids in human cancer therapy. Evid Based Complement Alternat Med. 2005;2(1):49–57.

48. Bhargava P, Marshall JL, Dahut W, Rizvi N, Trocky N, Williams JI, et al. A phase I and pharmacokinetic study of squalamine, a novel antiangiogenic agent, in patients with advanced cancers. Clin Cancer Res. 2001;7(12):3912–9.

49. Perni M, Galvagnion C, Maltsev A, Meisl G, Müller MBD, Challa PK, et al. A natural product inhibits the initiation of α-synuclein aggregation and suppresses its toxicity. Proc Natl Acad Sci. 2017;114(6):E1009–E17.

50. Moore KS, Wehrli S, Roder H, Rogers M, Forrest JN Jr, McCrimmon D, et al. Squalamine: an aminosterol antibiotic from the shark. Proc Natl Acad Sci U S A. 1993;90(4):1354–8.

51. Salmi C, Loncle C, Vidal N, Letourneux Y, Fantini J, Maresca M, et al. Squalamine: an appropriate strategy against the emergence of multidrug resistant gram-negative bacteria? PLoS One. 2008;3(7):e2765.

52. Hraiech S, Brégeon F, Brunel J-M, Rolain J-M, Lepidi H, Andrieu V, et al. Antibacterial efficacy of inhaled squalamine in a rat model of chronic Pseudomonas aeruginosa pneumonia. J Antimicrob Chemother. 2012;67(10):2452–8.

53. Alhanout K, Rolain JM, Brunel JM. Squalamine as an example of a new potent antimicrobial agents class: a critical review. Curr Med Chem. 2010;17(32):3909–17.

54. Qin Z, Pandey NR, Zhou X, Stewart CA, Hari A, Huang H, et al. Functional properties of Claramine: a novel PTP1B inhibitor and insulin-mimetic compound. Biochem Biophys Res Commun. 2015;458(1):21–7.

55. Adèle S, Frédéric L, Jean Michel B, Tania Nawfal D, Blin O, Rolain JM. Polyaminosteroid analogues as potent antibacterial agents against mupirocin-resistant Staphylococcus aureus strains. Anti-Infect Agents. 2019;17:1–6.

56. Masri A, Anwar A, Khan NA, Siddiqui R. The use of nanomedicine for targeted therapy against bacterial infections. Antibiotics (Basel). 2019;8(4):260.

57. Hussain S, Joo J, Kang J, Kim B, Braun GB, She Z-G, et al. Antibiotic-loaded nanoparticles targeted to the site of infection enhance antibacterial efficacy. Nat Biomed Eng. 2018;2(2):95–103.

58. Wang Y, Yuan Q, Feng W, Pu W, Ding J, Zhang H, et al. Targeted delivery of antibiotics to the infected pulmonary tissues using ROS-responsive nanoparticles. J Nanobiotechnol. 2019;17(1):103.

59. Pinto-Alphandary H, Andremont A, Couvreur P. Targeted delivery of antibiotics using liposomes and nanoparticles: research and applications. Int J Antimicrob Agents. 2000;13(3):155–68.

60. Wang L, Hu C, Shao L. The antimicrobial activity of nanoparticles: present situation and prospects for the future. Int J Nanomedicine. 2017;12:1227–49.

61. Salem W, Leitner DR, Zingl FG, Schratter G, Prassl R, Goessler W, et al. Antibacterial activity of silver and zinc nanoparticles against Vibrio cholerae and enterotoxic Escherichia coli. Int J Med Microbiol. 2015;305(1):85–95.

62. Singh P, Garg A, Pandit S, Mokkapati V, Mijakovic I. Antimicrobial effects of biogenic nanoparticles. Nanomaterials (Basel). 2018;8(12):1009.

63. Khan I, Saeed K, Khan I. Nanoparticles: properties, applications and toxicities. Arab J Chem. 2019;12(7):908–31.

64. Diwan A. NanoViricides Technology. Shelton; 2020.

65. Finch G, Havel H, Analoui M, Barton RW, Diwan AR, Hennessy M, et al. Nanomedicine drug development: a scientific symposium entitled "Charting a roadmap to commercialization". AAPS J;62014:698–704.

66. Butler MS, Blaskovich MA, Cooper MA. Antibiotics in the clinical pipeline in 2013. J Antibiot. 2013;66(10):571–91.

67. Payne DJ, Gwynn MN, Holmes DJ, Pompliano DL. Drugs for bad bugs: confronting the challenges of antibacterial discovery. Nat Rev Drug Discov. 2007;6(1):29–40.

68. Gunasekaran T, Nigusse T, Dhanaraju MD. Silver nanoparticles as real topical bullets for wound healing. J Am Coll Clin Wound Spec. 2011;3(4):82–96.

Phytocompounds

Jiasen Wang

Abbreviations

ATP	Adenosine Triphosphate
FDA	Food and Drug Administration
HPV	Human Papillomavirus
HSV	Herpes Simplex Virus
KOH	Potassium Hydroxide
QS	Quorum Sensing
RCT	Randomized Controlled Trial
TTO	Tea Tree Oil
WHO	World Health Organization

Introduction

Phytocompounds, also known as phytochemicals and botanicals, as their name suggests, are chemical compounds derived from plants. Prior to the modern age of medicine, phytocompounds have long been exploited through ingestible and topical applications ubiquitously across all ancient civilizations. Their formulations are documented on bamboo and papyrus manuscripts from ancient China and Egypt as early as 3000 BC [1]. A significant proportion of the most potent medications we use daily in the art of medicine are derived from botanicals, with the WHO estimating at one point in the early twenty-first century approximately 30% of FDA approved drugs possessed plant-based origins [2]. These include morphine, vincristine, paclitaxel, digoxin, and aspirin. Although developed countries have scientifically advanced techniques to distill the active compounds from plants, bacteria, and the natural world into medications we utilize daily, less developed countries largely rely on the traditional ethnomedicine that often comprises largely of plant-based compounds. The World Health Organization in 1983 estimated that 80% of the population in portions of the world continue to rely on traditional medicine [3]. However, although widely quoted this statistic has come under scrutiny in recent years as new studies demonstrate that the majority of households in Ghana, China, and India prefer modern medicine (>80%) as their primary modality for treatment, and less than 5% prefer traditional medicine. However, they are not exclusive of one another, and 20% of their citizens continue to utilize traditional medicine in some form [4]. The decreasing reliance on ethnomedicines and concurrent decreasing biodiversity through the destruction of rich ecosystems such as the Amazon Rainforest in South America will culminate in the permanent loss of many of the oldest medical traditions as their current practitioners lose patients, students, and resources [5, 6]. This trend emphasizes the urgency to further study phytocompounds.

J. Wang (✉)
McGovern Medical School, Department of Internal Medicine, Houston, TX, USA

© Springer Nature Switzerland AG 2021
S. K. Tyring et al. (eds.), *Overcoming Antimicrobial Resistance of the Skin*, Updates in Clinical Dermatology, https://doi.org/10.1007/978-3-030-68321-4_15

The abundance, diversity, and geographic seclusion of different species of plants across the world provide a large spectrum of potential therapies. Yet, there has been a surprising deficiency of high-quality clinical trials against the numerous pathogenic microbes of the skin. Frequently, the best evidence for the touted benefits and therapeutic efficacy of these medications is at the level of expert experience and testimony [7]. Still, numerous compounds have been tested and demonstrated to exhibit antimicrobial activity in vitro against microbes with dermatological relevance. However, when trialed in vivo, the same efficacy was rarely observed in the clinical setting. Thus, established synthetic compounds remain the primary modality and treatment of choice for dermatologic infections. Plant-based therapeutics are subsequently more commonly relegated to a secondary, adjuvant role. For example, tea tree oil (*M. alternifolia*), hyperforin (*H. perforatum*), and coriander oil (*Coriandrum sativum*) all display antibacterial activity but are not used as primary treatments for infectious illnesses [8–10].

Today, patients and consumers are driving increasing demand for "natural" products in dermatological care, continuing an overall surge in popularity of complementary and alternative medicine. Phytocompounds are marketed as "botanicals" and serve as a mainstay in this category of products. However, they are poorly regulated by the FDA, and it is near impossible to confirm all of the "detoxifying, hydrating, strengthening" and other effects these products advertise. Furthermore, these products may vary in their contents, degrade over time, and are not without side effects. The goal of this chapter is to provide a review of plant-based compounds in regard to their potential as agents against increasingly antimicrobial-resistant organisms with pathogenic potential in the integumentary system. We will focus on therapies that have been well studied, as well as those with promising potential and delve into the mechanisms of their activity, why they may be effective against multidrug-resistant organisms, and what potential dangers and drawbacks they may possess.

Preparations and Active Metabolites

Plants produce primary and secondary compounds throughout their photo-biochemical lives. Primary compounds are ubiquitous metabolites necessary for the growth and development of plant life. Secondary metabolites are those which may be unique to a species of plants and often endow an evolutionary advantage to aid in survival in their environment. For example, chemicals involved in defensive mechanisms, hormonal signaling, and color sediments are classified as secondary metabolites [11]. There are more than 200,000 known compounds which are secondary metabolites of plants, and they can be categorized based on their organic chemical structures. Table 15.1 delves into these classes and a selection of plant species in which they can be found [11, 12].

Phytocompounds derived from these secondary metabolites are the active ingredients in many of our medications today. One study estimates more than 50% of antimicrobial, cardiovascular, immunosuppressive, and anticancer therapeutic agents are derived from these secondary metabolites [13, 14]. With so many known secondary compounds with the candidacy for dermatologic antimicrobial therapy, the challenge becomes identifying the compounds with significant effectiveness against the numerous pathogenic microbes related to the skin. Screening medical plants used in traditional ethnomedicine is the most effective and efficient method to identify these active secondary metabolites, most with antimicrobial potency, and has largely been the source of the phytocompounds on the market today.

The most relevant and well-studied preparations are essential oils. When plant components are exposed to solvents through a variety of methods, they liquify, and their active metabolites are extracted into a directly skin-applicable vehicle with minimal disturbance in their chemical structures. They can then be incorporated into lotions, gels, creams, or other vehicles that may be more comfortable to the patient. Currently,

Table 15.1 Secondary metabolites of plants

Classes	Subclasses	Examples	Parent structure	Botanical sources
Phenolics – Largest group of plant metabolites. Share the presence of one or more phenol groups. Widespread and contribute to plant color, taste and flavor	**Simple phenolics** – ubiquitous among plants, many properties including antimicrobial and anti-inflammatory	Arbutin salicylates Gallic acid Hydroquinone		*Capsicum* spp. *Arctostaphylos uva-ursi* *Cynara scolymus*
	Tannins – polyphenols, used to precipitate protein. Most commonly used to convert raw animal hide into leather	Gallotannins Ellagitannins		*Geranium robertianum* *Quercus alba* *Punica granatum* (pomegranate) *Filipendula ulmaria* Green tea
	Coumarins – derivatives of benzo-α-pyrone	Umbelliferone Aesculetin Scopoletin		*Melilotus* spp. (sweet clover) *Dipteryx odorata* *Galium odoratum*
	Flavonoids – largest group of naturally occurring phenols	Catechins Anthocyanidins Flavan-3-ols		*Compositae* spp. *Rutaceae* spp. *Leguminosae* spp. *Glycyrrhiza glabra* (liquorice) *Ginkgo biloba* (Gingko)

(continued)

Table 15.1 (continued)

Classes	Subclasses	Examples	Parent structure	Botanical sources
	Chromones and xanthones – derivatives of benzo-γ-pyrone	Eugenin Furanochromones		*Polygala nyikentis* *Ammi visnaga* Clove and mustard seeds
	Stilbenes	Resveratrol		*Pinaceae* *Eucalyptus* *Madura*
	Lignans – dimeric compounds formed by the union of two molecules of a phenylpropene derivative	Dibenzylbutane derivatives Dibenzylbutyrolactones Monoepoxy lignans Biepoxylignans		*Asteraceae* *Pinaceae* *Rutaceae*

Alkaloids – Contain at least one nitrogen atom in a heterocyclic ring. Widely used in medicine, this class is very heterogeneous	Saponins Nicotine Caffeine	Acridones Aromatics Carbolines Ephedras Ergots Imidazoles Indoles Purines Pyrrolidines	
Saponins – compounds possessing a polycyclic aglycone moiety with either a steroid or triterpenoid attached to a carbohydrate unit			*Saponaria* family *Aceracaea* *Dioscorea* *zingiberensis* *Quillaja saponaria* *Glycyrrhiza* spp. *Digitalis purpurea* *Dioscorea villosa*
Terpenes – name is derived from "turpentine" meaning "resin" in old French. All derived from 5-carbon isoprene units, and are classified according to the number of isoprene units in the molecule			
Hemiterpenes – consist of a single isoprene unit	Angelic acid Isovaleric acid		*Angelica* *archangelica* *Vaccinium myrtillus*

(continued)

Table 15.1 (continued)

Classes	Subclasses	Examples	Parent structure	Botanical sources
	Monoterpenes – consist of two isoprene units, have molecular formula $C_{10}H_{16}$	Limonene Linalool Linalyl acetate Citronellal Carvone Camphor Menthol	Citronellal, Limonene, Menthol, Eucaliptol, Thymol, Camphor	*Lamiaceae* *Pinaceae* *Rutaceae* *Apiaceae* *Melaleuca* *Alternifolia*
	Sesquiterpenes – consist of three isoprene units, have molecular formula $C_{15}H_{24}$. Subclasses include acyclic, monocyclic, and bicyclic	Acyclic- e.g. Farnesol Monocyclic, e.g., bisabolol Bicyclic, e.g., caryophyllene	Farnesol, Nerolidol	*Vernonia colorata* *Arnica montana* *Atractylodis rhizoma*
	Diterpenes – consist of four isoprene units, have molecular formula $C_{20}H_{32}$. Further classified into acyclic and macrocyclic	Vitamin K1 Carotenes (vitamin A)	Abietadiene, Cassaic acid	*Jateorhiza palmata* *Teucrium chamaedrys* *T. scoradonia* *Gibberella* *Kalmia latifolia*

Sesterterpenes – consist of five isoprene units

Geranyl farnesol

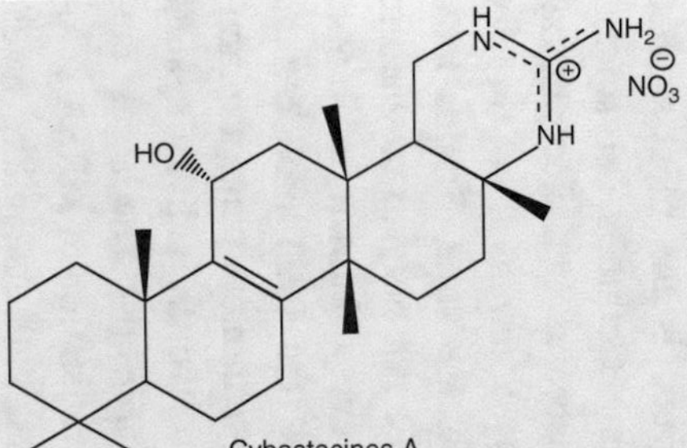

Triterpenes – consist of six isoprene units

Boswellic acids

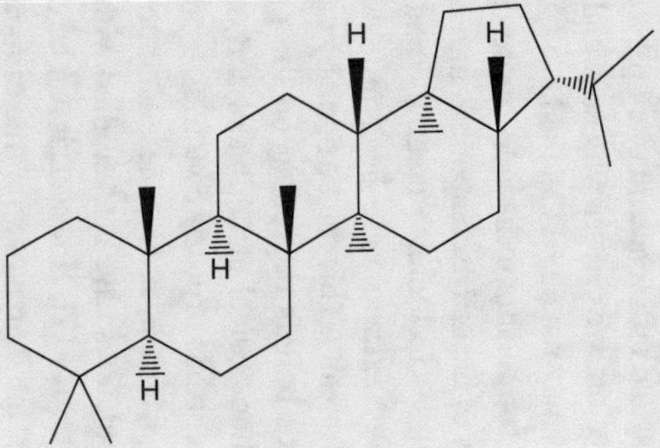

Cybastacines A

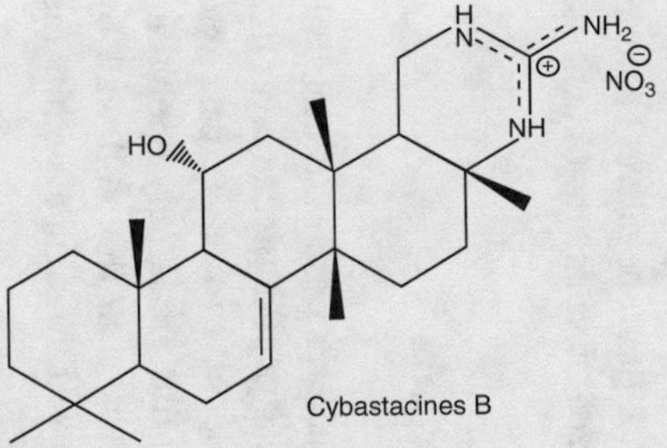

Cybastacines B

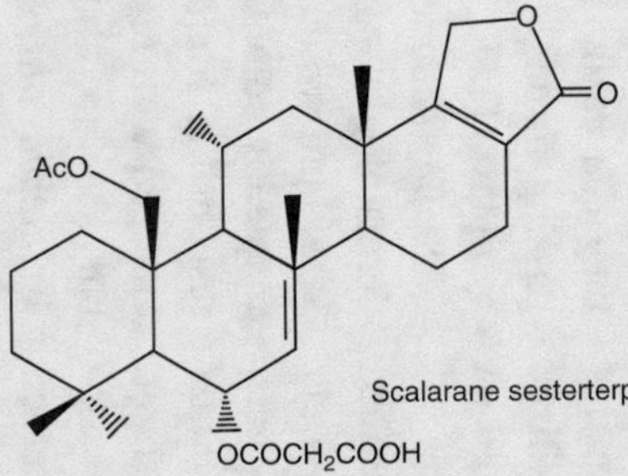

Scalarane sesterterpene

Camellia sasanqua
Theacaea spp.

Boswellia carterii

around 100 essential oils are recommended for dcrmatological indications, and 88 were identified to be recommended for skin infections [15].

However, essential oils contain all of the extractable complex organic metabolites which can number in the hundreds and even thousands [12]. While many of these metabolites are responsible for the medicinal anti-inflammatory and antimicrobial effects of essential oils, many are also responsible for undesirable negative effects such as phototoxicity and high allergenic potential. In addition, essential oils have several potential drawbacks which may hinder their effectiveness. Plants, like any other organism, are diverse intraspecies organisms and may vary in their chemical composition. Together with variations in nutrient sources, growing and harvesting techniques, and differences in plant parts utilized per batch of oil, we can see why essential oils on the market may not all be identical.

Other formulations include more purified derivatives of the active compounds into a variety of vehicles including creams and gels. Traditionally extracts have been utilized either orally or topically. This can be done by crushing, grinding, or boiling depending on the prescription by ethnomedical practitioners and recorded in pharmacopeias of many countries worldwide. Moroccan, Chinese, and Japanese Kampo among other formulations have been studied with promising results [16, 17]. However, it can be difficult to tease out the therapies with true clinical value from those which are supported by centuries of tradition and pseudoscience. In fact, a Cochrane review of traditional Chinese herbal therapies on the skin and soft tissue infections in 2014 found zero randomized controlled trials [18].

Antibacterial Phytocompounds

Bacteria with pathogenic potential frequently colonize the skin, contributing to normal skin flora. The most well-known and prevalent include *Staphylococcus aureus* and *Streptococcus pyogenes*. One study of 29,731 patients admitted to a tertiary care center found an 11% nasal colonization rate with MRSA [19]. While the mechanisms

by which bacteria and other microbes develop resistance have been well discussed throughout this book in earlier chapters, phytocompounds have unique mechanisms of action most of which are yet to be clearly elucidated. We will discuss the antibiotic effects of selected phytocompounds on gram-positive and gram-negative bacteria, along with hypothesized mechanisms of actions.

Gram-Positive Bacteria

The gram-positive bacteria possess a cell wall comprised of a 90–95% peptidoglycan layer that allows lipophilic molecules to easily pass into the cells. As essential oils are largely lipophilic, they can easily interact with this cell wall by passing through to exert influence within the cytoplasm [15].

Staphylococcus aureus is the most studied dermatologic pathogen. Cellulitis, erysipelas, acne, burn wounds, abscesses, and ulcers are all frequently colonized by *S. aureus* if not directly responsible for the disease state. Strains have emerged with resistance not only to methicillin but also to almost every known antibiotic. *Melaleuca alternifolia* (tea tree) produces an essential oil rich in the monoterpene terpinen-4-ol which displays noteworthy activity against resistant strains of *S. aureus* [8]. The largest randomized trial studied eradication of MRSA colonization in 214 hospital patients, pitting a test group with two treatment regimens over a period of 5 days. The trial group was assigned 10% *M. alternifolia* oil nasal cream applied thrice daily to the nares, 5% *M. alternifolia* body wash at least once daily, and a 10% *M. alternifolia* cream applied only to skin infections once daily. The control group was assigned a standard regimen of 2% nasal mupirocin applied thrice daily to the nares, 4% chlorhexidine gluconate body soap at least once daily, and 1% silver sulfadiazine cream applied to skin infections only [20]. 41% of patients in the trial arm successfully cleared compared to 47% in the standard therapy control arm. Interestingly, the study also found that while *M. alternifolia* formulations were much less effective at clearing MRSA colonization in the nares

(41%) versus mupirocin (78%), they were more effective at clearing the superficial skin sites and skin lesions. Additional studies have demonstrated their efficacy in treating MRSA colonized wounds and *P. acnes* and *S. epidermidis* related mild-moderate acne.

Tea tree oil and other phytocompounds with active monoterpenes appear to disrupt the plasma membrane by altering its fluidity and permeability, hindering its ability to regulate ions and molecules and conduct cellular respiration [8, 12]. Other terpenoid phytocompounds displaying promising in vitro action against *S. aureus* and other gram-positive bacteria include carvacrol found in *Origanum scabrum* and *vulgare* (oreganos), geraniol found in *Backhousia citriodora* (lemon myrtle) and *Cymbopogon martinii* (palmarosa), menthol found in *Mentha piperita* (peppermint), and eugenol found in *Laurus nobilis* (bay) and *Cinnamomum zeylanicum* (cinnamon) [15].

Hyperforin, a major compound of *H. perforatum*, commonly known as St. John's wort was found to have strong activity against a panel of gram-positive bacteria including *S. aureus* [10]. Coriander oil from *Coriandrum sativum* has also shown activity against gram-positive bacteria in addition to gram-negative bacteria, especially *E. coli*, and even fungi [9, 21].

Licorice or *Glycyrrhiza glabra* has also been extensively studied in vitro with reported antibacterial, antifungal, and antiviral effects [22]. Several compounds in aqueous and ethanol licorice extracts have been identified including glabridin, glabrol, and liquiritin which may inhibit bacterial growth. Additionally, toxins such as α-toxin produced by MRSA may be reduced by the activity of the phenol compound licochalcone E, and key virulence genes SaeR and Hla may even be inactivated by compounds found in licorice. While these reports are promising, these effects have yet to be proven in vivo [23].

Several other compounds have also demonstrated strong in vitro activity against numerous gram-positive bacteria. Chamomile (*Anthemis aciphylla* var. *discoidea*), bitter orange (*Citrus aurantium and zeylanicum*), and clove (*Syzygium aromaticum*) all displayed higher in vitro activity against gram-positive bacteria than tea tree oil, but have not been tested in vivo [15].

Group A β-hemolytic *Streptococcus pyogenes* and *Clostridium perfringens* are frequently implicated in a variety of skin infections of varying severity and urgency. While several studies have targeted these bacteria in vitro and successfully demonstrated the efficacy of tea tree oil, eucalyptol, and camphor against them, there remains a relative dearth of quality studies compared to *S. aureus*, especially clinical trials [15].

Gram Negatives

Gram-negative bacteria differ from gram-positive bacteria by the presence of a peptidoglycan cell wall 2–3 nm thick sandwiched between an inner cytoplasmic cell membrane and an outer bacterial cell membrane composed of a phospholipid bilayer. While the thick outer membrane protects the microbe from lipophilic molecules often found in essential oils, they remain vulnerable to small active solutes due to the increased presence of porins and pumps which serve as transmembrane channels. These transport proteins have been well discussed in Chap. 1 as a mechanism of resistance to several classes of antibiotics. As a result, gram-negative bacteria pose serious threats from a resistance standpoint. *E. coli* and *Pseudomonas aeruginosa* are two gram-negative bacteria frequently isolated from patients with chronic skin wounds and often with resistance profiles and comorbidities that pose unique treatment challenges. Extended-spectrum beta-lactamase *E. coli* is now frequently found in nonhospital patients, and *P. aeruginosa* contributes toward chronic but nonfatal skin infections such as green nail syndrome.

E. coli is analogous to *S. aureus* in that it is the most well-studied gram-negative pathogen of the skin from the standpoint of essential oil antibacterial activity. While rosewood (*Aniba rosaeodora*), chamomile (*Anthemis aciphylla* var. *discoidea*), and thyme (*Thymus vulgaris*) all displayed in vitro inhibition against *E. coli* and *Pseudomonas*, the minimum inhibitory concentrations (MIC) values required were higher than those for gram-positive bacteria [12]. This is likely due to the thick phospholipid bilayer outer membrane. Similar to activity against gram positives, the most anti gram-negative activity was identified in oils containing high levels of α-pinene and terpinen-4-ol such as tea tree oil. Other oils such as palmarosa oil and peppermint oil exhibited effects on *E. coli* cell morphology by elongating filaments and increasing their cell length from 3–5 um to 10–25 um, indicating cellular damage [12]. In addition, peppermint oil, rosemary oil, eucalyptus oil, and menthol were observed to eliminate R-plasmid activity, decreasing the spread of genes encoding resistance in *E. coli* [24].

Allium sativum (Garlic) is a common dietary staple that has been used extensively as a medicine across cultures ranging from China, India, and Egypt for at least 5000 years. Well studied for its traditional lauded properties of antihypertensive, anti-lipid, and antineoplastic effects, it has also been studied for its antimicrobial properties. Indeed, Pasteur noted its antibacterial properties, and it was even used occasionally in WWI and WWII as an anti-gangrene agent on wounds. Allicin and ajoene are sulfur phytocompounds found to have antibacterial properties against a wide array of bacteria including *E. coli* and *S. aureus* [25]. However, no randomized controlled trials have been identified, which may be due to the severity of bacterial skin infections and the efficacy of our modern mainstay antibiotics.

Biofilms

Biofilms are well recognized as a modality of resistance against antimicrobials and was the focus of discussion in Chap. 13. The multicellular consortiums convey several advantages for the organisms living within it including structural stability, firm adherence to the host surface, and resistance to antimicrobial and host immune response. The formation and behavior of the biofilm rely on a phenomenon termed quorum sensing (QS) – when the microorganisms reach a critical number, they begin to synthesize and release signaling molecules to communicate and cooperate [26]. Biofilms are estimated to be involved in 80% of human infections, yet difficult to detect [27]. In the skin, they are undetectable in biopsies due to breakdown of the glycocalyx during processing but may be visualized by an electron, epifluorescence, or confocal microscopy. One study found that 60% of chronic wounds contained biofilms compared to 6% of acute wounds [28]. Three of the most common species identified were *Staphylococcus aureus*, *Pseudomonas aeruginosa*, and *Enterococcus faecalis*.

Phytocompounds can play an important role in the fight against biofilms. Essential oils and plant extracts have been tested and active agents isolated which are most effective against biofilms. While select essential oils such as that of clove, ginger, coriander, cumin, menthol, thyme, and eucalyptus have demonstrated in studies to have some action toward biofilm eradication, the active compounds have been identified thus far to be terpenoids and phenylpropenes [29]. Terpenes and terpenoids such as thymol and carvacrol are especially efficacious [30]. Thymol, from thyme, and carvacrol disrupt membrane permeability to alter leakage of potassium and ATP. Phenylpropenes include eugenol, isoeugenol, vanillin, safrole, and cinnamaldehyde. Eugenol was found to have activity against *E. coli* and reduced biofilm formation [31].

Quorum sensing (QS), as a key mechanism in the development and maintenance of biofilms, is often a target of antibiofilm therapies. Targets aim to interfere by inhibiting signal generation and signal reception or by degrading signal molecules known as autoinducers (AIs) [32]. Anti-QS agents were first characterized in the red marine alga *Delisea pulchra* [33]. Investigations found it contained halogenated furanones which competitively inhibit and destabilize cytoplasmic transcription factors (e.g., LuxR in gram-negative bacteria) involved in QS [34]. However, as most furanones are halogenated, they may be too toxic and unfit for clinical use. Numerous plants have also been tested for anti-QS properties due to the similarity of their secondary metabolites to mimic AIs and downregulate QS regulating receptors and genes [35]. Identified phytoconstituents with anti-QS activity include alkaloids (e.g., tomatidine), organosulfur compounds (e.g., violacein), and phenolics (e.g., coumarins, flavonoids, quinones, and terpenoids). A more in-depth review of this topic is discussed in Chap. 12 of the textbook *A New Look into Phytocompounds* [36].

While these active compounds are effective in inhibition of the biofilms, they are less so in reducing and eradicating them. Several studies have hypothesized that there may be synergy with phytocompounds and established antibacterial medications. In the last decade, a few studies have tested this idea against biofilms of *S. aureus*, *P. aeruginosa*, *L. monocytogenes*, and *E. coli* with numerous antibacterial agents such as aminoglycosides (specifically streptomycin, tobramycin, and amikacin), beta-lactams (methicillin and oxacillin), vancomycin, and the fluoroquinolone ciprofloxacin. An overwhelming 75% of the compounds which demonstrated synergy was the terpenoid class [37]. Further research is required to investigate this interesting and promising avenue of therapy.

Antifungal Phytocompounds

Fungal infections of the skin include yeasts and dermatophytes. Rarely life-threatening unless found in the bloodstream, they are opportunistic organisms that have drastic impacts on quality of life, especially in immunocompromised patients.

Yeasts

Candida genera consist of around 150 species, and more than 17 are reported to cause candidiasis in humans. *C. albicans* is the most common culprit and can cause intertrigo, thrush, and vaginitis which is exacerbated in immunocompromised patients [38]. Given its extensive presence as a skin and oral pathogen, it has naturally developed resistance to first and second line antifungals such as azoles and terbinafine. The chronic and low-acuity infections of *Candida* make it an ideal candidate for phytocompound therapy. Indeed, most frequently used dermatologic oils and phytocompounds have been tested for activity against candida. *Santolina chamaecyparissus* (santolina) and *Thymus* spp. (thyme) essential oils are recommended for their strong in vitro evidence against fungi. Other essential oils have been tested including *Cananga odorata* (ylang-ylang), *Cinnamomum cassia* (cinnamon), *Coriandrum sativum* (coriander), and *Lavandula angustifolia* (lavender) [15]. All demonstrate strong in vitro activity against fungi but are yet to be tested for their clinical efficacy.

Lu et al. (2016) extensively reviewed the current literature of phytocompounds active against *Candida* spp. Phenylpropanoids, quinones, flavonoids, terpenoids, alkaloids, stilbenoids, and bisbenzyls were discussed to have varying degrees of activity, but all studies were in vitro. Allicin from garlic, diferuloylmethane from curcumin, and lycopene (a carotenoid) from fruits were noted to exhibit anti-candidal effects as well [39].

Organisms of the *Candida* species produce biofilms that can strongly augment their pathogenicity and resistance against antimicrobial agents. Fixed or sessile *Candida* cells in biofilms are up to 1000 times more resistant to azoles than their free-floating, planktonic counterparts [40]. In vitro testing of phytocompounds against *Candida* biofilms has failed to show significant antifungal activity when used alone but has demonstrated synergy with several antifungal compounds including the azoles, fluconazole and itraconazole, and echinocandins micafungin and caspofungin. The most active compounds potentiating these antifungals were those of the monoterpene (e.g., thymol and carvacrol) and sesquiterpene class (e.g., farnesol and artemisinins), together comprising 67% of those compounds identified. The other 33% included phenylpropanoids such as eugenol and cinnamaldehyde, the flavonoid baicalin, and the alkaloid berberine and decapeptides tyrocidines [37]. Essential oils of *Cymbopogon winterianus* (citronella) and *Cinnamon cassia* (cinnamon) have shown activity against candidal biofilm as well in vitro [41]. Gold nanoparticle complexes using cinnamaldehyde exhibited effective biofilm inhibition of gram-positive and gram-negative bacteria as well as *C. albicans* [42]. Other yeasts also produce biofilms, but candida has been the model in all in vitro studies due to its prevalence; thus further investigation is required.

Candida auris is an archetype of increasing microbial resistance and warrants special mention. Named after its discovery in Japan from the ear canal of an elderly patient suffering chronic otitis, it has now been isolated across the world as a pathogen of candidiasis and fungemia. Infamous for its consistent resistance to many azoles and echinocandins with multimodal mechanisms of resistance including biofilm formation and transmembrane protein pumps identified from genetic sequencing, phytocompounds are poised to be a viable alternative therapy. Unfortunately, no mention of this pathogen has been identified in phytocompound studies thus far. Yet as a member of the candida species, we can hypothesize that the phytotherapies discussed above will have similar efficacy against this pathogen.

Dermatophytes

Dermatophyte is an inclusive term for the three fungi genera *Microsporum*, *Epidermophyton*, and *Trichophyton*. Infections of the hair, skin, and nails lead to chronic but low-risk infections that can be quite a headache to treat. Especially when involving nails, they are extraordinarily resistant to topical therapy, and a complete regimen of oral terbinafine or griseofulvin may be upward of a year to completely treat the infection. Given the length of these systemic treatments, there are toxic adverse effects such as liver damage which may occur. Essential oils are thus a great alternative and have been studied extensively in the clinical setting. One study directly compared *M. alternifolia* (tea tree oil) to clotrimazole for onychomycosis in 117 patients. After 6 months of twice-daily therapy and debridements at 0, 1, 3, and 6 months, there was a similar rate of clinical cure at 60% for tea tree oil and 61% for clotrimazole. When cultured, 18% of tea tree oil achieved clearance compared to 11% of clotrimazole [43]. Another study compared tea tree oil at concentrations of 25% and

50% in preparations of ethanol and polyethylene glycol against placebo in the treatment against tinea pedis. 39% showed improvement in the placebo arm versus 72% in the 25% tea tree oil formulation and 64% in the 50% formulation [44]. Earlier trials had shown poor efficacy with tree tea oil against tinea pedis; however, the strength was only 10%, and thus a higher concentration may be key in treating dermatophytosis. This was further supported by a trial testing the efficacy of *Eucalyptus pauciflora* essential oil on tinea pedis, corporis, or cruris in 50 patients for 3 weeks. After 2 weeks all patients were clear on KOH scrapings, and after the completion of 3 weeks of therapy, 60% of patients had complete resolution of skin symptoms, and the other 40% reported improvement in their skin symptoms such as scaling, pruritus, and erythema. Repeat KOH scrapings were also negative at 2 months in all patients [45]. Similar to their mechanism of action against bacteria, compounds high in monoterpenes such as tea tree oil appear to exert their antifungal effects by changing the permeability and fluidity of the fungal cell membrane [46].

Garlic (*Allium sativum*), as described above with antibacterial activity, also has antifungal properties, likely due to the activity of the trisulfur compound ajoene. In a study of 34 patients with tinea pedis, a cream composed of 4% ajoene resulted in complete clinical cure in 79% of patients within a week. After 2 weeks 100% of the 34 patients had achieved resolution of their symptoms. While this study lacked a control arm, every patient was followed up in 90 days and did not report recurrence of their disease [47].

Malassezia and Others

Implicated in tinea versicolor and seborrheic dermatitis, *Malassezia* spp. is a common affliction across the world. *M. alternifolia* is the only essential oil that has been tested against *Malassezia* and other fungi such as *Madurella mycetomatis* with excellent in vitro activity. These studies have led to tea tree oil products to be highly successful and marketed around the world in hair products as shampoos and conditioners. Interestingly, grape seed extracts rich in the active compound flavan-3-ols from *V. vinifera* were studied against several strains of *Malassezia* with impressive activity. As the grape extracts are rich in potent antioxidants, they are already used in several topical cosmetic skin products marketed for antiaging effects and have been well tolerated without toxicity [48]. Two other studies tested essential oils against *Malassezia* infections in dogs. *Zataria multiflora* and *Thymus kotschyanus* were found to be active against *Malassezia*-related atopic dermatitis in dogs, and five essential oil mixtures of Mediterranean plants (*C. paradise, S. sclarea, O. basilicum, R. officinalis, C. limon, A. nobilis, L. hybrida*, and *T. vulgaris*) effectively cleared *Malassezia* otitis externa in dogs [49, 50]. With such promising efficacy from the phytocompounds reviewed against fungal pathogens, it is disappointing that there are no clinical studies on this topic.

Antiviral Phytocompounds

Viral infections are extraordinarily prevalent in the skin. The most common include the herpes simplex virus (cold sores, genital ulcers), the human papillomavirus (common and genital warts), and the molluscum contagiosum virus. All typically instigate benign infections that generally self-resolve but may be a significant hindrance on quality of life. Others such as varicella (chickenpox), zoster (shingles), and the now eradicated variola (smallpox) are more severe dermatological infections that require systemic treatment and may have fatal consequences if left untreated. Currently, only a few antiviral medications are available, and there is a need for more options with increasing resistance. Phytocompounds are excellent candidates in this regard, and several phytocompounds are already well-established therapies in viral skin infections such as podophyllotoxin and salicylic acid. Viruses are divided into enveloped and non-enveloped viruses, the differentiating factor being the presence of a lipid membrane coating enveloped viruses such as HSV. Similar to the

increased efficacy of essential oils and other phytocompound formulations against gram-positive bacteria, the same principle applies to viruses – enveloped viruses appear to be much more susceptible to essential oils and other lipid-based formulations. HPV, as a non-enveloped virus, appears to be much more resistant to essential oil formulations [12]. However, other mechanisms such as local immunomodulation of several phytocompounds do not require active interaction with the virus itself to display antiviral efficacy.

Podophyllotoxin from American mayapple or mandrake root (*Podophyllum peltatum*) is a first-line topical treatment of condyloma acuminatum. A systematic review found that a 0.5% solution or gel was 45–83% effective in clearing symptoms within 3–6 weeks, but recurrence rates ranged between 13% and 100% [51]. However, adverse effects such as headache, local pain, and irritation were identified to decrease compliance. Addressing this issue, a randomized controlled trial tested podophyllotoxin in a solid lipid nanoparticle gel vehicle in 97 patients with recurrent condyloma acuminatum, and there was a 97.1% response rate. Compared to the standard gel arm which had a response rate of 90.6%, the nanoparticle gel improved response as well as lowered the rates of adverse events [52]. This appears to be an avenue of research that deserves to be further investigated. Mechanistically, podophyllotoxin appears to destabilize microtubules and tubulin cellular structures to enact their antiviral properties; resistance has not been studied yet. Additionally, podophyllotoxin is also very effective for molluscum contagiosum. A study with 0.5%, 0.3%, and 0% placebo cream was tested in 150 adult patients randomly controlled over 3 days per week over 4 weeks. Results showed a complete clearance of 92% in the 0.5% cream group, 52% in the 0.3% cream group, and 16% in the placebo group [53]. Studies confirming efficacy and evaluating safety in pediatric patients has not yet been performed.

The best antiviral candidates are those that are virustatic – halting proliferation by inhibiting key steps in viral replication. Alternatively, antivirals can be virucidal and exhibit their activity by denaturing structural proteins comprising the envelope or capsid. Numerous essential oils have been studied to elucidate their mechanisms of action against viruses and appear to lean heavily toward virucidal mechanisms. For example, *Artemisia arborescens* oil is strongly virucidal against HSV-1 and HSV-2 [54]. Another study demonstrated that the envelope of HSV-1 was disrupted when treated with *O. vulgare* (oregano) oil and *S. aromaticum* (clove) oil [55]. Furthermore, the active compound eugenol found in clove oil demonstrated strong in vitro activity against HSV-1 and HSV-2. In these studies of HSV, it was determined that essential oils exhibited their effects the most on free viruses prior to adsorption onto the cell surface and penetration into the cytoplasm. This suggests that the main mechanism of action involves interaction with the viral envelope or surface protein in a manner that prevents cellular entry into their target host cell [12].

Salicylic acid is another phytocompound utilized frequently in dermatology for the treatment of acne and verrucas as well as in other applications such as chemical peels. Although first isolated from the herb meadowsweet (*Filipendula ulmaria*) in 1839 and determined to be a derivative of the salicylate class of compounds which are plant hormones, it has been used in various formulations extracted from willow tree leaves several thousand years ago by Hippocrates for the treatment of fevers and headaches. Today salicylic acid is commonly found in over-the-counter acne products due to its comedolytic effects and over-the-counter wart remover kits due to its keratolytic and immune-stimulating properties which may be responsible for its antiviral activity. A 2012 meta-analysis of randomized controlled trials confirmed that although there was a wide range of reports on the efficacy of salicylic acid (0–80%) in clearing warts, it is indeed superior to the placebo (RR 1.56, 95% CI 1.20–2.03) [56]. This variation is likely due to nonoptimal applications together with variations in length and compliance of therapy at home. Additionally, it is often utilized in conjunction with cryotherapy which may confound results. Yet a couple of studies have shown that the effects of salicylic acid persisted even as an isolated therapy. The advantages of painless application and minimal adverse effects if applied properly with concentrations adjusted for the location of the wart make it a great topical antiviral therapy. Given these considerations, it has also been studied for activity against molluscum contagiosum, but results have been disappointing compared to the effectiveness of other treatments such as cantharidin from the perspective of lesion clearance and adverse effects.

Phytocompounds utilized as traditional therapies against verruca vulgaris in Europe include topical arborvitae (*Thuja occidentalis*) and fresh juice of greater celandine (*Chelidonium majus*). Systemic phytocompounds against verruca vulgaris include extract of purple coneflowers (*Echinacea purpurea*) by Native Americans and Siberian ginseng (*Eleutherococcus senticosus*) in traditional Chinese medicine [7]. However, studies have yet to validate and measure the efficacy of these traditional therapies. The most common and standardized method to measure antiviral properties of promising phytocompounds in vitro is via plaque reduction assay on *vero* (a lineage of cells from an African green monkey) kidney cells infected with the virus of interest. Essential oils have been extensively tested for antiviral properties through this method and have identified several compounds with promising in vitro activity against HSV-1, including lemon (*Citrus limon*), lavender (*Lavandula latifolia*), and santolina (*Santolina insularis*) [57]. Interestingly, while tea tree oil did not demonstrate ideal activity in vitro against HSV-1, it has been tested in clinical trials with reported efficacy. In a trial of 18 patients with recurrent herpes labialis, 6% tea tree oil was tested against placebo, and the mean time to clearance with tea tree oil was 9 days compared to 12.5 days with placebo [58]. Other case reports demonstrate activity against warts as well [59].

Green tea (*Camellia sinensis*) extracts have been found to have strong activity against condyloma acuminatum, especially if the extract contains a high concentration of a class of polyphenols known as sinecatechins. One of these polyphenols, epigallocatechin, has been found to be especially effective against condylomas, and recently an ointment with this compound has trademarked as polyphenon E by a Japanese pharmaceutical company. This compound has been well studied in four RCTs. In phase III trials, 10% and 15% formulations were tested against the placebo with the vehicle alone. The active ointment had an efficacy of 54–57% after thrice daily application for 16 weeks compared to 34–35% with placebo and fewer than 10% experienced recurrence of the warts. Adverse side effects were quite tolerable with only 5% of patients discontinuing the therapy due to intolerable adverse effects including pruritus and pain [60, 61]. Unfortunately, the mechanism of action has yet to be elucidated, but it may be associated with its antioxidant and immune-enhancing activity. Polyphenon E cream is now FDA approved and marketed as Veregen®.

Risks and Adverse Effects

Phytocompounds and botanical medicines generally fall under the umbrella branch of complementary and alternative medicines. The main reasons for this are their perceived safety and efficacy in conjunction with a lack of regulation and high-quality clinical studies. For example, garlic, a dietary staple found worldwide is consumed daily and touted for its wide-ranging medicinal properties including those discussed earlier in this chapter. It may be impossible to regulate. The World Health Organization has made strides in encouraging the regulation and standardization across the world in this respect, and 124 member countries reported having instituted regulations of herbal medicines in 2018, a tremendous increase from 65 countries with regulations in 1999 [2]. However, regulations are far and wide in their stringency, ranging from exclusive regulations of herbal compounds to treating botanicals with the same status of conventional pharmaceuticals. The ease of access to phytocompounds also complicates regulation as essential oils and botanical extracts can be easily self-distilled or made at home after obtaining the plant part from the local grocer, florist, or one's own backyard. However, given the rich history and broad-ranging applications of phytocompounds, it is therefore natural that the myriad of adverse and toxic effects which they induce has been well reported and studied, especially in the field of dermatology.

Several modalities of toxicity can be observed. Virtually all botanicals have the potential to provoke irritant and allergic contact dermatitis. The most well-known allergic contact dermatitis is caused by the urushiol oleoresin from the genus *Toxicodendron* which poison oak and ivy belong. Other allergic contact dermatitis inducing substances include sesquiterpene lactones (especially the α-methylene-γ-lactone moiety) found in the Asteraceae or Compositae family such as the species *A. montana*. Compositae mix and sesquiterpene lactone mix can be utilized in patch testing to determine sensitization if there is high risk or suspicion for Compositae dermatitis [62].

Another modality of toxicity is through photosensitization. Phytophotodermatitis occurs after an inert compound is activated by exposure to UV light after contact with the skin. It is most commonly caused by the families of *Apiaceae* and *Rutaceae* (citrus) which contain high levels of furocoumarins made of angular angelicins and linear psoralens such as 5-methoxypsoralens (5-MOP, bergapten) that react with oxygen in the presence of UVA (peak 320–340 nm) to produce a keratolytic and DNA-damaging compound. Berloque dermatitis is especially well-known due to the prevalence of 5-MOP utilized in older perfume fragrances but is now rare as it is a recognized irritant and removed as a common ingredient. As part of the plant's defense systems, both urushiol and furocoumarins or their derivatives can be found throughout the plant kingdom. Given the large number of compounds often found in plant extracts and essential oils, there is a high chance sensitivity may develop in a patient if used for an extended period of time.

The cytotoxicity of essential oils has been studied in vitro with proxy tissue substitutes such as human fibroblasts, dermal epithelial cells, and tumor cell lines when studying antibacterial and antifungal effects. Monkey kidney cells are occasionally used for studying antiviral properties. Most studies found that essential oils exert cytotoxic effects at 5.0–1950 μg/ml, antibacterial effects at 20–20,000 μg/ml, and antiviral effects even at 1–200 µg/ml [12]. Thus from these in vitro results, we would expect most oils to be cytotoxic before antibacterial but achieve good effects against viruses. However, it appears the substitute tissue may not be a good proxy for the in vivo setting as the monocellular culture models do not accurately simulate the complex skin barrier. Thus, adjustment scales have been created to better correlate in vitro and in vivo toxicity, one of which was the system by Halle and Gores in 1987, and can be utilized to decrease in vivo animal testing [63]. When this scale is applied to *M. alternifolia* tea tree oil studies, we expect the toxicity of tea tree oil to be low to mild in humans. Several patch test studies support this and report that up to 5% of patients may experience irritation and 0.15–1.8% of patients may experience allergic contact dermatitis from patch test results. However, these tend to exaggerate real-life experiences. Various formulations on the market may decrease allergenicity, and the only reports of adverse effects were very mild in clinical trials with *M. alternifolia*. There does appear to be a dose-dependent correlation, as formulations with concentrations of 25–100% increased the risk of contact dermatitis to 2–8% of patients [58].

Phytocompounds as antimicrobials may be limited by their effectiveness as studied in vitro and concentration achievable at the site of action. This is complicated by the difficulty in maintaining optimal absorption and transport of active constituents below the maximum dosage without adverse effects. While phytocompounds have great antimicrobial potential in the skin, care must be taken to raise clinical awareness that their utilization is not without risk.

Challenges Facing Phytocompounds and Current Research Trends

Although synthetic derivatives and immunomodulators have become the first line of future dermatologic remedies, phytocompounds remain in a comfortable position. The ecologic diversity of plants and rich ethnomedical pharmacopeias

ensure that there will always be an endless supply of compounds for research into their medical antimicrobial properties.

Once an efficacious compound is discovered, there may be unforeseen challenges that arise. When paclitaxel was discovered to be an effective anticancer agent in the 1960s from the bark of the pacific yew *Taxus brevifolia*, the harvesting of bark was fatal for the tree and threatened to endanger the species as demand far outpaced supply. Fortunately, responsible harvesting practices were followed. Later, when total chemical synthesis was achieved in the 1990s, the raw wood was no longer required [64]. Another significant challenge is the standardization of phytocompounds due to the presence of complex and diverse secondary metabolites which vary depending on the age, geographic location, and part of the plant species utilized to create the medication. Indeed, adulteration with corticosteroids such as clobetasol has been a documented problem in China. This may lead to the perceived efficacy of a phytocompound where there may be in reality minimal, and continued use may lead to dangerous and significant adverse effects if utilized long term [65].

The current direction of phytocompound research is highly promising. The journal *Phytomedicine* consistently publishes high-quality research of botanicals, and the WHO consistently compiles and releases the pharmacopeias of the world's traditional ethnomedical therapies. Together with the availability of new technologies enabling high throughput in vitro testing against a variety of infectious diseases, phytocompounds are poised to make breakthroughs in the coming years and decades. The bottleneck may be clinical trials, which are required to bring standardization and approval to many of the botanical compounds discussed in this chapter. While the efficacy of our current antimicrobials may alleviate the immediate pressure for new therapies, rising resistance will make it necessary to pursue phytocompounds as alternative sources of effective antimicrobial therapies with novel mechanisms of action. More recent clinical studies are testing not only the efficacy of the phytocompound alone against a microbial pathogen but adjuvant with an established antimicrobial. For example, *Turnera ulmifolia* has been found to synergize with aminoglycosides against MRSA by inhibiting the efflux mechanisms associated with resistance [66]. Another modality of resistance in which phytocompounds have demonstrated a promising role is the fight against biofilms [37]. Although to date there has not been any single phytocompound identified capable of eradicating biofilms alone, numerous studies provide evidence of botanicals enhancing known antimicrobial compounds' activity against biofilms.

Summary

Phytocompounds are plant-derived chemicals with a broad spectrum of medicinal activity. In this chapter, we have reviewed phytocompounds that are effective for the treatment of bacteria, fungi, and viruses that exhibit infectious potential in the skin. While some are millennia-old household remedies such as garlic, others are newly discovered and hold great potential in the present and future battle against ever more prevalent resistant microbes. Active ingredients have been identified and extracted for the most potent botanical agents, but the extent of the ecologic diversity of botanicals implies that there are many effective therapies yet to be discovered. Essential oils are the easiest and most standardized techniques for in vitro testing, but care must be taken to avoid toxicity and sensitivity. Other advantages include the availability of phytocompounds – they may be much more accessible in low-resource countries or in environmental disasters and even war. Innovative and novel ways to apply these chemicals are also being introduced. In vitro research is demonstrating synergistic effects of phytocompounds together with established antibiotics, and novel vehicles with nanoparticles are promising improved efficacy and decreased adverse effects. However, more clinical trials studying phytocompound applications in dermatology are required to confirm their clinical role against infectious diseases.

References

1. Ahmad Khan MS, Ahmad I. Chapter 1 – Herbal medicine: current trends and future prospects. In: Ahmad Khan MS, Ahmad I, Chattopadhyay D, editors. New look to phytomedicine. London: Academic Press; 2019. p. 3–13.
2. World Health Organization, editor. WHO global report on traditional and complementary medicine, 2019. Geneva: World Health Organization; 2019. 226 p.
3. Parveen A, Parveen B, Parveen R, Ahmad S. Challenges and guidelines for clinical trial of herbal drugs. J Pharm Bioallied Sci. 2015;7(4):329–33.
4. Oyebode O, Kandala N-B, Chilton PJ, Lilford RJ. Use of traditional medicine in middle-income countries: a WHO-SAGE study. Health Policy Plan. 2016;31(8):984–91.
5. Decaëns T, Martins MB, Feijoo A, Oszwald J, Dolédec S, Mathieu J, et al. Biodiversity loss along a gradient of deforestation in Amazonian agricultural landscapes: biodiversity thresholds. Conserv Biol. 2018;32(6):1380–91.
6. Barlow J, Lennox GD, Ferreira J, Berenguer E, Lees AC, Nally RM, et al. Anthropogenic disturbance in tropical forests can double biodiversity loss from deforestation. Nature. 2016;535(7610):144–7.
7. Reuter J, Merfort I, Schempp CM. Botanicals in dermatology. Am J Clin Dermatol. 2010;11(4):247–67.
8. Cox SD, Mann CM, Markham JL, Bell HC, Gustafson JE, Warmington JR, et al. The mode of antimicrobial action of the essential oil of Melaleuca alternifolia (tea tree oil). J Appl Microbiol. 2000;88(1):170–5.
9. Lo Cantore P, Iacobellis NS, De Marco A, Capasso F, Senatore F. Antibacterial activity of Coriandrum sativum L. and Foeniculum vulgare Miller Var. vulgare (Miller) essential oils. J Agric Food Chem. 2004;52(26):7862–6.
10. Schempp CM, Pelz K, Wittmer A, Schöpf E, Simon JC. Antibacterial activity of hyperforin from St John's wort, against multiresistant Staphylococcus aureus and gram-positive bacteria. Lancet. 1999;353(9170):2129.
11. Hussein RA, El-Anssary AA. Plants secondary metabolites: the key drivers of the pharmacological actions of medicinal plants. In: Builders PF, editor. Herbal medicine. London: IntechOpen; 2019.
12. Reichling J, Schnitzler P, Suschke U, Saller R. Essential oils of aromatic plants with antibacterial, antifungal, antiviral, and cytotoxic properties – an overview. Complement Med Res. 2009;16(2):79–90.
13. Newman DJ, Cragg GM. Natural products as sources of new drugs over the last 25 years. J Nat Prod. 2007;70(3):461–77.
14. Gordaliza M. Natural products as leads to anticancer drugs. Clin Transl Oncol. 2007;9(12):767–76.
15. Orchard A, van Vuuren S. Commercial essential oils as potential antimicrobials to treat skin diseases. Evid Based Complement Alternat Med. 2017;2017:1–92.

16. Ait-Sidi-Brahim M, Markouk M, Larhsini M. Chapter 5 – Moroccan medicinal plants as antiinfective and antioxidant agents. In: Ahmad Khan MS, Ahmad I, Chattopadhyay D, editors. New look to phytomedicine. London: Academic Press; 2019. p. 91–142.

17. Higaki S, Mommatsu S, Morohashi M, Yamagishi T, Hasegawa Y. Susceptibility of Propionibacterium acnes, Staphylococcus aureus and Staphylococcus epidermidis to 10 Kampo Formulations. J Int Med Res. 1997;25(6):318–24.

18. Wang YF, Que HF, Wang Y-J, Cui XJ. Chinese herbal medicines for treating skin and soft-tissue infections. Cochrane Wounds Group, editor. Cochrane Database Syst Rev. 2014

19. Marzec NS, Bessesen MT. Risk and outcomes of methicillin-resistant Staphylococcus aureus (MRSA) bacteremia among patients admitted with and without MRSA nares colonization. Am J Infect Control. 2016;44(4):405–8.

20. Dryden MS, Dailly S, Crouch M. A randomized, controlled trial of tea tree topical preparations versus a standard topical regimen for the clearance of MRSA colonization. J Hosp Infect. 2004;56(4):283–6.

21. Delaquis PJ, Stanich K, Girard B, Mazza G. Antimicrobial activity of individual and mixed fractions of dill, cilantro, coriander and eucalyptus essential oils. Int J Food Microbiol. 2002;74(1):101–9.

22. Pastorino G, Cornara L, Soares S, Rodrigues F, Oliveira MBPP. Liquorice (Glycyrrhiza Glabra): a phytochemical and pharmacological review. Phytother Res. 2018;32(12):2323–39.

23. Wang Q, Qian Y, Wang Q, Yang Y, Ji S, Song W, et al. Metabolites identification of bioactive licorice compounds in rats. J Pharm Biomed Anal. 2015;115:515–22.

24. Schelz Z, Molnar J, Hohmann J. Antimicrobial and antiplasmid activities of essential oils. Fitoterapia. 2006;77(4):279–85.

25. Sharifi-Rad J. Plants of the genus Allium as antibacterial agents: from tradition to pharmacy. Cell Mol Biol. 2016;62(9):57–68.

26. Abisado RG, Benomar S, Klaus JR, Dandekar AA, Chandler JR. Bacterial Quorum sensing and microbial community interactions. Garsin DA, editor. mBio. 2018;9(3):e02331–17.

27. Wolcott R, Dowd S. The role of biofilms: are we hitting the right target? Plast Reconstr Surg. 2011;127:28S–35S.

28. James GA, Swogger E, Wolcott R, deLancey Pulcini E, Secor P, Sestrich J, et al. Biofilms in chronic wounds. Wound Repair Regen. 2008;16(1):37–44.

29. Jafri H, Ansari FA, Ahmad I. Chapter 9 – Prospects of essential oils in controlling pathogenic biofilm. In: Ahmad Khan MS, Ahmad I, Chattopadhyay D, editors. New look to phytomedicine. London: Academic Press; 2019. p. 203–36.

30. Ceylan O, Ugur A. Chemical composition and antibiofilm activity of Thymus sipyleus BOISS. subsp. sipyleus BOISS. var. davisianus RONNIGER essential oil. Arch Pharm Res. 2015;38(6):957–65.

31. Zhang Y, Wang Y, Zhu X, Cao P, Wei S, Lu Y. Antibacterial and antibiofilm activities of eugenol from essential oil of Syzygium aromaticum (L.) Merr. & L. M. Perry (clove) leaf against periodontal pathogen Porphyromonas gingivalis. Microb Pathog. 2017;113:396–402.

32. Musk DJ Jr, Hergenrother PJ. Chemical countermeasures for the control of bacterial biofilms: effective compounds and promising targets. Curr Med Chem. 2006;13(18):2163–77.

33. Manefield M, Rasmussen TB, Henzter M, Andersen JB, Steinberg P, Kjelleberg S, et al. Halogenated furanones inhibit quorum sensing through accelerated LuxR turnover. Microbiology. 2002;148(4):1119–27.

34. Lowery CA, Dickerson TJ, Janda KD. Interspecies and interkingdom communication mediated by bacterial quorum sensing. Chem Soc Rev. 2008;37(7):1337–46.

35. Rasmussen TB, Givskov M. Quorum sensing inhibitors: a bargain of effects. Microbiology. 2006;152(4):895–904.

36. Husain FM, Al-Shabib NA, Noor S, Khan RA, Khan MS, Ansari FA, et al. Chapter 12 – Current strategy to target bacterial quorum sensing and virulence by phytocompounds. In: Ahmad Khan MS, Ahmad I, Chattopadhyay D, editors. New look to phytomedicine. London: Academic Press; 2019. p. 301–29.

37. Zacchino SA, Butassi E, Cordisco E, Svetaz LA. Hybrid combinations containing natural products and antimicrobial drugs that interfere with bacterial and fungal biofilms. Phytomedicine. 2017;37:14–26.

38. Sardi JCO, Scorzoni L, Bernardi T, Fusco-Almeida AM, Mendes Giannini MJS. Candida species: current epidemiology, pathogenicity, biofilm formation, natural antifungal products and new therapeutic options. J Med Microbiol. 2013;62(1):10–24.

39. Lu M, Li T, Wan J, Li X, Yuan L, Sun S. Antifungal effects of phytocompounds on Candida species alone and in combination with fluconazole. Int J Antimicrob Agents. 2017;49(2):125–36.

40. Ramage G, Rajendran R, Sherry L, Williams C. Fungal biofilm resistance. Int J Microbiol. 2012;2012:528521.

41. de FD de Almeida L, de Paula JF, de Almeida RVD, Williams DW, Hebling J, Cavalcanti YW. Efficacy of citronella and cinnamon essential oils on Candida albicans biofilms. Acta Odontol Scand. 2016;74(5):393–8.

42. Ramasamy M, Lee J-H, Lee J. Development of gold nanoparticles coated with silica containing the antibiofilm drug cinnamaldehyde and their effects on pathogenic bacteria. Int J Nanomedicine. 2017;12:2813–28.

43. Buck DS, Nidorf DM, Addino JG. Comparison of two topical preparations for the treatment of onychomycosis: Melaleuca alternifolia (tea tree) oil and clotrimazole. Complement Ther Med. 1998;6(3):167–8.

44. Satchell AC, Saurajen A, Bell C, Barnetson RS. Treatment of interdigital tinea pedis with 25% and 50% tea tree oil solution: a randomized, placebo-

controlled, blinded study. Australas J Dermatol. 2002;43(3):175–8.

45. Shahi SK, Shukla AC, Bajaj AK, Banerjee U, Rimek D, Midgely G, et al. Broad spectrum herbal therapy against superficial fungal infections. Skin Pharmacol Physiol. 2000;13(1):60–4.

46. Hammer KA, Carson CF, Riley TV. Antifungal effects of Melaleuca alternifolia (tea tree) oil and its components on Candida albicans, Candida glabrata and Saccharomyces cerevisiae. J Antimicrob Chemother. 2004;53(6):1081–5.

47. Ledezma E, Sousa LD, Jorquera A, Sanchez J, Lander A, Rodriguez E, et al. Efficacy of ajoene, an organosulphur derived from garlic, in the short-term therapy of tinea pedis. Mycoses. 1996;39(9–10):393–5.

48. Simonetti G, D'Auria FD, Mulinacci N, Innocenti M, Antonacci D, Angiolella L, et al. Anti-dermatophyte and anti- *Malassezia* activity of extracts rich in polymeric flavan-3-ols obtained from *Vitis vinifera* seeds: grape seed extracts against dermatophytes and *Malassezia*. Phytother Res. 2017;31(1):124–31.

49. Nardoni S, Pistelli L, Baronti I, Najar B, Pisseri F, Bandeira Reidel RV, et al. Traditional Mediterranean plants: characterization and use of an essential oils mixture to treat Malassezia otitis externa in atopic dogs. Nat Prod Res. 2017;31(16):1891–4.

50. Khosravi AR, Shokri H, Fahimirad S. Efficacy of medicinal essential oils against pathogenic Malassezia sp. isolates. J Mycol Méd. 2016;26(1):28–34.

51. Lacey CJN, Woodhall SC, Wikstrom A, Ross J. 2012 European guideline for the management of anogenital warts. J Eur Acad Dermatol Venereol. 2013;27(3):e263–70.

52. Xie F, et al. Treatment of recurrent condyloma acuminatum with solid lipid nanoparticle gel containing podophyllotoxin: a randomized double-blinded, controlled clinical trial. Nan Fang Yi Ke Da Xue Xue Bao. 2007;27(5):657–9.

53. Syed TA, Lundin S, Ahmad M. Topical 0.3% and 0.5% podophyllotoxin cream for self-treatment of molluscum contagiosum in males. Dermatology. 1994;189(1):65–8.

54. Saddi M, Sanna A, Cottiglia F, Chisu L, Casu L, Bonsignore L, et al. Antiherpevirus activity of Artemisia arborescens essential oil and inhibition of lateral diffusion in Vero cells. Ann Clin Microbiol Antimicrob. 2007;6(1):10.

55. Siddiqui Y, Ettayebi M, Haddad A, Al-Ahdal MN. Effect of essential oils on the enveloped viruses: antiviral activity of oregano and clove oils on herpes simplex virus type 1 and Newcastle disease virus. Med Sci Res. 1996;24:185–6.

56. Kwok CS, Gibbs, S, Bennett, C, Holland, R, Abbott R. Topical treatments for cutaneous warts. Cochrane Database Syst Rev. 2012;(9).

57. Koch C, Reichling J, Schneele J, Schnitzler P. Inhibitory effect of essential oils against herpes simplex virus type 2. Phytomedicine. 2008;15(1):71–8.

58. Carson CF, Hammer KA, Riley TV. Melaleuca alternifolia (Tea Tree) oil: a review of antimicrobial and other medicinal properties. Clin Microbiol Rev. 2006;19(1):50–62.

59. Millar BC, Moore JE. Successful topical treatment of hand warts in a paediatric patient with tea tree oil (Melaleuca alternifolia). Complement Ther Clin Pract. 2008;14(4):225–7.

60. Tatti S, Swinehart JM, Thielert C, Tawfik H, Mescheder A, Beutner KR. Sinecatechins, a defined green tea extract, in the treatment of external anogenital warts: a randomized controlled trial. Obstet Gynecol. 2008;111(6):1371–9.

61. Stockfleth E, Beti H, Orasan R, Grigorian F, Mescheder A, Tawfik H, et al. Topical Polyphenon® E in the treatment of external genital and perianal warts: a randomized controlled trial. Br J Dermatol. 2008;158(6):1329–38.

62. Reider N, Komericki P, Hausen BM, Fritsch P, Aberer W. The seamy side of natural medicines: contact sensitization to arnica (Arnica montana L.) and marigold (Calendula officinalis L.). Contact Dermatitis. 2001;45(5):269–72.

63. Halle W, Halder M, Worth A, Genschow E. The registry of cytotoxicity: toxicity testing in cell cultures to predict acute toxicity (LD50) and to reduce testing in animals. Altern Lab Anim. 2003;31(2):89.

64. Young, et al. Evaluating the impact of paclitaxel on Taxus brevifolia distribution. J Appl Ecol. 1997;34(11):87–95.

65. Fong HHS. Integration of herbal medicine into modern medical practices: issues and prospects. Integr Cancer Ther. 2002;1(3):287–93.

66. Coutinho HD, Costa JG, Lima EO, Falcão-Silva VS, Siqueira Júnior JP. Herbal therapy associated with antibiotic therapy: potentiation of the antibiotic activity against methicillin – resistant Staphylococcus aureus by Turnera ulmifolia L. BMC Complement Altern Med. 2009;9(1):13.

Summary: Overcoming Antimicrobial Resistance of the Skin

Yasmin Khalfe and Stephen K. Tyring

Abbreviations

AMR   Antimicrobial resistance
NSC   National Security Council
WHO   World Health Organization

Summary

A public health crisis that existed before the COVID-19 pandemic and will likely persist beyond the pandemic is antimicrobial resistance (AMR). AMR is an emergent health threat responsible for the death of approximately 35,000 Americans and over 700,000 people globally each year. A continued rise in resistance is projected to kill 10,000,000 annually by 2050 [1]. According to Dr. Tedros Adhanom Ghebreyesus, Director General of the World Health Organization (WHO), AMR is "one of the most urgent health threats of our time."

In 2014, the President's Council of Advisors on Science and Technology reported on the combat against AMR. The council recalled how drastically life changed with the development of antimicrobials, stating: "For an American in the 21st century, it is hard to imagine the world before antibiotics. At the beginning of the 20th century, as many as nine women out of every 1,000 who gave birth died, 40 percent from sepsis. In some cities as many as 30 percent of children died before their first birthday. One of every nine people who developed a serious skin infection died, even from something as simple as a scrape or an insect bite. Pneumonia killed 30 percent of those who contracted it; meningitis killed 70 percent. Ear infections caused deafness; sore throats were not infrequently followed by rheumatic fever and heart failure. Surgical procedures were associated with high morbidity and mortality due to infection." The account describes infectious disease in stark contrast to what exists today and gives insight to what the world was like over 100 years ago.

This picture changed dramatically in the twentieth century due to three major developments: improvements in public health, vaccines, and antibiotics. Public health measures such as cleaner water and food supplies, as well as better sewage disposal, were implemented. Food safety had proven to be a challenge in the late nineteenth century, as the US population had moved from rural to urban settings, and food supplies became less safe as farms and gardens were not as readily available. There was little to no control over the

Y. Khalfe (✉)
School of Medicine, Baylor College of Medicine, Houston, TX, USA

S. K. Tyring
Department of Dermatology, University of Texas Health Science Center, Houston, TX, USA

Center for Clinical Studies, Houston, TX, USA

© Springer Nature Switzerland AG 2021
S. K. Tyring et al. (eds.), *Overcoming Antimicrobial Resistance of the Skin*, Updates in Clinical Dermatology, https://doi.org/10.1007/978-3-030-68321-4_16

quality of food, milk, or juice sold at markets. As was illustrated in Upton Sinclair's book from 1906, *The Jungle*, the meat packing industry at the beginning of the twentieth century was infamous for including anything in sausages and canned meats that happened to "fall in," from diseased animals and rats to fingers of employees. Publication of this book led to the Meat Inspection Act of 1906 and eventually to the Food and Drug Administration in 1930, primarily due to efforts by Dr. Harvey Wiley. Modern methods of preserving food and beverages, however, began with Gail Borden in 1853 with condensation and Dr. Louis Pasteur in 1864 with pasteurization.

Another pioneer in public health was Dr. John Snow who showed the value of a clean water supply and the general notion of public health during a cholera epidemic in London in 1854. Dr. Snow famously identified a single water pump in Soho as the waterborne source of cholera and had the pump handle removed to prove his point. He also introduced many other concepts of public health, including "clusters of infection" on maps, statistical analysis of disease spread, and contact tracing. Additionally, the widely held public health concept of hand washing began in 1847 when Dr. Ignaz Semmelweis began exhorting his fellow physicians at the Vienna General Hospital to wash their hands before delivering babies in order to prevent "childbed" (puerperal) fever. The primary cause of the "morbid poison" was found in the twentieth century to be *Streptococcus pyogenes*. At that time about 5 in 1000 women died in deliveries by midwives or at home. The death rate in Europe and the United States by physicians working in the "best" maternity hospitals was 10–20 times higher. The reason was found to be because the faculty physicians and their medical students at these facilities began the day by performing barehanded autopsies on the women who had died the previous day of childbed fever. Without washing their hands, they then went to the wards to examine pregnant women and deliver babies. Many of Semmelweis' colleagues were outraged by his suggestion that they were the cause of childbed fever, and he was met with enormous resistance and criticism. As a result, Semmelweis lost his appointment at the Vienna General Hospital, suffered a mental health breakdown, and died in an insane asylum. In 1867, Dr. Joseph Lister elaborated the theory of antiseptic surgery, including handwashing, in Scotland. It was only when Dr. Robert Koch linked a germ, *Bacillus anthracis*, to a specific infectious disease, anthrax, that the true mechanistic benefit of handwashing was recognized and further accepted.

Aside from the great strides in public health measures, the development of antimicrobials, and antibiotics in particular, has saved millions of lives and is one of the world's greatest innovations. Deaths from infectious diseases declined markedly over the course of the twentieth century and contributed to a substantial increase in life expectancy. However, while there were major improvements in infection-related deaths during the twentieth century, the United States and the world are now at dire risk of this progress being lost. As early as 1954, Dr. Alexander Fleming warned of the potential problem of AMR in his Nobel Prize address stating, "It is not difficult to make microbes resistant to penicillin in the laboratory by exposing them to concentrations not sufficient to kill them, and the same thing has occasionally happened in the body." If prescribed antibiotics are not taken for the proper length of time, if the drug quality is poor (a particular problem in less affluent countries), or if the medicine is taken reflexively rather than when needed (a common dilemma for American pediatricians confronted by anxious parents demanding therapy for a child's viral illness), the issue of resistance becomes a concern.

Inevitably, bacteria and other microbes evolve in response to their environment and can develop mechanisms to resist being killed by antimicrobials. For many decades, the issue was manageable as the growth of resistance was slow and the pharmaceutical industry continued to create new antibiotics. Over the past decade, however, this brewing problem has become a crisis. The evolution of antibiotic resistance is now occurring at an alarming rate and is outpacing the development of new countermeasures capable of thwarting infections in humans. This situation threatens patient care, economic growth, public health, agriculture, economic security, and national security [2].

In response to this, agreements and legislation have been formed to address the building AMR issues. Twenty leading pharmaceutical companies have formed the $1 billion AMR Action Fund to combat antimicrobial resistance by supporting the development of new antibiotics. In addition, two new policy proposals have been introduced in Congress. The Disarm Act of 2019 would increase federal reimbursement for new antibiotics, and the Pasteur Act of 2020 would give qualified new antibiotic makers a guaranteed reimbursement level.

Still, overcoming AMR today is no longer a matter of finding a new mechanism of action for an antimicrobial agent. Many other factors have come into consideration, such as our understanding of biofilms and the microbiome. Long before infectious diseases were understood, phytocompounds such as artemisinin from wormwood and quinine from cinchona trees were used as antimicrobial agents against malaria; today, phytocompounds are now being investigated further for a number of infectious diseases. New drug delivery systems are also now being tested, including systems that utilize nanoparticles.

The growth of AMR and emergence of novel infectious diseases in the past few decades have been exacerbated by antimicrobial overuse in humans, livestock, and agriculture. As seen with the COVID-19 pandemic, the lack of existing vaccines for infectious diseases makes the availability of effective antimicrobials incredibly important. Rather than treating infections, vaccines decrease the desperate need for treatments and cures by contributing majorly to disease prevention.

While no infectious disease in history has been responsible for more morbidity and mortality than smallpox, no single intervention has saved more lives than the smallpox vaccine. Variolation or inoculation was the method first used to immunize an individual against smallpox (variola) with material taken from a patient or a recently variolated individual, in the hope that a mild, but protective, infection would result. The procedure was most commonly carried out by inserting/rubbing powdered smallpox scabs or fluid from pustules into superficial scratches made in the skin. The patient would develop pustules identical to those caused by naturally occurring smallpox, usually producing a less severe disease than naturally acquired smallpox. Eventually, after about 2–4 weeks, these symptoms would subside, indicating successful recovery and immunity. The method was first used in China and the Middle East before it was introduced into England and North America in the 1720s. Although this method was occasionally successful, safety was a major issue, because of the risk of the patient developing smallpox. The safe and effective vaccination method was introduced by Dr. Edward Jenner in England by using pustules from the much milder cowpox to vaccinate against smallpox. After 170 years and a heroic effort of the WHO and CDC, led by Dr. Donald Henderson from 1967 to 1977, the last patient with wild-type smallpox was treated in 1977. When smallpox was officially declared eradicated in 1979, it marked the greatest single achievement in medical, public health, or vaccine history. Over the past two centuries, scientist have developed vaccines against a myriad of other diseases, and millions of children and infant lives have been saved by stopping infectious diseases from having the chance to cause devastation [3].

Ironically, as the COVID-19 pandemic rages and the world waits for a COVID-19 vaccine, it is tragic that fewer children are being vaccinated against other deadly diseases. According to the WHO, estimates show that at least 80,000,000 children less than 1 year of age could miss routine vaccinations due to the pandemic. WHO, UNICEF, and Gavi, the Vaccine Alliance, have found that routine vaccinations are stalled in at least 68 countries [4]. These groups announced a goal to raise at least $7,400,000,000 for Gavi to protect 300,000,000 children in these 68 lower-income countries through 2025. Sadly, even in developed countries in North America and Europe, unfounded fear of vaccines by adults will inevitably prevent children from receiving available vaccines and any COVID-19 vaccine(s).

Likewise, 30,000 to 60,000 people, mostly adults, die each year of non-pandemic influenza in the United States. Most of these needless deaths are due to lack of vaccination, which implies that even when a COVID-19 vaccine becomes available, many people will also refuse to be vaccinated. The lack of vaccination against preventable diseases ultimately leads to further antimicrobial use and exacerbates AMR. Additionally, antibiotic overuse during the COVID-19 pandemic could further accelerate AMR, and accordingly the WHO has published guidance on judicious use for patients with COVID-19 [5]. The fear of vaccination along with the overuse of antimicrobials are a cause for concern given the re-emergence of multiple infectious diseases and growth of resistance. Therefore, one of the most important criteria needed to overcome AMR is education.

The effect of politics on infectious diseases is also notable. For example, the political situation in Venezuela caused the country to plunge into an economic crisis resulting in the collapse of its healthcare system. One measure of the collapse is the 40% increase in infant mortality since 2008, primarily due to infectious diseases, especially malaria, measles, and diphtheria, as well as infectious causes of diarrhea and acute bronchitis [6]. Likewise, infectious diseases have had a striking effect on US politics. During the influenza pandemic of 1918–1919, one of the 50,000,000 deaths had a particularly marked effect on American politics today. That death was of Friedrich Trump, a man who came to Canada from Germany in 1885 and made his fortune by opening bars and brothels when the Klondike Gold Rush began. After the Gold Rush, he returned to Germany and married Elizabeth Crist but was ordered to leave the country because he failed to do military service. He and his wife then moved to New York City with his fortune, estimated to be approximately $32,000 (>$500,000 in today's money). Unfortunately, he died in 1918 at the age of 49 due to pneumonia from the influenza pandemic. His widow and his son, Frederick Christ Trump, invested wisely in real estate, thus transforming thousands into millions and then billions of dollars. This fortune then allowed his grandson, Donald J. Trump, the means to become the President of the United States. Paradoxically, the pandemic that allowed the Trump family to become rich and Donald to become president is now being followed by the COVID-19 pandemic that is threatening his presidency.

From a federal standpoint, the US government was ill prepared for a pandemic such as the COVID-19 crisis. The top US agency charged with preparing for this pandemic or the next influenza pandemic, the Assistant Secretary for Preparedness and Response, had spent more resources on stockpiling for anthrax or radiological/nuclear threats than on influenza or other pandemics according to the US Department of Health and Human Services medical countermeasures budgets. Additionally, the expiration of federal programs aimed at tracking infectious diseases has been a center of controversy during the COVID-19 pandemic. One of these programs, called Predict, was founded in 2009 as part of the Emerging Pandemic Threats program that was initiated due to the 2005 H_5N_1 bird flu scare [7]. With this, some experts have argued that a disaster preparedness and response unit should be reestablished as part of the National Security Council (NSC) in addition to the Office of Pandemics and Emerging Threats [8].

Lastly, the indirect economic costs of infectious diseases and AMR are striking, as currently seen by the COVID-19 pandemic. This crisis caused by infectious disease has taken a significant toll on the world, leaving millions of people unemployed. The influenza pandemic of 1918–1919 is the most recent precedent for the current pandemic's effects on economies and world trade. This pandemic was estimated to have killed 50,000,000 people worldwide; more soldiers in WW1 died of the influenza pandemic than died of bullets, bombs, and poison gas. In an earlier example in history, *Yersinia pestis* in the form of the Black Death killed one third of Europe's population from 1347 to 1351 and had a disastrous effect on Europe's economy and trade. During the same period, the Black Death adversely affected the largest empire in world history, the Mongol Empire. The plague cutoff trade and travel between China, Russia, and Persia, severing connections between the major parts of the empire, causing it to collapse between 1335 and 1368. As evidenced by these examples, infectious diseases have had major effects on local economies, trade, migration, colonization, and conquest throughout history. The spread of diseases caused by rising AMR and emerging infectious agents can easily lead to social and political upheaval.

As a medical specialty heavily involved with infectious diseases, dermatology is a field in which AMR and emerging infectious diseases are crucial issues. During the COVID-19 pandemic, dermatologists have played a crucial role in treating patients with cutaneous manifestations of this unknown disease (Figs. 16.1 and 16.2). A broad spectrum of skin manifestations has been reported, and these signs have been identified in up to 20% of adult cases of COVID-19 [9]. Additionally, dermatologists commonly care for immunocompromised patients or prescribe immunosuppressants such as corticosteroids and biologic agents. With this, dermatologists have had to navigate guidance on whether these patients are at greater risk of infection by COVID-19 based on relatively low amounts of available information and studies at the time of the ever-evolving pandemic. Dermatologists have

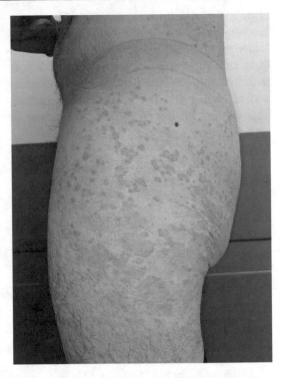

Fig. 16.2 Urticarial lesions due to COVID-19

played a crucial role in the midst of this international health crisis, and it is imperative that they continue to learn and develop knowledge on how to diagnose and treat this novel infection, as well as other emerging diseases.

In relation to AMR, dermatologists treat many skin conditions that warrant the use of antimicrobials. From dermatologic surgery to cutaneous diseases caused by bacterial, viral, fungal, or parasitic infections, dermatologists employ antimicrobials daily in their practice. In fact, dermatologists prescribe more antibiotics per provider than any other specialty [10, 11]. Consequently, dermatologists should be aware of local resistance development patterns and lower the risk of AMR by using directed therapy for the appropriate microbe, adjusting drug dosages to an effective level, prescribing antimicrobials judiciously, and providing education on AMR.

As seen with the COVID-19 pandemic, understanding newly emerging diseases is crucial for all physicians. The emergence of novel infectious diseases is a public health threat that is further exacerbated by AMR. While antimicrobials have

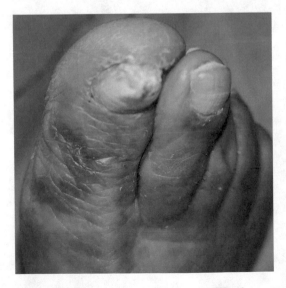

Fig. 16.1 Chilblain-like lesions due to COVID-19

allowed for huge strides in public health over the last century, the danger of resistance is a real and major concern that must be addressed immediately. It is imperative that dermatologists have an understanding of emerging infectious diseases and resistance development to effectively treat patients and combat AMR that has arisen in recent years.

References

1. No Time to Wait: Securing the Future from Drug-Resistant Infections. United Nations Interagency Coordination Group on Antimicrobial Resistance 2019. https://www.who.int/antimicrobial-resistance/interagency-coordinationgroup/final-report/en.
2. Report to the President on Combating Antibiotic Resistance. President's Council of Advisors on Science and Technology; 2014. https://obamawhitehouse.archives.gov/sites/default/files/microsites/ostp/PCAST/pcast_carb_report_sept2014.pdf.
3. Stern AM, Markel H. The history of vaccines and immunization: familiar patterns, new challenges. Health Aff (Millwood). 2005;24(3):611–21.
4. WHO: At least 80 million children under one at risk of diseases such as diphtheria, measles and polio as COVID-19 disrupts routine vaccination efforts, Warn Gavi, WHO and UNICEF. World Health Organization; 2020. https://www.who.int/news-room/detail/22-05-2020-at-least-80-million-children-under-one-at-risk-of-diseases-such-as-diphtheria-measles-and-polio-as-covid-19-disrupts-routine-vaccination-efforts-warn-gavi-who-and-unicef.
5. Kuehn BM. Alarming antimicrobial resistance trends emerge globally. JAMA. 2020;324(3):223.
6. Friedrich MJ. Venezuela's infant death rate rises amid worsening humanitarian crisis. JAMA. 2019;321(11):1041.
7. McNeil D, Kaplan T. U.S. will revive global virus-hunting effort ended last year. The New York Times. 30 August 2020, p. A4.
8. Wilensky G. The importance of reestablishing a pandemic preparedness office at the White House. JAMA. 2020;324(9):830–1.
9. Shinkai K, Bruckner AL. Dermatology and COVID-19. JAMA. 2020;324(12):1133–4.
10. Centers for Disease Control and Prevention Outpatient antibiotic prescriptions: United States, 2018. https://www.cdc.gov/antibiotic-use/community/pdfs/Annual-Report-2018-H.pdf. Updated June 23, 2020.
11. Barbieri JS, Bhate K, Hartnett KP, Fleming- dutra KE, Margolis DJ. Trends in oral antibiotic prescription in dermatology, 2008 to 2016. JAMA Dermatol. 2019;155(3):290–7.

Correction to: Overcoming Antimicrobial Resistance of the Skin

Stephen K. Tyring, Stephen Andrew Moore, Angela Yen Moore, and Omar Lupi

---

Correction to:
S. K. Tyring et al. (eds.), *Overcoming Antimicrobial Resistance of the Skin*, Updates in Clinical Dermatology, https://doi.org/10.1007/978-3-030-68321-4

A revised manuscript for chapter 1 received from the editor and the same has been updated.

Production team inadvertently missed to fix the citations in chapter 2 and 12. This has now been updated.

The updated versions of the chapters can be found at
https://doi.org/10.1007/978-3-030-68321-4_1
https://doi.org/10.1007/978-3-030-68321-4_2
https://doi.org/10.1007/978-3-030-68321-4_12

Index

© Springer Nature Switzerland AG 2021
S. K. Tyring et al. (eds.), *Overcoming Antimicrobial Resistance of the Skin*, Updates in Clinical
Dermatology, https://doi.org/10.1007/978-3-030-68321-4

Printed in the United States
by Baker & Taylor Publisher Services